DR ATKINS'
VITA-NUTRIENT
SOLUTION

DR ATKINS' VITA-NUTRIENT SOLUTION

NATURE'S ANSWER TO DRUGS

DR ROBERT C. ATKINS

POCKET
BOOKS

LONDON · SYDNEY · NEW YORK · TOKYO · SINGAPORE · TORONTO

This edition published by Pocket Books, 2002
An imprint of Simon & Schuster UK Ltd
A Viacom Company

1 3 5 7 9 10 8 6 4 2

www.simonsays.co.uk

Simon & Schuster Australia
Sydney

A CIP catalogue record for this book is available from the British
Library

ISBN 0-7434-2997-4

Typeset by Palimpsest Book Production Limited
Polmont, Stirlingshire
Printed and bound in Great Britain by
Omnia Books Ltd, Glasgow

This book is not meant to replace the advice and treatments
prescribed by your health care provider. It is not meant to encourage
treatment of illness, disease, or other medical problems by the
layman. Rather, it is meant to inform you and open you to new
health choices that are now available to those who seek broader
knowledge. Any application of the recommendations set forth in the
following pages is at the reader's discretion and sole risk. If you are
under a physician's care for any condition, he or she can advise you
about information described in this book.

CONTENTS

————<○>————

PART II

THE VITA-NUTRIENTS

PART III

TARGETED VITA-NUTRIENT THERAPY

Introduction

THE CAT'S OUT OF THE BAG

Solution – or Revolution?

While most of my previous books bear the word 'revolution' in their titles, it's ironic that the title of this book merely indicates that I have a solution, when, in fact, the thrust of this book is a truly revolutionary idea. Though the impact of this solution is indeed revolutionary, the total upheaval implied by the word won't be necessary. Happily, much of the groundwork is already in place and changes are occurring, albeit slowly. Still, when it comes to fighting disease, putting a halt to undue suffering and enjoying a higher quality of life, I tend to get impatient.

Mainstream medicine's most prominent voices have long advised us that vita-nutrients have no inherent power to treat or prevent disease, and that we don't need to make a special effort to obtain these substances for our bodies. What we have not been taught, however, is that a monumental body of evidence belies this contention. Collected by scientists at the world's most eminent institutions and published in our most prestigious journals, it definitively establishes that vitamins, minerals, amino acids and all the other natural sources of nourishment that I call 'vita-nutrients' can safely and effectively replace many of the drugs and invasive procedures that medicine imposes on us.

In short, the cat is out of the bag. Scientists have proved the therapeutic value of nutrients and have placed us at the threshold of a new era in medicine.

When I started to write this book, I didn't fully realize just how close we are to crossing that threshold. Nor did I recognize the extent of the company I keep – the thousands of doctors and research scientists from the finest quarters of conventional medicine who, like me, have opted to treat their patients with an extremely broad range of nutritional supplements.

I had intended to report on the successful vita-nutrient treatments that we've devised over the past twenty years at the Atkins Center for Complementary Medicine, which have helped tens of thousands of people prevent and overcome illness. But in order to take full advantage of the important work of many others in this growing field, I decided instead to assemble a small, devoted team of nutritionists, researchers and writers who could help me explore both the published research and personal knowledge of some of our most progressive and creative nutrition practitioners. What we learned was so exciting that one day one of my co-workers exclaimed, 'Dr Atkins, I think this book could change the world.' A few months later the comment was, 'This book will change the world.' While I realized, of course, that one book can't possibly attain a goal this momentous, I confess that I'll be disappointed if it doesn't help in at least some small way.

WHAT THIS BOOK WILL REVEAL TO YOU

Part One of this book will show you why the vita-nutrient solution isn't just a means of preventing deficiency states. In fact, it's the treatment of choice for most of the chronic illnesses that plague us today. By addressing the true causes of disease instead of temporarily alleviating symptoms, it enables longer-lasting, more effective healing. Part Two will reveal the full disparity between the role nutrients can and should play in overcoming illness, along with the way the medical profession can restrict its options. Here I describe the therapeutic capabilities of over one hundred vita-nutrients and nutritional herbs. You'll learn that familiar vitamins and herbs that you see listed on the side of a cereal box represent only a fraction of the natural healing substances that are available to all of us. These vita-nutrients can be such powerful health resources that I have come to consider them 'the tools of healing'.

In Part Three we'll put together all of this information by creating a personalized programme to help you regain or improve your health. This system, which is based on the principle of targeting your nutritional supplements, will help you create your own tailor-made programme, much like the ones we use at the Atkins Center. These will not only correct the deficiencies that cause specific health problems, but will also play health-restoring roles unrelated to deficiencies. Whether your problem is diabetes, heart disease, cancer, arthritis or an infection, you'll formulate a vita-nutrient solution that will help you get well – without resorting to the drugs and invasive procedures with consequences that are often as serious as the ailment itself. Empowered by a new level of health care choices, you should do very well indeed.

AN INTERACTIVE SOLUTION

I believe that this newfound power comes hand in hand with a duty to share it – with your family, with friends and, yes, with your doctors. The vita-nutrient solution is a community solution, although it is by no means a substitute for professional medical care. You will need a doctor at your side to watch over your well-being and monitor your progress.

Even though the vast majority of medical professionals care about their patients' health and are always open to a promising new treatment, they are often unwilling to ignore the pronouncements of medicine's policy makers – who as a group have never been as enthusiastic about natural treatments as they are about pharmaceuticals. The grass-roots support on which nutritional medicine has always had to rely must overcome consensus medicine's resistance to change. Find out if your doctor will guide you or will at least support your efforts to find a nutrient-based health programme. You might even ask him or her to read this book, which is copiously footnoted with solid mainstream research citations and references for that very purpose. If a doctor dismisses nutrition or tells you that supplements may interfere with medications, I hope this book will convince you to consider finding a different physician.

Happily, though, old attitudes are eroding, and eventually a new breed of doctor will be born from the seeds sown by the vita-nutrient solution. We have no stronger force than an idea whose time has come. But this particular idea can do more: it will liberate us from degenerative diseases, improve our physical and mental capabilities, and redefine the parameters of what we consider to be good health. The science proves it; so does clinical experience. Nutrition will be a large part of medicine's future, and that future can be here now.

PART I

NUTRIENTS
VS
DRUGS

CHAPTER 1

THE TREATMENT OF CHOICE

Have you ever read or received advertisements proclaiming 'Breakthrough!!! Natural treatments your doctor won't tell you about! Safer revolutionary treatment for heart disease, cancer, fatigue . . . or what-have-you'? Perhaps you wondered if the words heralded something important; or perhaps you remained sceptical.

While the details of such ads may or may not be true, there is one thing I can assure you: There *are* breakthroughs that can restore your health from debilitating illness or, if you are healthy, make you even healthier. They are natural, safe and nutritious – and they have not been adopted by mainstream medicine.

THE GRATIFICATIONS OF NUTRITIONAL MEDICINE

For the past quarter century I have devoted my medical career to developing and teaching others about complementary medicine, a somewhat revolutionary school of thought in which the doctor tries, whenever possible, to replace risky medical and surgical interventions with safe, gentle and nourishing efforts to restore the patient's health. The focal point of this activity is the Atkins Center for Complementary Medicine, where I and my staff of health professionals treat thousands of patients with a wide spectrum of health problems that range from the life-threatening to simple prevention. In that time span, I have witnessed the ability of vita-nutrient therapy to overcome illnesses of just about every kind. This kind of treatment is growing so exponentially that even now I am constantly amazed at its impressive successes.

To give you the flavour of the exhilarating satisfaction I get from practising this new kind of medicine, listen to the story of my patient Marie Speller. An eleven-year-old who had been recently diagnosed with juvenile diabetes, she had been prescribed two varieties of insulin. Doctors are traditionally taught that juvenile diabetes carries with it a life sentence requiring insulin. However, I had learned from treating other diabetic patients that if one of the lesser-known vita-nutrients, calcium AEP, is given during the first year of this illness, the illness can be reversed. I put Marie on a vita-nutrient programme, and we were able to lower her insulin dose, week by week, until six months later she stopped taking the drug completely. Her blood sugar levels were virtually normal and have remained so for the past two years, at which time her pancreas responded to a carbo-hydrate meal with a normal output of insulin.

When I first saw Ron Barlow, he could not pass his high school exams and had to be put in a special tutorial class. Why? Because the radiation therapy he received to remove a cancerous growth in his brain had damaged that organ. Records showed that dozens of other youngsters treated as Ron had been had never gone to college.

I gave Ron every vita-nutrient I knew that helped brain function. A few weeks later, the young man, who had never got as much as a 'D' on an exam since his radiation, received an 'A' on his midterm. His teachers were astounded. Ron was later accepted at a good college, where he is now doing very well.

CASE HISTORIES PROVIDE SCIENTIFIC DATA

While these stories are certainly dramatic, others may be more illustrative because they are typical of 80–90 per cent of patients with similar problems. For example, Jack Spanfield came to the

Atkins Center at age forty-three with an eleven-year history of ulcerative colitis. Its painful symptoms include frequent bloody diarrhoea, mucus and cramps. Jack had failed to benefit from the strongest of medications and required two painkilling enemas every day when I first examined him. After two weeks of targeted vita-nutrient therapy and a sugarless diet, he began to improve. Within six weeks his bowel function was completely normal, and within three months he was off all medications.

Marian Longstaff, a seventy-four-year-old woman, had had psoriasis for seventeen years. Even with considerable doses of prednisone, she was suffering from itchy, scaly patches on her scalp, knees, elbows and arms. She improved within six weeks on a vita-nutrient programme, and in seven months the scales, the itching and the prednisone were all gone.

Isabel Palmer, a forty-one-year-old woman, had diabetes, asthma, migraine headaches and high blood pressure. After a few months on vita-nutrients targeted specifically to all of these conditions, every problem was gone or virtually gone.

Karen Wickman, a forty-eight-year-old woman with a complete absence of hair (alopecia areata), complained of fatigue, memory loss and high cholesterol, for which she took a statin drug. After a few months of taking vita-nutrients she could buy in a health food store, her cholesterol dropped sixty points, even without the medications. Her memory and alertness improved, and best of all, her hair started growing in!

Ronald Dawson, age thirty-six, had migraines so severe that he had been on disability for four years. Within a month of starting vita-nutrients, he was off three different kinds of strong medications and his migraines had stopped.

The great majority of patients I see at the Atkins Center could also tell you stories of how they benefitted by upgrading their nutritional intake. Yet most had been told by well-trained specialists that nothing else – besides drugs – could help them. Don't believe anyone who tells you that! It simply means that nothing can be done within medicine's officially sanctioned surgical and pharmaceutical boundaries. Beyond these narrow confines, however, is a universe of scientifically validated treatments – vitamins, minerals, fatty acids, amino acids, enzymes and other biochemical substances that exist naturally in our bodies or diet – which the medical establishment chooses not to recognize.

Taking nutritional supplements is not new. But what *is* new now is that medical science itself, through research and experiment, is beginning to legitimize the nonpharmaceutical prescriptions used for so long by progressive health practitioners. Together, published studies and real-world clinical evidence prove that a wide range of these nourishing compounds can overcome illness as well as (and usually better than) the best drugs and invasive surgeries that money can buy.

The patients I have described refused the conventional wisdom of the medical establishment. In so doing, they recovered far beyond anyone's expectations, simply by eating properly and taking nutrient supplements. From headache to hypertension, diarrhoea to diabetes, most modern-day illnesses are diet-related disorders. They result from eating incorrectly and not ingesting enough of the nourishing, naturally present biochemicals that optimize vital bodily functions. Successful treatment of illness results from replenishing the supply of these substances through diet and nutritional supplements.

TREATMENT OF CHOICE DEFINED

The vita-nutrient solution isn't just a supporting actor for successful therapy; in most instances the vita-nutrients themselves should be the treatment of choice. This concept is so important that I should define it here. The phrase refers to the first option that a doctor selects to treat the condition in question. It is the 'gold standard' against which other treatments must be compared.

In medical school I was taught that 'treatment of choice' status should be given to therapies that have the highest benefit-to-risk ratio. Medical educators recognized that the number one choice should both favourably affect the illness (the benefit) and should have relative freedom from side effects (the risk). It's easy to understand why the benefit-to-risk ratio is the hallmark for choosing one therapy over others. But what many fail to recognize is that when this same criterion is applied, virtually all patients would be far better off with nutritional treatments.

In an ideal world, the medical profession would select treatments of choice strictly on these sensible criteria. Nutrients, however, are rarely given the consideration they deserve – even as a second line of defence. As a result, we are all victims of a tragic double standard that favours prescription drugs, along with their high cost and risk of unwanted (but not unexpected) side effects.

I would match a vita-nutrient solution against a combination of pharmaceuticals any day. Take the need to fight water retention, something many women would like to do every month and, more seriously, a major goal when treating high blood pressure or congestive heart failure. My treatment of choice would be taurine, an amino acid that promotes fluid excretion by restoring a natural balance between potassium and sodium, the minerals that govern how much fluid our tissues retain. As a bonus, it contributes to maintaining a regular heart rhythm and the heart's ability to contract, among many other physiological functions. In its required therapeutic dosage, taurine has absolutely no undesirable side effects.

By contrast, mainstream medicine's treatment of choice for fluid retention is the diuretic, a drug that also encourages excretion – not by allowing our cells to function more healthfully, but by impairing the kidneys' ability to reabsorb and hold on to vitally necessary minerals. In the process, diuretics elevate blood sugar, cholesterol and triglycerides; disrupt heart rhythm; increase uric acid levels; and drain the body of trace minerals and other nutrients.

All things considered, which treatment would you prefer?

To give another example, heart disease, the Western world's number one killer, arises in large part from atherosclerosis, the condition that results when our bodies deposit plaque within the walls of our vital arteries. Conventional medicine identified cholesterol as the enemy and has been waging a public health campaign to reduce the national cholesterol count by all means possible, including the widespread dispensation of cholesterol-lowering drugs. These medications may reduce the proportion of fats in the bloodstream, but should we accept a victory at any price? Drug treatments have proved successful only two times in eighty trials. Most of these studies have shown that more people die sooner from causes other than heart disease if they take these medications than if they aren't treated at all.

I certainly don't agree with the use of pharmaceuticals to lower cholesterol, because it may be only the harbinger, not the cause, of heart disease. Cholesterol is too valuable for us to remove it deliberately from our diets. To lower its concentration in the blood, however, nothing is more effective than pantethine, a derivative of the B-complex nutrient pantothenic acid. At least eight studies agree that pantethine impressively lowers triglycerides, low-density lipoprotein (LDL, the 'bad' cholesterol), and total cholesterol while increasing high-density lipoprotein (HDL, the artery-cleansing 'good' cholesterol).

You will not read about pantethine in standard cardiovascular textbooks, and you'll be hard-pressed to find a doctor familiar with it. Instead, cardiac specialists typically wait until the anticholesterol drugs fail, then begin to consider surgical solutions – a heart bypass, angioplasty, maybe a heart transplant. Their records of success are no more impressive than those of the cholesterol-lowering drugs. If the field of cardiology took into account only the work of its own scientists, it would soon discover other choice solutions: nutrients like magnesium, coenzyme Q_{10}, and carnitine. These substances strengthen the heart and, as part of a total therapy, can eliminate the need for a heart operation.

Literally dozens of other nutrients offer smarter fixes for the health problems that prescription drugs presume to address. Not all of them are documented as solidly as I'm sure they will be one day, but in the absence of published research evidence, we have the equally persuasive and conclusive experience of hands-on health practitioners. These are far-thinking professionals who prescribe nutritional supplements almost daily and see the results directly on their patients.

ENABLERS VS BLOCKERS: COMPLEMENTARY THERAPY

Vita-nutrients and pharmaceuticals need not be rivals. The fact is, both accomplish many of the same things – they can decrease blood sugar, raise your spirits, make you drowsy, control heart rate, minimize inflammation or any number of other responses. The difference is in how they work. Nutrients are enablers: they give your body a chance to do what it needs to do by facilitating a natural physiological process, thus causing the body to function better. Usually the impact isn't immediate; they perform best over the long term. In contrast, drugs, which can master acute situations, become problematic when used chronically. Why? Because they are disablers, or blocking agents. They work by preventing a normal process from taking place, usually an enzyme performing a vital role. For drugs to work, there must be a disease; only in a disease state can one hope to benefit from blocking an essential life function. Think about this: *Drugs, by their inherent nature, can play no role in health care – only in sickness care.*

Though drugs almost always carry an inherent risk (which is seldom true for nutrients), their use isn't necessarily hazardous or detrimental. With diametrically opposed mechanisms of action, medications and vita-nutrients can and should work in harmony. Long ago I selected the term 'complementary medicine' to designate a health care system that takes advantage of this happy synergy. In many instances we need to block or abruptly change a bodily function. At other times we need to achieve a response that no nutrient can perform. Many of my patients must continue to take prescription drugs, but because I emphasize nutrient therapy, most of them require fewer medications, and in smaller, far safer dosages. The best medical care will always emphasize enabling our bodies to heal themselves. How can it be appropriate for the first treatment of choice to be something that's potentially harmful when there are safer, equally effective alternatives?

Why, then, do so many of our doctors prescribe pharmaceuticals so exclusively that they give you the impression that enabling substances do not exist? One answer is that the pharmaceutical approach is all that is being taught to our doctors-in-training. For more insight, a brief understanding of the history of nutrition may be helpful to you.

A BRIEF HISTORY OF NUTRITION

Modern medical education has never truly appreciated nutrition, even though it is just as crucial as anatomy, physiology, biochemistry and pharmacology to understanding human health. Because nutrition is the only one of these basic disciplines that medical schools do not typically offer in their curricula, nature's pharmacy has received the short end of the therapeutic stick from the start. Even with the explosion of nutritional research in the last decade, the newest edition of *Cecil's Textbook of Medicine,* the authoritative reference work that is a medical student's bible, still fails to mention the Harvard studies that prove that vitamin E cuts the incidence of heart disease by almost 50 per cent. Nor does it mention more than a handful of the studies you'll read about in this book.

How did this come about? A hundred years ago or so, nutritional scientists believed that germs and other microbes caused all of our sickness and disease. The existence of very small molecules with essential health-promoting roles (later dubbed vitamins) was a new, even revolutionary theory. By the first decades of the 1900s, researchers had confirmed that people could be afflicted with deficiency diseases, and in rapid succession we learned that vitamin A cured night blindness, vitamin D prevented rickets, scurvy disappeared with a small dosage of vitamin C, and so on. The recognition of deficiency diseases was a major breakthrough that established nutrition as a medical science. Ironically enough, though, these remarkable discoveries would later create major obstacles to the broader approach to health care that works so effectively today.

From the beginning, nutritional research was always focused on the concept of 'deficiency'. A nutrient's value was measured only in terms of the consequences of its absence. If the lack did not lead to a deficiency disease, the nutrient tended to be dismissed as valueless and unimportant. It certainly didn't qualify to be labelled 'essential', a title reserved for the vitamins and minerals that the body could not manufacture on its own and could not do without. Some substances provided beneficial effects only under certain circumstances, which called for the invention of a 'conditionally essential' category that, in my view, established the basis for today's nutritional pharmacology. The conditions under which nutrients became 'essential' generally are associated with sickness, which plants the notion of nutritional therapy squarely in the medical profession's lap.

Unfortunately, mainstream medical science failed to recognize this point, and decades passed before anyone posed the more pertinent questions: What roles does a given nutrient play in the body? How much of it do we need? What is the optimum amount of this nutrient? (Every constituent of our body – sodium, iron, glucose – has an optimum level.) The answers would probably reveal that most of us fall in the low end of the nutrient intake curve, ingesting only marginal amounts that are barely above what mainstream medicine considers a deficiency. True, the normal intake of vitamin B_1 might be sufficient to prevent beriberi, but is it enough to prevent a learning disability or cardiomyopathy? As you'll learn later on, giving B_1 supplements to children whose stores are low can increase their capacity to learn by 25 per cent. Nevertheless, medical orthodoxy won't even consider the possibility that the inability to concentrate could in fact be a symptom of a suboptimum B_1 level.

BEYOND DEFICIENCY

Once researchers established all the deficiency diseases they were willing to consider, medicine's interest in nutrients waned. By the 1940s the story seemed so finished that Oxford University turned down a large endowment to conduct nutrition research. The gist of the school's response? 'We've already identified all the essential nutrients. What more is there to do?'

The task of educating the public was taken up by lay nutritionists such as Gaylord Hauser, Adelle Davis and Carlton Fredericks (each of whom personally contributed to my pursuit of nutrition in medicine). They spread the word that nutritional supplements were proving to be safe, and higher amounts could often bring about striking health benefits. In clinical experience, Frederick Klenner, MD, showed that extremely high doses of vitamin C could treat a wide variety of ailments. (Subsequently, Nobel Prize winner Linus Pauling, PhD, influenced millions of people to take such doses preventively.)

But it was the publication of *Biochemical Individuality* in 1956 that marked the birth of modern therapeutic and preventive nutrition. Roger Williams, PhD, the author of this landmark book, showed that our nutritional needs are as unique as our fingerprints and that an off-the-rack, one-diet-fits-all nutrient standard missed the point entirely. Alcoholism, diabetes, mental illness, arthritis and many other health problems can result when we fail to obtain optimal amounts of nutrients, Williams argued. He even went so far as to suggest that people take vitamins and minerals in doses well beyond the recommended dietary allowances (RDAs), which by then had become the definitive standard of human nutritional needs.

Perhaps the lay nutrition movement infuriated the arbiters of official nutritional policy. They dug in their heels, maintaining the position that we get all the nutrients we need from food. Supplements, they claimed, were unnecessary unless the person was undergoing unusual stress or dietary restrictions. Thus the nutritional old guard continues to stick to its original deficiency-oriented beliefs, in spite of the fact that international research demonstrates one major clinical success after another. The debate is hardly academic. Such intransigence, to give an example, has kept expectant mothers from consuming the amount of the B-complex nutrient folic acid necessary to prevent fatal or crippling spinal birth defects.

If we are to realize the full power of nutrition-based medicine, we must look beyond deficiency. Only then can we solve the riddles of cancer, heart disease and our other degenerative diseases. It is an achievable goal, but only if we understand that most of the power of vita-nutrients is derived from doses that have nothing to do with merely correcting a deficiency. When essentiality is applied as the yardstick, we're limited to a handful of vitamins and minerals, less than half of the amino acids, and two essential fatty acids. In the past two decades, however, we've discovered a host of nonessential (by the official definition) nourishing substances that play roles in the body so vital that, for all intents and purposes, we would all suffer without them. They are the nutritional equivalents of the car or electricity. We would not die without them, but without them we cannot regain good health, once it is lost. These vita-nutrients, for the proficient user, are indeed the tools of healing.

CHAPTER · 2

◆

WHEN OUR
NUTRITION FAILS US

DIET-RELATED DISORDERS

I have proposed that the presence or absence of deficiency does not define the extent of a vita-nutrient's worth. However, when there are deficiencies, its value increases many times over. Unfortunately, modern eating habits make deficiencies increasingly more probable. Though food alone may once have been sufficient for optimal health, today we face a variety of unnatural hazards that deplete our bodies of nutrients that were once readily available.

FOOD FALLS SHORT

Food production plays a key role in depriving our bodies of important nutrients. Our soil is routinely depleted by the agricultural practice of using inorganic fertilizer instead of biologically active compost. This practice, introduced over 150 years ago, decreases the nutritional value of plant life grown in that soil and weakens the plants' immune systems by depriving them of the nutrients they need to remain strong. This, in turn, makes them susceptible to destruction by aphids and other pests, creating crops that may not be able to survive without being sprayed with cancer-causing and soil-depleting pesticides. These pesticides have been implicated in causing neurodegenerative diseases such as Parkinson's and Alzheimer's.

Further, several essential elements are depleted from many soils by overfarming, acid rain or the many geological forces that dictate soil mineral content. Iodine-deficient soils lead to goitre epidemics, zinc-deficient soils lead to stunted growth and poor immune function, and most important, selenium-deficient soils lead to premature aging, cancer and heart disease. But any soil, even that of the seemingly highest quality, could well be relatively deficient in some vital nutrient.

The most prevalent practice in vegetable distribution is to pick them before they are ripe and then treat them with sulfites and other chemicals to give the appearance but not the taste or nutritional value of ripe vegetables. 'Fresh' fruits and vegetables are not fresh at all unless they are picked when ripe and eaten immediately. Today, however, this is seldom possible, and as a result we are losing an enormous amount of nutritional value from the foods we eat.

Food goes through many processes before we eat it, and these also contribute to substantially reducing its nutrient content. Canning is a nutritional disaster, but slicing and dicing, freezing and thawing, freeze-drying, separating, extracting and a host of other procedures also deprive the food of valuable nutrients. Nutritional value is lost day by day simply in transporting the food to the supermarket and to our kitchens. And after we bring it home, we unwittingly apply the ultimate *coup de grâce*: we bake it, boil it, microwave it and reheat the leftovers. It has been estimated that 80–95 per cent of the micronutrients originally found in food are lost before we finally eat it.

THE REFINING PREDICAMENT

Perhaps most detrimental of all is the practice of refining our food. In this process, the whole food is separated into component parts, thereby discarding some of its nutrient-rich components.

Refining is our most threatening food process because more and more of us are its victims. The percentage of our diet that comes from refined foods is at an all-time high, and by an ever-increasing margin.

Foods that nourish the animal kingdom share a remarkable characteristic: they all contain the vitamins, minerals and accessory factors necessary for the one who eats them to metabolize and utilize them fully. Nature does not require us to forage for a second food in order to extract the nutritional value from the first food. In other words, partitioning food and discarding the nutrients necessary to metabolize the part of the food you do eat creates a nutritional shortage, forcing you to take in other foods to get those nutrients, thereby draining your reserves of those nutrients. In that way, the refining process turns foods into antinutrients – into foods that not only do not nourish us, but rob us further of the nutrients we need to remain healthy.

The first documented example of the harm wrought by refining is in the polishing of rice. Historically the highly nutritious rice husks (or polishings) were discarded in making white rice, the nutritional staple of so many Oriental cultures. A plethora of white rice-only diets produced an epidemic of beriberi that could be dramatically cured by a small quantity of rice polishings. Thus the negative effects of refining nutrients out of foods was established and has proven just how essential those nutrients are.

SUGAR: THE ANTINUTRIENT

The quintessential antinutrient is sugar. It is 100 per cent carbohydrate and therefore contains no vitamins or minerals. Nevertheless it needs to be metabolized instantly. The stores of all the many nutrients involved in processing its constituent sugars, glucose and fructose, into ready energy are depleted in this process. As a result, these nutrients must be supplied from other dietary sources. Corn syrup, the simple sugar most rapidly increasing in usage, poses the same problem. To cite just one example, the critical glucose-metabolizing mineral chromium is severely depleted by consuming either sweetener.

Flour is a close second to sugar and corn syrup in health-threatening effects. However, its negative effect is more significant because its consumption is encouraged by the endorsement of the food pyramid that is based on grains and recommends six to eleven servings every day. While unmilled whole grains are indeed a significant source of essential minerals and other micronutrients, the milling process removes some 70–90 per cent of these nutrients, leading to the same antinutrient effect ascribed to sugar. 'Enriching' the grains by adding an incomplete smattering of synthetic B vitamins and inorganic iron does little to change the results. The vital minerals selenium, chromium, magnesium, zinc, manganese and copper are not replaced, nor are key nutrients like essential fatty acids and B_6. Yet the perpetrators of the food pyramid make no effort whatsoever to distinguish between whole grains and white flour, even though all nutritionists on the advisory panels are totally aware of the enormous nutritional depletion involved in the refining process. Worst of all, we are now consuming carbohydrates such as pasta, cereal, bread and crackers more than ever before, mistakenly believing we are making a healthy choice.

OTHER ASSAULTS

Many other factors combine to jeopardize our nutritional health. The environment – pollution, pesticides, petrochemicals, electronic emanations from our contemporary technology – all increase our needs for nutrients that, by acting as antioxidants, are necessary to detoxify our systems from this chemical burden. The widespread use of antibiotics has created a generation of people with shortages of beneficial bacteria that help keep pathogenic yeast in check. High stress levels as well as drug and alcohol consumption also increase nutrient need well beyond current recommendations. As we age, we may have inadequate hydrochloric acid or pancreatic enzymes to assimilate the nutrients in our food. Finally, a variety of illnesses affect our nutrient intake, and a variety of medications block their function. Thus it is strikingly apparent that we are not getting and cannot get optimal nutrition only from the foods we eat. Supplements are necessary, and many studies confirm that fact.

The Vita-Nutrient Naysayers

Virtually every study comparing supplement takers with a matched group that does not take supplements shows that those taking nutrients are far healthier. Those of the nutritional old guard who believe that our nutrients must be provided by the food we eat accept that dogma on faith, stubbornly unmoved by the avalanche of multinational published research that demonstrate one major clinical application of nutritional therapy after another. One would wonder why.

Although the 'food must supply the nutrients' position came about for honest albeit unscientific reasons, I do not feel it is perpetuated by naiveté. The cozy interdependence of the major food industry giants and many nutrition department heads at major institutions has been well documented. Consider also the fact that the profit margins within the food industry are highest when packaged, processed, long-shelf-life food is purchased and are lowest when fresh produce, meat, fish, eggs and milk are purchased. The quintessential high markup items are cereals, pasta, crackers and packaged bread. Is it a coincidence that this nutritional rogues gallery has been proposed to be the basis of our food pyramid? If you were the chief executive of one of the food conglomerates, would you not pursue a business strategy leading to greater consumption of high-profit cereal-type foods than low-profit fresh foods?

For the past half century the most effective strategy has been to convince nutritionally naive citizens and public officials that cereal is good for you. But considering the fact that scientific data shows these highly allergenic refined carbohydrates to be more harmful than beneficial, such convincing takes some doing. No problem – all you have to do is endow enough nutrition departments. The department heads, in turn, will put the desired spin on scientific observations, keep economically incorrect scientific papers out of the peer-reviewed journals they control, dictate the areas appropriate for further research, and most important, give the government honchos no alternative ideas to consider. The successful strategy has long been that when scientific evidence is lacking, stack the panel with 'experts' who not only know their bread, but also know which side it's buttered on.

THE COUNTERMOVEMENT BECOMES A REVOLUTION

With this background in mind, it is easy enough to understand why the concept of therapeutic vita-nutrition will be labelled controversial – even though scientific evidence has established its worth and even though remarkable advances have been taking place every day. Against this backdrop of a nutrition science seemingly created for the benefit of the food industry, there arose a countermovement of health professionals who were learning that nutrients had therapeutic effects. I became a part of that movement, and I am pleased to have helped thousands of doctors join the groundswell of those who recognize vita-nutrients to be the tools of healing. Nutrition is now poised to replace pharmaceuticals as the primary treatment of choice in medicine.

The countermovement may have begun with the first double-blind test in psychiatry: the use of the vitamin niacin to treat schizophrenia. Drs Abram Hoffer and Humphrey Osmond, who published the study, soon attracted many followers who called themselves 'orthomolecular psychiatrists'. The term 'orthomolecular' was coined by Nobel Prize winner Linus Pauling, PhD, who defined it as prescribing the optimal amount of each substance normally present in our bodies. Although the practitioners of this new field limited their scope to vitamins, minerals and amino acids, the concept provided a stark contrast to the prevailing medical practice of treating patients with substances not normally found in our bodies – indeed, not found even in nature. The orthomolecular concept caught and captured my attention and ultimately led me to write this book.

MY OWN TRANSFORMATION

Let me pause for a moment to answer a question that I ask of nearly every guest I interview on my radio broadcast: 'How did you get into this kind of medicine?'

My story starts in 1963. After completing my study of internal medicine and cardiology at Cornell, Columbia and Rochester Universities, I totally accepted mainstream medicine. Because I was overweight, I decided to embark on a diet that I had read in the *Journal of the American Medical Association*. This diet (which many of you now know as the Atkins diet) worked extremely well and allowed over 99 per cent of people who followed it to lose weight without hunger and with increased energy. By 1972 I had introduced ten thousand patients to the diet, and their successes were consistently and predictably replicated. I wrote my first book, *Dr Atkins' Diet Revolution,* and it became a huge best-seller that was printed in nine languages. I received tens of thousands of letters from all over the world confirming the diet's nearly universal success. But at the height of its popularity, a remarkable event took place that changed my life for ever.

In 1973 the American Medical Association called for a special nutrition consensus panel to issue a press release and position paper critical of the low-carbohydrate diet. Though consensus panels customarily review the work in question and acknowledge all scientific studies pertinent to the subject being critiqued, this one did neither. It said, in essence, that what I had been observing and documenting for nine years could not have happened. They denied that my patients had lost weight, claiming that people lose only water weight on such a diet. They denied their improved state of health and laboratory findings by announcing that people would surely get worse. In other words, the panel proclaimed that Dr Atkins could not be telling the truth. And because it was made up of AMA appointees, its opinion was unchallenged in the world of mainstream medicine.

Naturally I was shocked. Either my entire professional life, patient records, letters, confirming studies in the scientific literature and acknowledgments from other doctors getting similar results were a total fantasy, or the AMA was trying to convince the public of something that was not true.

That event turned out to be my career-changing turning point. Very few doctors ever question the pronouncements of a medical consensus panel, and I had been no different. However, after this harrowing incident I became instantly programmed to question these edicts at every turn. I found examples of improper recommendations wherever I looked – recommendations for unnecessary and futile surgery, recommendations to use

dangerous medications instead of safer agents, recommendations for invasive and risky diagnostic procedures that provide
less information than safer tests – and perhaps worst of all,
total refusal to consider vita-nutrient therapies. Mainstream
medicine's rejection of orthomolecular medicine led directly to
my personal investigation of it and subsequent acceptance of
its principles.

Once I learned how consistently people benefited from vitamins, minerals and amino acids, I sought to develop therapeutic
combinations of these nutrients that would serve to replace side
effect–laden pharmaceuticals commonly used to treat our most
widespread illnesses. Using the medical library for therapeutic
inspirations, I began to work with combinations of vitamins
and minerals to treat patients with conditions such as arthritis,
coronary disease, high blood pressure, fatigue, insomnia and
acute infections. As these combinations proved themselves equal
to the drugs they replaced, but without their adverse side effects,
I had them tableted into combinations with specific therapeutic
purposes. They provided the building blocks for a nutrient
prescribing system I call 'Targeted Nutrition'. I do not think I
was ahead of my time; I was merely taking advantage of an
idea whose time has come.

THE VITA-NUTRIENT INFORMATION EXPLOSION

Today the published research on vita-nutrient therapy has
increased some twentyfold since my first library search was
conducted. That means that over 90 per cent of the work that
establishes nutrients as true competitors to pharmaceuticals has
been completed in the last two decades. Most of it, in fact,
has been done in the past five years. I rely on these studies, not
only to encourage the broad acceptance of vita-nutrient therapy,
but also, for my own growth, to learn of new ways to treat
patients effectively.

The plethora of research, along with the medical practices of
doctors who are using nutrition-based therapeutics, is rapidly
bringing about an expansion of the orthomolecular paradigm.
I believe that the natural offshoot of this paradigm – the vita-
nutrient solution – will redefine the scope of nutritional therapy.

Any biochemical substance normally found in our bodies may be considered a nutritional substance, and the question we must ask will be: 'Does the person have the optimal amount of each of these substances?'

When the standard for essentiality was whether or not the body could manufacture the substance independently, our list of potential therapeutic nutrients was quite limited. However, now that we have learned that a host of substances that our bodies make from other nutrients can themselves play enormously important health roles, both the arena and the benefits have expanded. Today we recognize scores of these healing tools that work by nourishing us. All are products of an information explosion that is capable of changing the face of medicine for ever.

PART II

THE VITA-NUTRIENTS

VITA-NUTRIENTS, ONE BY ONE

I've always felt that doctors today should be congratulated for the illnesses they prevent rather than for the ones they cure. The beauty of complementary medicine is that it focuses equally on preventing and curing disease. It works, in essence, by capitalizing on our bodies' own in-house pharmacy, which is designed to replenish what is depleted and create what is missing. Using vita-nutrients in the proper dosages will bolster our bodies' pharmacy by helping to obtain optimum results without uncomfortable and unnecessary side effects.

Because these nutrients work synergistically, you will notice that I often recommend taking one vita-nutrient in conjunction with another in order to boost its overall potential. Remember, though, that while nature's own healing formulas are far safer than the potent pharmaceuticals prescribed today, it is nevertheless important to adhere to my 'supplement suggestions' and guidelines, which you will find throughout each vita-nutrient section.

Part Two, which is the heart of the book, is designed to familiarize you with all the vita-nutrients available today. These natural substances are the foundation of my practice at the Atkins Center. I describe each in terms of what it can do for you and what I have learned about it from my patients, along with supporting evidence from published medical studies. I am confident that once you have read about the wonders of these nutrients, you will question the practice of using pharmaceuticals as our only available weapons against disease. Furthermore I feel certain that the facts you will learn about vitamins, minerals, amino acids, essential fats, accessory nutrients, hormones and herbs will dramatically change your attitude towards health care today. It is the beginning of a revolution that will change the doctor–patient relationship and lead to a healthier and more natural lifestyle.

Before we get going, though, there are a few terms I should

explain that are indispensable to understanding the valuable roles
these nutrients play. The most important are 'free radicals' and
'antioxidants'.

FREE RADICALS AND ANTIOXIDANTS

Oxygen is a double-edged sword. Without it we can't stay alive,
but a surplus can be deadly. Happily, the body has a way to
handle these oxygen-derived by-products – known as 'free radicals' – which allows us to both maximize oxygen and remain
alive. The answer lies in valuable protector nutrients known as
antioxidants. If our cells did not contain these substances, we
would die within a matter of sec-onds.

You are sitting in front of your hearth, enjoying a roaring
fire. Without a screen, the sparks flying off the fire would
damage your rug and furniture. The bigger the fire, the bigger
the screen you'll need. No one would think of risking their fine
furniture by not using a big enough screen.

So it is with free radicals and antioxidants. The sparks flying
off the fire are just like the free radicals that fly through our
cells when we burn food for energy. The screen is the counterpart of the antioxidant nutrients and enzymes in our cells that
protect us from these damaging by-products. The more free
radical sources you are exposed to – smog, emotional and physical stress, pesticides, indoor pollution, cigarette smoke, burnt
foods, excessive intake of liquid vegetable oil, aerobic exercise
– the more protector nutrients, or antioxidants – you'll need.
Even if you are not exposed to any of these things, normal
metabolic processes will still produce a significant amount of
free radicals.

The most important antioxidants are vitamin C, vitamin E,
carotenoids, zinc, selenium and glutathione. N-acetyl cysteine,
taurine, lipoic acid, CoQ_{10}, milk thistle, curcumin, grape seed
extract and other nutrients act as cellular protectors as well.
Even if you cannot afford the more esoteric antioxidant nutrients, you should try to take a combination of the 'primary'
group. Why? Antioxidant nutrients work best as a team, and
the more well balanced the team, the better the results.

The results we gain with an optimized intake of antioxidants are impressive. Research shows that antioxidants will not only reduce the risk for many diseases, but also slow down the aging process. While disease and aging are complicated matters, they always involve an excess of free radicals. Cancer, heart disease, arthritis, Alzheimer's disease and premature aging are just a few of the ailments that result when the body does not have adequate free radical defence.

But don't let these sobering facts about oxygen's by-products negate the importance of the number one life essential, oxygen. It is essential for keeping our tissues healthy, and a lack of it is incompatible with survival. Remember this principle: *It is the combination of oxygen with antioxident nutrients that will maximize its most positive health benefit.* Oxygen is like the electricity that runs your appliances, and antioxidants are the protective shields that insulate it and keep it from burning down your house. You need them both.

I hope you see why I singled out the constant cellular battle between free radicals and antioxidants. Win this battle. If you do, you'll enjoy a healthy life, free of disease, where every day can be enjoyed to the fullest.

CHAPTER 3

VITAMINS

VITAMIN A: *Infection fighter, skin protector*

Ancient Egyptians used cooked liver as a remedy for night blindness, but many centuries passed before we understood why. And in 1915, when we found the answer – vitamin A – the modern age of nutrition dawned. In the eighty years since, we've discovered even more ways in which this nutrient assures our health.

Although night blindness is the officially recognized deficiency disease of vitamin A, many maladies are inextricably linked with how much of the nutrient circulates in our bodies. As one of our major antioxidants, it's an invaluable ally against heart disease and other degenerative conditions.[1] It's needed for healthy reproduction, hormone stability in women, proper growth, blood sugar balance and defence against infections, to cite just a few of its responsibilities.

THE ORIGINAL INFECTION FIGHTER

Vitamin A earned its reputation as the 'infection vitamin' long before vitamin C usurped the title. Despite C's powerful ability in this area, vitamin A is just as necessary a part of the infection-fighting process. It shores up the immune system in myriad ways, with much of its work occurring in the mucous membranes that line the gastrointestinal tract.

At the first hint of a cold, I start to take between 50,000 and 100,000 IU of vitamin A daily, along with large doses of vitamin C and zinc. This nutrient prescription, I think, is one of the reasons I haven't missed a single day of work because of an illness for more than three decades. Taking large short-term doses also improves recovery from stronger respiratory and sinus infections. And an oral supplement programme combined with direct skin treatments will slow a herpes outbreak.

Childhood Infections The bloodstream's level of retinol, as vitamin A is more technically known, is one of the major factors that account for why children in industrialized countries don't die from such seemingly benign viral infections as the measles, unlike the kids in underdeveloped nations. Meeting vitamin A needs throughout the world could save 1.2–2.5 million lives every year. The number of deaths from respiratory disease would plunge by 70 per cent; the number of deaths from diarrhoea-related diseases would drop by 39 per cent.[2]

Surprisingly enough, vitamin A deficiencies still exist in the United States and in other industrialized nations, although perhaps they are not as critical as they are in the rest of the world. Of twenty Long Beach, California, children who had the measles, one small study found, half were deficient in vitamin A – yet all of them were well fed. Children are extremely susceptible to vitamin A deficiencies, partly because infections drain their little bodies' retinol stores. However, just a single 20,000 IU dose can quicken their recovery from chicken pox and virtually eliminate its possible complications.[3] Further, infants would face fewer life-threatening lung infections if they were fed vitamin A supplements regularly.[4] In view of the subtle adverse consequences of childhood vaccinations, I find myself recommending a strategy based on childhood supplementation with vitamin A and other nutrients; it's equally effective and far safer.

AIDS Retinol reinforces the immune system's resistance to any infectious disease, even AIDS, where the impact has been studied extensively. Some scientists assert that even a modest supplement programme of vitamin A, between 13,000 and 20,000 IU per day, may slow the disease's advance.[5] People with AIDS are at least two hundred times more likely than their otherwise healthy counterparts to have low levels of the vitamin, even when their vitamin intake from food is adequate. Doctors can predict the life expectancy of someone with AIDS just by measuring blood concentrations of retinol.[6]

Skin Problems As I talk to patients with skin disorders and scan the literature in search of new therapies, it sometimes seems that traditional dermatologists will prescribe a cortisone-derived cream for just about every skin disorder they encounter. Old habits die hard, I suppose – but then, I may have an equally narrow focus. For almost 100 per cent of the skin conditions I treat, I prescribe vitamin A. I also recommend it preventively to keep skin healthy.

As the pharmaceutical industry knows full well, vitamin A is ideally suited to nourish and heal the skin. Look at the passionately promoted products at the cosmetic counter. Their active ingredients, frequently, are retinoids, the synthetic versions of vitamin A. Nature holds the patent on the real thing, which forces the companies to develop these inadequate imitations. I may be unduly sceptical, but I think natural vitamin A, because it is safer, is a better product.

The treatment of acne is a good example of vitamin A's value. If you're prone to persistent pimply eruptions, I'd bet a blood test would reveal that you're in the low end of the vitamin A range. The skin typically clears on a strong supplement programme, using a dosage between 200,000 and 500,000 IU per day for three or four months.

That's a big dose, one that requires a doctor's oversight because of the likelihood of side effects. I doubt, however, that its toxicity comes close to that of isotretinoin, one of the patentable pharmaceuticals. Women who are even remotely likely to get pregnant, for example, can't take the drug because it magnifies the risk of birth defects astronomically.

No one who has acne needs to worry about any possibility of treatment-related side effects. I've discovered through my practice how to complement the impact of natural vitamin A, making lower doses as effective as higher amounts. First, sugars and refined carbohydrates must be eliminated from the diet. By including vitamin E, zinc, pantothenic acid, GLA and the beneficial bacteria as part of the acne therapy, you can get by with only 100,000 IU of vitamin A, a much safer dosage.

Psoriasis also improves from taking vitamin A supplements. Of the medical trials I've reviewed, the most effective protocol used is 100,000 IU, along with some additional vitamin D.[7]

Pulmonary Disease Vitamin A's critical value to the skin is but one aspect of its benefit to all epithelial tissue. Epithelium is the layer of cells that form the outermost layer of the skin. If you think about this, both the digestive and the respiratory tract are in contact with the external environment. I had always used vitamin A as part of the Atkins Center protocol for emphysema, a form of chronic obstructive pulmonary disease (COPD). Scientific studies show that people with severe pulmonary disease exhibit low vitamin A levels; those patients who take vitamin A supplements exhibit improved lung function.[8]

Digestive Ailments Because of its close connection to mucous membranes and epithelial cells, vitamin A proves to be a worthwhile treatment addition for certain intestinal illnesses. It has helped my several hundred colitis and Crohn's disease patients, and its value for treating and preventing duodenal ulcers was emphasized by the Harvard study showing that men with the highest vitamin A intake had a 54 per cent lower risk of ulcer than those whose intake was lowest.[9]

Cancer Although it is often overshadowed by the more widely known beta-carotene, vitamin A continues to impress scientists as a cancer preventive and treatment.[10] One reason is that it apparently goes a long way towards halting a tumour's reemergence following surgery. One study tested the vitamin on 307 people who underwent operations for lung cancer. Some of them took 300,000 IU of the vitamin daily for a year; the others did not. After twelve months the vitamin takers remained free of new tumours for a longer period of time and developed far fewer tumours than the people who did not use supplements.[11]

Without vitamin A's round-the-clock vigil, other cancers are also much more likely to attack, including prostate cancer[12] and certain forms of leukaemia. The cells that make up the surface layer of our skin, called epithelial cells, seem to depend heavily on it, too, for protection from malignancies. People who develop these skin cancers, including basal cell carcinoma and squamous cell carcinoma, frequently have significantly lower than average blood levels of retinol.[13]

Longtime tobacco chewers often will notice the growth of a whitish coating on the soft mucous membranes inside their mouths. The appearance of this condition, called leukoplakia, often foreshadows cancer, but vitamin A has, in some experiments, caused it to vanish. Administering 32,000 IU daily for six months reduced the formation of new lesions and allowed for complete remissions in more than half of the tobacco chewers who took it.

Women's Health Concerns Retinol can be one of a woman's most needed nutrients. Some of premenstrual tension's bothersome symptoms disappear under the vitamin's influence and may not return even after discontinuing the supplement programme. In one study, 50,000 IU per day reduced heavy menstrual bleeding;[14] in other research, a larger daily amount (150,000 IU) was useful in treating benign breast disease.[15] Taken along with folic acid and boron, vitamin A contributes to minimizing hot flushes and other menopausal symptoms.

It is not always true that higher doses bring better results. It is said that amounts above 8,000 IU may cause birth defects, but I have not seen any convincing studies to back up this warning. Women who are pregnant or who plan to have a child should consider limiting their A supplementation to no more than 8,000 IU per day unless there is compelling reason to use more. Avoiding the vitamin completely, however, is not wise. Women need a good supply of it, not only to make hormones, including progesterone, but to nourish the foetus and reduce the risk of pregnancy-related complications, such as low birth weight.[16] In studies of retinol-deficient mothers-to-be, researchers have found no ill effects from daily dosages as high as 6,000 IU.[17]

Don't just guess at how much retinol you and your baby will

need. Ask your obstetrician to authorize lab tests for vitamin A (and while you're at it, many of the other nutrients, especially folic acid).

Wound Healing Whether injured by a sunburn or a surgical incision, skin heals better with vitamin A supplements, because the nutrient stimulates the release of a compound that facilitates tissue repair. It also generates collagen synthesis in the wound, improves the quality of new tissue and lowers the risk of an infection.[18] Along with zinc, vitamin A should be taken routinely immediately before and after any kind of surgery.

Blood Sugar Disorders Although a carbohydrate-restricted diet and certain sugar-metabolizing supplements control diabetes-like problems quite well, every little bit helps when you confront the world's most serious metabolic disease. Because of a relatively recent study suggesting that vitamin A might add to blood sugar stability, I make sure to include the nutrient in antidiabetes protocols. A study based on fifty-two healthy people found that those who consumed more than 10,000 IU of vitamin A per day metabolized glucose better than those who took in less than 8,000 IU. Researchers conclude that the nutrient allows the body to use insulin more efficiently, helping the hormone to get blood sugar into the body's cells.[19] If the finding is replicated, retinol will represent a major step towards beating insulin resistance, the disorder behind both Type I and Type II diabetes, high blood pressure, high triglycerides, hypoglycemia and obesity.

Supplement Suggestions

An average adult should consume about 5,000 IU of vitamin A every day. For a retinol-deficiency-related illness, you may need to take up to 100,000 IU per day. Cod liver oil and liver are the best sources, followed by butter, egg yolks, cream and whole milk. Cereals and skimmed milk, even when fortified with the nutrient, are not good sources.

For a supplement source, vitamin A palmitate is the version commonly found in multivitamin formulations, and it usually meets our needs. Vegetarians should note that it is synthetic and not derived from any animal. If your body's vitamin A stores must be replenished in a hurry, as would be necessary at the outset of an acute respiratory infection, use the mycellized version, which bypasses the liver and is absorbed easily, thus reducing the likelihood of a toxic accumulation. Even in amounts of 100,000 IU a day for months at a time, mycellized vitamin A has never caused any documented side effects. This safety record does not mean, however, that therapeutic dosages need not be monitored by a doctor.

Mycellized A performs impressively against sinus and other acute infections, especially when combined with mycellized vitamin E. Its liquid doesn't taste great, but it's worth tolerating for quick, impressive results. Other forms, such as retinol palmitate and emulsified preparations, have also logged impressive results.

CAROTENOIDS · *Cancer and heart protectors, antioxidant*

Understand the carotenoid story, and you'll be well on the way to grasping how nutrients maintain and enhance health. Some six hundred of these plant pigments exist naturally, yet you're probably familiar with only one – beta-carotene. For decades this most important carotenoid was the 'darling' of the nutrition community. Hundreds of studies were published demonstrating that people with higher beta-carotene levels had impressive protection against all forms of cancer, heart disease, macular degeneration and a range of other degenerative diseases. Hoffman–La Roche, the leading supplier of the nutrient, confidently funded a series of studies that were expected to make their product, synthetic beta-carotene, a 'must' in the lives of everyone who wanted cancer protection. Between 1994 and 1996 the studies were published, and synthetic beta-carotene laid the biggest egg since Dewey lost to Truman. Everyone asked why. How could dietary beta-carotene be of such spectacular value, while beta-carotene capsules actually seemed to make cancer prevention somewhat worse?

You'll get the key to the answer by noting this section refers to carotenoids, not just to beta-carotene. Although it is the most examined member of the carotenoid family, beta-carotene still is only one member. As we are beginning to understand, the carotenoids are a nutritional collective that work best in a fashion similar to the B complex. Their therapeutic worth may be only as good as the weakest link in the chain, and an overload of one could compromise the work of the others.

The rather disquieting research findings from 1994 came from studies that tested synthetic beta-carotene, a chemical clone made in the laboratory that is not as easily absorbed into our cells as the real thing. The artificial version is inferior for two primary reasons:

- It does not contain any of the other natural carotenoids.
- Its overwhelming presence may interfere with our cells' absorption of the other natural carotenoids in food. For example, we know that the synthetic form lowers the blood's concentration of lutein, another carotenoid with its own unique health-promoting power.

The earlier conclusion that beta-carotene itself shielded us from disease was based in large part on research that didn't involve synthetic beta-carotene, but rather used natural supplements or natural food sources of the nutrient – kale, squash, tomatoes, broccoli, spinach and so on. This distinction usually isn't mentioned. The therapeutic might of the real and artificial versions can differ significantly. As a relatively recent study illustrated, synthetic beta-carotene could not reverse cancerous changes in stomach cells. Natural beta-carotene could.[1]

Equally important is the usually disregarded fact that the carotenoids are fat-soluble nutrients. For optimal absorption and use in our bodies, they need to be consumed with some fat-containing food.

To harness the power of one carotenoid, then, the secret is to use them all. Though we'll explore the qualities of individual complex members here, it is essential to use them together. With the enormous power of the entire spectrum of natural carotenoids, we can expect to benefit from all the disease-preventing, health-promoting potential of this nutrient complex.

BETA-CAROTENE

It's often noted that beta-carotene is most easily transformed into vitamin A. This certainly is true, but by functioning as an antioxidant in its own right, beta-carotene accomplishes far more without converting into the vitamin.

Cancer Disregarding the artifact of taking synthetic beta-carotene, scientists have learned that people with the lowest intake of beta-carotene have a higher incidence of cancer, especially when this nutritional deficiency coexists with a low level of vitamin A.[2] In tissue that bears cancerous growths, beta-carotene levels are measurably lower.[3] Its protection extends to many forms of cancer, particularly that of the lung, stomach and breast.[4,5] Beta-carotene has also been shown to slow the activity of colon cells and, in doing so, to reduce the risk of colon cancer.[6]

To work at its best, beta-carotene needs not just the other carotenoids, but other antioxidants. In partnership with vitamin C, for instance, it can reduce the risk of cervical dysplasia[7] and other premalignant lesions. In another study, supplements of 40 mg taken with retinol (a form of vitamin A) and vitamin E produced an improvement in 71 per cent of people who had leukoplakia, a prime example of a premalignant lesion in the mouth.[8]

In a natural form with the full array of other carotenoids, I have a lot of confidence in beta-carotene. At the Atkins Center this treatment is a major, nearly invariable part of our therapy for established or disseminated cancer, and we find that 90 per cent of our cancer patients do better than they would be expected to do if they had relied on mainstream medicine alone. The majority of successful alternative cancer practitioners seem to agree about the value of natural beta-carotene.

Heart Disease The antioxidant action of beta-carotene plays a very important role in the prevention of heart and artery disease. A study of 333 patients who took 50 mg of beta-carotene showed that the nutrient reduced major cardiovascular events by 50 per cent in comparison with people who did not take the supplement.[9] Beta-carotene was also found to have a protective effect in angina patients, who experienced far less chest pain on diets that were high in natural beta-carotene. Beta-carotene is also known to increase the level of the protective HDL cholesterol.[10]

Cholesterol cannot clog arteries until it oxidizes, and many studies have shown that beta-carotene can prevent this dangerous reaction from taking place. Although vitamin C appears to be the first line of defence in protecting cholesterol from going bad, beta-carotene plays an equally important role as the essential backup nutrient.[11]

Immune Reinforcement Beta-carotene also strengthens the immune system. Here is where I take advantage of its conversion into vitamin A, one of our major infection fighters. (It is important to note, though, that beta-carotene stimulates the immune system independent of its ability to turn into another vitamin.) I prescribe natural beta-carotene routinely for all of my patients with chronic viruses and with acute and chronic infections. According to the research, doses of beta-carotene greater than 30 mg taken for more than two months produced a significant enhancement of immune system function.[12] A lack of the nutrient is notably prominent among people with AIDS. One study found that over 70 per cent of AIDS patients were deficient or in the lowest quarter of the normal range of beta-carotene levels,[13] and another study found a thirteenfold reduction of the nutrient in children with AIDS.[14] More to the point, dosages of 180 mg per day have helped AIDS patients reverse the depletion of their immune cells.

LUTEIN AND ZEAXANTHIN

Because they're so frequently exposed to the oxidizing light rays of the sun, our eyes need all the antioxidant protection they can get. Vitamin C and certain bioflavonoids are two mighty guardians in our retinas' delicate cells. Beta-carotene helps, but lutein and zeaxanthin are the dominant carotenoids that protect our eyes; they are concentrated especially in the macula, our true centre of sight at the back of the retina. Because of their yellowish colour, lutein and zeaxanthin are particularly adept at absorbing the damaging blue rays from the light spectrum. Lutein also seems to be better than beta-carotene at heading off free radical harm to fats inside the eyes.

If consumed regularly from kale, collard greens, spinach and other leafy green vegetables, the two carotenoids are an unbeatable combination. Not only can they ward off cataracts,[15] but they can also cut by 57 per cent the risk for macular degeneration, a deterioration of central vision that's responsible for about one-third of all new cases of blindness every year.[16]

LYCOPENE

The pigment that colours tomatoes and watermelons, lycopene is perhaps the strongest and most underrated carotenoid. Like beta-carotene, it protects LDL cholesterol from oxidizing and building up on artery walls. Some research suggests it may be even more important than beta-carotene for heart health.[17]

Lycopene may also extend up to ten times more cancer protection than its more famous carotenoid partner, according to lab estimates. It's particularly effective against cancer of the breast, lung, endometrium and prostate.[18] Smokers with low lycopene levels had four times more lung cancer than those with the highest levels.[19]

Of some five hundred carotenoids tested in a study of prostate cancer risk among a group of 47,894 men, only lycopene, the most abundant carotenoid found in the prostate, demonstrated any protective ability. For the men who ate two daily servings of tomato-containing foods (although not whole tomatoes or tomato juice), the prostate cancer risk was reduced by 35 per cent.[20] Fats or oils are necessary for dietary lycopene to be absorbed. What a long way we've come from a century ago, when people thought tomatoes were poisonous!

SUPPLEMENT SUGGESTIONS

When people say, 'Eat your veggies', they're really saying, 'Take in a full spectrum of carotenoids'. All leafy, dark green vegetables contain the carotenoids, as do yellowish or orangish vegetables like squash and carrots. Lycopene is found most abundantly in tomatoes, guavas, watermelon and pink grapefruit. Strawberries, though red, do not contain it. Remember, fat-free diets do not allow us to absorb the carotenoids optimally.

For the strongest therapeutic advantage, though, you'll need to take dosages much greater than can be obtained from food. Everyone, I feel, should be taking a natural broad-spectrum carotenoid supplement. The only exceptions to this might be people who cannot metabolize carotenoids well, such as alcoholics or anyone else with an impaired liver.

Don't be alarmed if the palms of your hands turn yellow orange when you drink a lot of carrot juice or consume high carotene dosages. You have not developed beta-carotene toxicity. Yellowish skin is simply a sign that you are harmlessly storing the carotenoids in the fat under your skin.

While vitamin A in doses above 8,000 IU is not recommended during pregnancy, the carotenoids are perfectly safe. I have yet to see or read about toxicity of natural carotenoids at any dose.

The ideal form of carotenoid supplements are those derived from algae, such as *Dunaliella salina*, or whole-food concentrates. The *D. salina* is standardized to its beta-carotene content. An average adult may opt to take 10,000–25,000 IU for preventive care. I usually prescribe 75,000 IU for people with cancer, and many German oncologists use considerably more. (In fact, they check their patients' hands to make sure that their palms are golden yellow!)

For optimal protection against cancer or macular degeneration, I would bolster *D. salina*'s carotenoids with additional lycopene, lutein and zeaxanthin.

B COMPLEX: *The energy team*

As they uncovered the links between various aspects of health and certain chemicals in our food, the nutritional pioneers of the 1920s and 1930s had to backtrack quite a bit. Upon discovering the apparent nutritional key to one vital bodily process, they returned to the same food and found an entirely different substance involved in the same, or similar, body function.

Eventually they realized that they were dealing with a cluster of related nutrients, the ones we now know as the B-complex vitamins. In the next pages you will read about B_1, B_2, B_3, B_6, folic acid, B_{12}, pantothenic acid and biotin.

Though each member of this nutritional family has unique therapeutic properties, they all share two common points:

- They are responsible for producing energy by extracting fuel from the carbohydrates, proteins and fats in our food.
- They exist together in nature.

Might the B-complex nutrients appear together for a reason, perhaps to carry out their shared purpose? If so, would the absence of one or more of them interfere in some way with our energy metabolism and, ultimately, our health? These suppositions are in fact true, and they go a long way towards explaining why processing and refining disturb food's fragile nutritional balance and contribute to most of our degenerative diseases.

Because the B vitamins are so intertwined, separating them would diminish the functioning of the complex as a balanced whole and violate the imperative to keep them together. By keeping them together, we can take advantage of their individual traits without creating new imbalances that have their own specific consequences. I'll be returning to this theme repeatedly while pointing out the individual advantages of each B nutrient.

VITAMIN B_1 (THIAMIN): *Brain energizer*

The person who doesn't require additional thiamin is a rare find. If you eat cooked food, you need more than you currently get. As much as half of the vitamin B_1 in uncooked foods falls prey to the stovetop. And if you eat a lot of refined, processed flours and grains, 'fortified' or otherwise, the high heat will find little to kill off. Both pregnancy and lactation amplify the body's B_1 requirement, as does the consumption of sugar and other refined carbohydrates, exercise, an overactive thyroid gland and drinking alcohol or tea. The requirement also increases with age. Older people can't metabolize the vitamin the way they once could, so they must consume more of it.[1]

Beriberi, the disease that is the result of a thiamin deficiency, sounds like an exotic ailment of days gone by, an affliction of the developing world. Nevertheless it still exists today. Doctors know it as alcohol-related cardiomyopathy, because it usually develops from severe alcoholism. The heart muscle is its principal target, and it loses its ability to contract effectively. However, the disease doesn't ignore the nervous system, the digestive system or any other part of our physiological makeup.

Heart Disease For every alcohol-addicted person with full-blown alcohol cardiomyopathy, another hundred heavy drinkers suffer a lesser degree of heart impairment from an insufficiency of B_1.[2] Still, you need not drink to excess to drain your body of B_1 or to suffer the cardiac consequences. Preventing heart disease is a tougher task when you don't have enough of the vitamin. Diuretic drugs, commonly prescribed to treat high blood pressure, congestive heart failure and water retention, further deplete the body of thiamin, along with many other nutrients.

Replenishing the body's stores of thiamin is absolutely essential for reversing the loss of heart muscle function, as well as treating cardiomyopathy and congestive heart failure. Regular doses of B_1 dramatically improved cardiac function in a small 1995 experiment involving thirty people with severe heart failure who had been taking the diuretic medication furosemide.[3]

Learning Disabilities Another hallmark of beriberi is brain dysfunction, but mental impairment becomes apparent long before a low thiamin level can be classified as an official deficiency. Raising the blood measurement to a healthier range, conversely, can be a safeguard against mental impairment.

B_1 supplements can help children with deficiencies of the vitamin expand their learning capacity up to 25 per cent, according to school-administered standard testing.[4] In some instances severe behavioural problems have disappeared entirely. High doses, other research found, can enable the mentally retarded to concentrate better and make greater use of their mental abilities.[5] Even college students given 50 mg of thiamin daily for two months showed faster reaction times and were found to be more clearheaded, composed and energetic.[6]

Emotional Disturbances Aggressive and addictive behaviour, as well as other personality disorders and mental illnesses, share several nutritional common denominators, including a thiamin deficiency. Up to 30 per cent of the people admitted to hospital psychiatric wards are deficient in B_1, according to research estimates. I've seen people with certain kinds of depression respond very well to thiamin therapy. A daily dosage of 400 mg helps maintain healthy levels of the brain chemicals such as acetylcholine, which are responsible for elevating mood.[7]

Alzheimer's Disease Among people afflicted with this debilitating loss of memory, blood levels of B_1 are typically significantly below normal. The activity of a certain enzyme used to gauge the body's thiamin level also drops – by as much as 50 per cent. Unfortunately, bringing the blood concentration to a healthier range cannot undo the damage that the disease has already inflicted, although one researcher asserts that a certain subgroup of Alzheimer's patients do respond to prodigious dosages.[8] The low success rate in this regard makes me believe that the vitamin is better as a preventive than as a treatment.

Neural Disorders and Pain Thiamin improves nerve function and diminishes pain in several different neurological conditions. The most common reason I give B_1 injections is to alleviate peripheral neuropathy, a frequently painful disorder characterized by numbness or an uncomfortable tingling in the hands and feet. The shot works more than half the time, as long as the other B-complex vitamins accompany thiamin.

In addition, according to a German study, a twelve-week course of thiamin and other B vitamins was able to help patients with diabetic neuropathy, a nerve degeneration caused by poorly controlled blood sugar.[9] The thiamin was in the form of allithiamine, and prodigious doses (320 mg) were used. The supporting nutrients B_6 and B_{12} were also given in high doses.

Thiamin supplementation, balanced with the other B-complex

members, also lifts pain from shingles, migraine headaches and some arthritic conditions. For relief from some of fibromyalgia's unexplained muscle pains, supplements can help, but a special 'activated' form of B_1, thiamin pyrophosphate, is required. The more common kinds of B_1 are fine for soothing garden-variety cramps and muscle soreness. In fact, unusually high oral doses (between 1 and 4 grams) have succeeded where pharmaceutical painkillers had failed. Studies have shown that large doses eased pain for 78 per cent of a sizable group of headache patients; joint pain also improved for almost three-quarters of the participants.[10]

Lead Poisoning B_1 has already been established as an indispensable requirement for enhancing learning capacity. Further evidence of its role in childhood nutritional medicine is provided by its ability to counteract lead poisoning. The risk of a toxic buildup of this poisonous metal isn't borne exclusively by unattended babies who eat peeling paint chips. Lead poisoning is one of the major environmental hazards that children living in industrialized nations face, causing learning difficulties, nerve damage, and other neurological problems.[11] Because the body retains every bit of the toxic metal that it acquires, the danger extends into adulthood. Even a slightly lower than adequate B_1 level permits more lead to build up, but supplementation helps to decrease the accumulation.

Immune Weakness Some children who are prone to recurrent fevers and other ailments typical of a weak immune system respond beautifully to B_1 therapy. Many of these kids have unusually high levels of folic acid and vitamin B_{12} in their bodies.[12] The finding again proves the important principle that B vitamins work best when they're balanced and can pose problems when out of whack.

SUPPLEMENT SUGGESTIONS

Except as warranted for pain or other specific illnesses, 50–100 mg thiamin will cover most people's daily needs. Remember, though, that it must be balanced with a similar amount of its

B-complex companions. Standard thiamin hydrochloride, the form most frequently used in over-the-counter supplements, will serve you well for general health purposes. It's easily absorbed, and I rarely feel compelled to administer more than 300 mg a day. When the body's B_1 content must be increased more rapidly, thiamin pyrophosphate makes a better choice. Better still is allithiamine, the most readily absorbed form available.

Don't let this discussion, or the ones that follow, turn you away from the principle of insisting on taking the B complex as a unit. (On page 325 I describe a useful example of such a formula.) If you have one of the specific problems I discuss here, you may wish to supplement your supplement by taking the B complex along with 100–200 mg of allithiamine or the pyrophosphate form.

VITAMIN B_2 (RIBOFLAVIN):
Antioxidant, energizer and team player

Not all nutrients are superstars, nor need they be. For each nutritional equivalent of David Beckham, there are several secondary players that don't grab the limelight or set individual records. They interact with and support the superstars in ways that allow the attention grabbers to shine.

Vitamin B_2 (riboflavin) is the consummate team player on the B-complex roster. Without it the B team could not possibly make the A list for metabolizing food, safeguarding cells and forestalling deficiencies of other nutrients.

Some of B_2's value comes from its ability to speed up the conversion of vitamin B_6, the B-complex superstar, to its active form in the body. At the same time, it's one of the major nutrients involved in regenerating glutathione (see page 181), one of our most important antioxidants. The two are so intimately tied that scientists often measure the body's glutathione level to gauge riboflavin levels.[1] The B vitamin's antioxidant action is vital to a natural approach to preventing and treating cataracts (although extremely high dosages of 500 mg and more have actually caused retinal damage to experimental animals).[2] Riboflavin also limits the cell damage inflicted by a stroke or heart attack and mini-mizes respiratory injuries from various toxins.[3] Further, treatment of sickle cell anemia improves when riboflavin, which guards our red blood cells, is included.

A lack of riboflavin can impair the body's absorption of iron and weaken the thyroid gland.[4] To fully correct an underactive thyroid, some people often require daily B_2 injections of 500 mg – an amount that approaches the outer bounds of safe use (when administered alone) and a dosage far beyond what I normally prescribe.

Critical illnesses elevate the need for riboflavin to a greater extent than normal. One study of 102 intensive-care patients found that a reduced B_2 level significantly raised the risk of dying.[5] Even a slightly low level could impede recovery, some researchers assert, but few hospitals bother to monitor their patients' B_2 status. Other research indicates that a B_2 deficiency increases the likelihood of depression or another mental health problems.[6]

SUPPLEMENT SUGGESTIONS

Most doctors know only the superficial signs of a B_2 deficiency, including cracks at the corners of the mouth and difficulty in adjusting to darkness or bright lights. My suspicions are aroused when I find out that someone eats a diet high in carbohydrates. Whole grains, it is true, are a good source of the nutrient, but refined flours, even if fortified, are not. Eggs, meat, poultry, fish and nuts provide a more certain supply.

Supplements are the most dependable source. For general use, all one needs is 25–50 mg a day. Increase the dosage to help address any riboflavin-associated concerns. I'd like to remind you one more time to keep the amount in proportion with the other B-complex nutrients.

VITAMIN B₃: *Niacin: restores sanity, controls cholesterol, niacinamide: repairs joints, controls diabetes*

NIACIN (NICOTINIC ACID)

Niacin is the one vitamin that mainstream medicine considers to be a drug. It may be, in fact, the most effective cholesterol-normalizing 'drug' of all. But using it as a drug violates one of the basic tenets of prescribing B vitamins: they must be given as a team. Here, the companion nutrients are ignored, and with that comes a list of needless side effects. An acceptable risk for a drug, perhaps, but not appropriate for a valuable nutrient.

Vitamin B₃ is a member of the B complex that is critical for energy production and well-being on many levels, especially heart health and optimal circulation. It is involved in over fifty reactions that turn sugar and fat into energy. It is also needed for amino acid metabolism and is involved in converting fats into compounds known as eicosanoids, hormonelike agents that control our bodies' metabolic pathways.

Vitamin B₃ comes in two forms: niacin and niacinamide. While both will meet the body's requirement for B₃, their therapeutic powers differ. Niacin helps lower cholesterol and triglycerides, while niacinamide helps osteoarthritis and may prevent diabetes.

Niacin: Unequaled Cholesterol Control For people who already have had a heart attack, niacin improves the chance of staying alive better than prescription medications.[1] That was the conclusion of a study, the Coronary Drug Project, that pitted the nutrient against two cholesterol-lowering drugs, clofibrate and cholestyramine, to determine which best deters a nonfatal heart attack and lengthens long-term survival following a heart attack. Even several years after treatments had stopped, the death rate was lower only for those who had taken niacin.[2]

In one fell swoop, niacin combats four major risk factors for heart disease:

1. High LDL cholesterol. This 'bad' form of cholesterol amasses on the inside of artery walls, restricting blood

flow and resulting in hardening of the arteries (athero-sclerosis). Niacin supplements force LDL levels to drop, usually by some 10–25 per cent.

2. Low HDL cholesterol. A low concentration of the 'good' cholesterol is one of the strongest predictors of cardio-vascular disease, because HDL helps to cleanse the blood-stream of LDL. Niacin raises HDL significantly, up to 31 per cent, according to one study.[3]

3. Elevated lipoprotein(a). A sticky by-product of LDL, lipoprotein(a) has emerged in the last few years as an inde-pendent risk factor for heart disease – as dangerous as high blood pressure, smoking, obesity and total choles-terol. It contributes to arterial blockages and makes blood more likely to clot. A higher level poses a greater risk. No medication now available has any effect on high amounts of lipoprotein(a). But niacin, along with vitamin C, reduces its risk.

4. High triglycerides. Another independent risk factor newly acknowledged to be of extreme importance, these blood fats signal the presence of an insulin disorder, Type II diabetes, and hypertension. Sharply curbing your con-sumption of sugar and other carbohydrates is the best way to tackle high triglycerides, but niacin supplements offer strong support, cutting them by anywhere from 20–50 per cent.[4]

So Why Don't Doctors Prescribe Niacin? Because niacin was first treated as a pharmaceutical agent, the harmony of the body was ignored and it was prescribed initially in high dosages of 3 grams and up. But in this range it caused diabeteslike blood sugar elevations, frequent liver problems, uric acid elevations and an almost certain red hot skin flush. So it was presented to only a small number of patients with lipid disorders, and some 42 per cent of them discontinued it because of these irri-tating or medically risky adverse effects.[5] It was not until recently that researchers began taking a new look at niacin, and now we have ways to get its benefits minus its disadvantages.

If taken at a comfortable dosage of 100 mg a day with a gradual increase to 1,000 mg a day, far less than that used in earlier studies, niacin achieved success[6] that no other nutrient and no other medication can match. In this dosage it raises the bloodstream's proportion of artery-cleansing HDL cholesterol by 20 per cent. A recent study for using a wax-matrix sustained-release niacin in doses of 1,500–2,000 mg found it both ideally effective and well tolerated.[7]

Niacin achieves its life-extending feat in ways other than by lowering blood lipids. Besides forcing LDL readings to plummet, it also makes this potentially dangerous fat more buoyant and less likely to be damaged and stick to artery walls.[8] Niacin also deters excessive clotting of blood that can lead to heart attacks and strokes.[9]

Clearing blood vessels does more than reduce the risk of cardiovascular disease. By optimizing circulation throughout the body, niacin helps to solve a variety of problems that stem from poor blood flow, including Raynaud's phenomenon (where the hands become extremely sensitive to the cold) and intermittent claudication (a painful leg condition prompted simply by walking). The better blood flow to the brain achieved with a modest dose of 100 mg of niacin also helps stave off senility.

How to Get the Most Out of Niacin The new era of niacin therapy began when more modest doses were proven effective, but it has been strengthened immeasurably by two other major breakthroughs. The first is the eminently logical strategy of using all of niacin's companion nutrients along with this single B vitamin. Nutritionally oriented doctors have long known that the entire B complex should also be generously provided. The second is the development of a compound of the vitamin called inositol hexanicotinate (IHN). Although inositol is itself a vita-nutrient, it was compounded synthetically in the hope of achieving niacin's success without its liabilities. It has succeeded well enough to threaten to change doctors' prescribing practices.

Because IHN, once taken into the bloodstream, breaks down into six molecules of niacin plus one of inositol (a lipid bene-factor in its own right), it accomplishes what niacin does but without the so-called niacin flush – a harmless tingling, itching warmth that flows over the skin when doses of 50 mg or more are taken. Although the flush, a result of histamine release triggered by niacin, is quite harmless and wears off when niacin is taken regularly, very few people will stand for it. Further, IHN does not share regular niacin's tendency to irritate the liver. Taking niacin with meals further minimizes the problem, as does taking a single aspirin tablet with it.

I now prescribe IHN fairly routinely for all my patients whom I feel will benefit from niacin. And improving cardiac risk factors is not the only reason I use it.

Niacin for the Brain Niacin's other crowning achievement, its ability to reverse schizophrenia, has both therapeutic and historical significance. In fact, a study done in 1952 by Drs Abram Hoffer and Humphrey Osmond was the first example of a double-blind test in psychiatry and the beginning of a programme of nutritional therapeutics called 'orthomolecular medicine'. The impetus was provided by the success of their test. Niacin and niacinamide doubled the two-year recovery rates from this mental disease after just five weeks.[10]

I have always found that niacin has a gently tranquillizing effect, and I prescribe it or niacinamide when anxiety is a presenting problem. Animal studies confirm that B_3 has a sedative effect. In another application, 500 mg of niacin per day helped considerably in treating patients who have anorexia and bulimia. And other research suggests that there is a link between niacin and cancer prevention.[11]

Niacin's Flip Side Niacin appears to raise blood sugar in people who have diabetes, although only moderately so.[12] Diabetics, however, need the nutrient's arterial protection more than other people do. The possibility of a glucose disturbance can be avoided entirely by taking lower doses of niacin along with chromium. The combination is as effective at lowering cholesterol as are high doses of niacin alone,[13] since chromium benefits both blood sugar and cholesterol.

NIACINAMIDE

Because of its different type of action, niacinamide, the other natural form of the vitamin, will not cause skin flushing – but neither will it improve cholesterol readings and blood circulation. I do not use it for cardiovascular purposes, but there are conditions that respond to this form of the B vitamin better than to niacin or inositol hexanicotinate.

Diabetes Since the 1940s science has known that people with Type I diabetes require smaller injections of insulin if they take niacinamide regularly. The nutrient can also prevent some of the pancreatic damage that ruins the body's ability to make its own insulin. The damage begins at a young age, which explains why Type I is also called juvenile-onset diabetes. It also explains why the earlier we can protect the pancreas, the more successfully we might prevent the disease.

That's what researchers had in mind when they gave the nutrient preventively to some eighty thousand children (ranging in age from five to seven) in New Zealand. Niacinamide slashed the incidence of Type I diabetes by more than 50 per cent.[14] In another study of fifty-six adults who were newly diagnosed with Type I, a daily dosage of 25 mg per kilogram of body weight (1,750 mg for the average adult) protected their pancreatic cells from harm and improved their ability to manufacture insulin.[15]

Osteoarthritis Niacinamide also diminishes osteoarthritis pain and improves joint mobility. Doses of 3 grams per day, in divided portions, worked well in a study performed by Wayne B. Jonas, MD, the director of the newly formed US government Office of Alternative Medicine. It takes about three months for the positive results to appear with niacinamide therapy, and improvement will continue well into the second and third years of supplementation.

Other Conditions Like niacin, niacinamide exerts a gentle sedating effect that's useful in treating a variety of emotional and neuropsychiatric problems, including anxiety, depression, attention deficit disorder, alcoholism and schizophrenia. In high doses the nutrient acts like an antioxidant and, in laboratory cell cultures, has worked against the HIV virus.[16]

SUPPLEMENT SUGGESTIONS

Meat, poultry, dairy products, seafood, nuts and seeds all provide vitamin B_3. With most of these foods on the enemies list of high-carbohydrate, low-fat proponents, it's easy to understand why an estimated 20–30 per cent of us fail to consume even the paltry recommended daily allowance. Supplements, then, are not supplemental: they satisfy a basic need.

Inositol hexanicotinate, niacin and niacinamide are generally safe in moderate doses. Some side effects may appear, especially if you're seeking the vitamin's therapeutic assistance in amounts larger than 500 mg a day. Take a good B-complex supplement to support the extra B_3, follow my guidelines, and you shouldn't have to worry.

• *Niacin* The original vitamin B_3 is generally safe, if used properly. The flushing sensation is harmless and expected. It lessens day by day, as your body gets used to it. Taking the supplement with some food or an aspirin tablet minimizes the reaction, as does starting off with a daily 100 mg dose and gradually increasing to higher amounts, which might have to be as much as 1,000 mg a day. Because the large dosages necessary for treating schizophrenia or lipid disorders work like a medication, they should be supervised by a health care practitioner. If you need to take that much, you should already be under a doctor's care. Timed-release formulations of niacin still allow the development of liver toxicity, which is why I prefer the inositol hexanicotinate.

• *Inositol hexanicotinate* I'm now using this form of niacin for most people who need niacin because it carries all of vitamin B_3's benefits and none of its risks. In the absence of a heart ailment or as a general preventive supplement, you will do fine by taking 100–500 grams per day. To improve your heart's health, 800–2,400 mg usually is necessary. I've never needed to prescribe a larger amount. Unlike timed-release forms of niacin, timed-release inositol hexanicotinate is safe. Some people notice a relaxing, anxiety-easing influence upon taking supplements. Others might call it drowsiness.

• *My one real precaution with either inositol hexanicotinate or niacin is just the flip side of its therapeutic effect* If you are taking vasodilating drugs, be aware that these vitamins will enhance the medications' effect. Rather than stopping the drug, first talk to your doctor and announce your desire to reduce or eliminate your pharmaceutical needs through the nutrient. If you're on cholesterol-lowering medications, the same holds true.

• *Niacinamide* High doses may cause nausea or extreme drowsiness for some people. For basic health maintenance, a daily 100 mg tablet should suffice. If you have Type I diabetes, take 300–600 mg daily. If you've been diagnosed recently with Type I diabetes or if you're trying to relieve osteoarthritis pain, your doctor should prescribe 1,500–2,000 mg.

VITAMIN B_6 (PYRIDOXINE): *The most essential B vitamin*

You don't need to search very hard to find good examples of how detached our dietary policy makers are from the latest nutrient research. The case of vitamin B_6, however, is one of the best illustrations. For a nutrient so integrally involved in a woman's hormonal health, diabetes and heart disease prevention, arthritis treatment and immune system strength, the RDA is a paltry 2 mg. However, the totality of scientific studies would place 50 mg as a more appropriate recommendation for daily B_6 dosage – and that's for generally healthy people. In treating certain illnesses, I usually recommend 100–200 mg a day, and in specific cases I've recommended as much as 1,500 mg.

Pyridoxine appears in more of my targeted nutrient therapies than any other vitamin. One reason is that it's involved in so many biochemical reactions essential to sustaining life. Another is the fact that even by government standards, the average person is so alarmingly deficient in it. Among residents of nursing homes, for example, B_6 is the most severe and most frequently observed vitamin deficiency. Milling and refining rob whole grains of almost all of their B_6, and virtually nothing is restored. Yet we are being told to eat more and more of these grains.

THE HEART OF B$_6$

Because so many biochemical aspects of health require pyridoxine, it's hard to limit our focus to a finite list of ways in which B$_6$ helps us. The vitamin is indispensable for manufacturing prostaglandins, the hormonelike compounds whose innumerable functions include dilating blood vessels and opening bronchial passages. A skewed prostaglandin balance can lead to tissue damage, inflammation, schizophrenia or even cancer. A short supply of vitamin B$_6$ is often the weakest link in the prostaglandin production process.

Diabetes To learn how long someone's body has been exposed to the tissue-damaging effect of high blood sugar, a doctor tests for something called glycosylated haemoglobin. Higher readings of this blood marker correspond to a greater extent of diabetes-related cellular harm. Vitamin B$_6$ reduces glycosylated haemoglobin, which suggests that the disease's cell damage decreases, too. Taking supplements helps stabilize blood sugar, encourages cells to metabolize blood glucose, and fights eye damage and vision loss from diabetic retinopathy. Regular use also lowers the level of xanthurenic acid, an injurious chemical by-product of a B$_6$ deficiency that causes diabetes in lab animals.

Heart Disease Diabetes, of course, drastically raises the risk of heart disease. Better blood sugar control, however, is only one of several major ways that pyridoxine protects our cardiovascular health. It's one of the three B-complex nutrients (along with folic acid and vitamin B$_{12}$) that so simply and swiftly eliminate our most recently recognized heart risk factor – homocysteine, an amino acid whose elevated level in the blood corresponds to greater rates of strokes and heart attacks.[1]

Additionally, a lack of the nutrient increases heart attack risk for reasons independent of homocysteine, according to Cleveland Clinic researchers. Without it, blood thickens and tends to clot, which can block off an artery.[2] The vitamin also acts as a diuretic, helping to reduce water retention and, as a result, lower high blood pressure. As a Harvard study of fifteen thousand American doctors illustrated, the men with the lowest

B_6 levels had 50 per cent more heart attacks than their better-nourished peers.[3]

Immune System Weakness Especially as we age, vitamin B_6 is critical to a strong natural defence from viral and bacterial infections.[4] A lack of it diminishes our best measurement of immune system functioning, the number of T cells. People with AIDS need the nutrient in an amount far beyond what they could possibly obtain from food. Even when they eat what a conventional dietitian would consider an adequate amount, AIDS patients still have a B_6 deficiency.

Hormone Disturbances Women have a special need for vitamin B_6, because it performs an integral role in maintaining a balance of female hormones. By helping to convert oestradiol, a form of oestrogen, into oestriol, its least harmful and least carcinogenic form, B_6 counteracts one cause of cancer in women. For similar reasons it must be included (along with choline, inositol and methionine) in any therapy for uterine fibroids, endometriosis or fibrocystic breast disease. As a natural diuretic, the vitamin brings welcome relief when premenstrual tension starts to flare.

Pregnancy-Related Problems A woman needs more B_6 when she's pregnant and when she's taking birth control pills. Both deplete the body of pyridoxine. Restoring a healthier amount often alleviates the depression that sometimes sets in as a side effect of oral contraceptives.[5]

The average mother-to-be often doesn't consume enough B_6 to meet her own and her baby's requirements. A daily 30 mg supplement will just begin to meet the demands of both. As a bonus, the vitamin relieves pregnancy-related nausea and decreases the risk of gestational diabetes and the high blood pressure of preeclampsia.[6]

Candidiasis Of the women who contend with an overgrowth of the *Candida albicans* yeast, two-thirds don't metabolize pyridoxine properly. The yeast prevents the body from converting B_6 into its active form, pyridoxal-5-phosphate. Until you get rid of the yeast infection, you may need to take direct supplements of this 'activated' B_6.[7]

Kidney Stones Combined with magnesium orthophosphate, B_6 cuts down on the formation of calcium oxalate, the main ingredient of most kidney stones (any source of magnesium will help).[8] This is just one example of the many ways that the vitamin helps the body to metabolize minerals correctly.

Brain and Nerve Impairment Epilepsy[9], attention deficit disorder, schizophrenia, depression and autism are among the neural and mental disorders whose successful treatment depends at least in part on pyridoxine. In a review of eighteen different clinical studies on autistic children given high doses of B_6, half of them benefitted; many became normal.[10] It also plays a pivotal role in making norepinephrine and serotonin, brain chemicals responsible for feelings of well-being.

In older people, higher B_6 levels are associated with better scores on memory tests.[11] Along with CoQ_{10} and iron, it helps people with Alzheimer's disease[12] and may be useful against Parkinson's disease, although some research indicates it may interfere with L-dopa and other Parkinson's medications.

Joint and Hand Pain My arthritis treatment wouldn't be as effective as it is without B_6. Alleviation of hand pain from carpal tunnel syndrome also depends on B_6 more than on any other single nutrient. For both treatment breakthroughs, I have to thank John M. Ellis, MD, and his 1973 book on the therapeutic uses of vitamin B_6.[13] Ellis' original work is by no means outdated; research still confirms that people with rheumatoid arthritis are often deficient in B_6.[14]

Skin Disorders Asthma, acne and seborrheic dermatitis respond to B_6 treatments. So does malignant melanoma, especially if the vitamin is applied directly on the skin.

SUPPLEMENT SUGGESTIONS

Pyridoxine is completely nontoxic, as long as you follow one rule of thumb: match high doses with similar amounts of the other B-complex vitamins and with a magnesium supplement. In the absence of these supporting nutrients, doses above 500 mg per day run the definite risk of sensory neuropathy, a numbness or tingling in the arms or legs, which in these cases is temporary. Taking the companion nutrients and lowering the B_6 dosage reverses this side effect. Today, I still see an occasional person who notices some numbness with relatively small doses, but the vast majority do just fine.

A good number of us can't adequately convert B_6 to pyridoxal-5-phosphate, the activated form that the body requires. For this reason, at least 20 per cent of your daily B_6 dose should be in the activated form. It's particularly useful, I've found, when repetitive stress injuries and carpal tunnel syndrome don't respond to standard B_6 supplements. The activated form is more potent, too, requiring approximately one-fifth the dosage, or between 25 and 100 mg daily.

To enhance the therapeutic effect, take B_6 alone with one meal and then with the other B vitamins at another meal later in the day. For general health protection, I'd like to see everyone take 50 mg a day. For any of the specific conditions associated with a lack of B_6, a better dosage range is 100–400 mg.

FOLIC ACID: *Our most significant deficiency*

Taking folic acid could stop 10 per cent of all heart attack deaths and could single-handedly prevent some 75 per cent of a common, crippling birth defect. In short, folic acid is the one vitamin we need more than any other.

As Roger Williams taught us long ago, a nutrition programme is only as good as the weakest link in the chain. This tenet is so important that it bears frequent repeating. Among our many weak links, folic acid is the weakest. Increasing our intake would prevent a significant number of stroke and cancer deaths and at the same time allow sufferers to find relief from arthritis, colitis, dementia, chronic fatigue, skin disorders, menopausal symptoms and postpartum depression.

The Feats of Folate

Fifty years ago, little was known about this B-complex vitamin. Scientists understood that folic acid deficiency, along with a lack of vitamin B_{12}, caused megaloblastic (pernicious) anemia and that just a tiny amount, 400–800 mcg, overcame the anemia. However, too much folic acid given alone could mask a vitamin B_{12} deficiency. After determining a minimum and a maximum amount, the medical leadership closed the book on folic acid.

But that was then. We know better now, thanks to some progressive researchers who weren't ready to shelve the matter. As they experimented with doses way beyond the microgram level, they ended up not only penning additional chapters, but rewriting the entire book about folic acid's therapeutic uses.

Birth Defects By taking a far greater daily dose of folic acid, women around the world will be able to prevent an extremely serious, very common kind of birth defect. When the neural tube, which forms an embryo's central nervous system, develops improperly, a baby will be born with one of several horrifying conditions; two of them are spina bifida, in which the spinal cord doesn't close completely, and anencephaly, in which a large portion of the brain is missing.[1]

Folic acid – in daily doses of 4 milligrams, not micrograms – can prevent some 75 per cent of these tragic birth defects. The medical research, including a landmark 1991 study of 1,195 women from seven countries, is voluminous and consistent.[2] Women must understand clearly that they need to maintain a strong intake of the vitamin – not just after becoming pregnant, but throughout their childbearing years. Foetal needs are critically important in the first few weeks after conception, when a woman may not know she is pregnant. When her folic acid status is low, other complications of pregnancy, including spontaneous abortion, low birth weight and premature rupture of the membranes, become more prevalent. Don't be reassured by the mainstream's proposed strategy of offering folic acid to mothers with a history of neural tube defects; some 95 per cent of infants with this defect are born to mothers who previously had healthy babies or to first-time mothers.

Additionally, it should be noted that new mothers shouldn't shelve their supplements once out of the delivery room. Folic acid is valuable for relieving postpartum depression (indeed, it's the Atkins Center's main treatment for the condition). Using 20 mg or more, we've racked up an impressive success rate.

Heart Disease When the history of heart disease is rewritten, the chapters on cholesterol will conclude with this sentence: 'High homocysteine is a greater risk factor, but it can be corrected easily with folic acid supplements.'

A blood protein largely overlooked until the past few years, homocysteine has taken centre stage on the pages of the world's medical journals. If the scientific community can ever wrest control from the politically influential doctors who advise on public health policy, homocysteine would inherit the mantle from cholesterol as Public Enemy No. 1, not only for its link to cardio-vascular disease, but also for its association with a wide spectrum of other illnesses.

Medicine finally is acknowledging that a higher than normal blood measurement of homocysteine is a bona fide risk factor – independent of all others – involving almost every form of atherosclerosis. The risk for heart disease triples when the substance's blood level exceeds 15.8 µmol/L – a reading still considered by many to be within the 'normal' range.[3] The odds, moreover, vary in direct proportion to the homocysteine concentration: drop your homocysteine levels by five points, and you reduce your risk by 40 per cent.

Study after study confirms homocysteine's contribution to modern-day epidemics. People who suffer heart attacks, according to one conclusive study, have lower amounts of both dietary and plasma folic acid.[4] The risk for stroke is even greater than for heart disease and greater still for peripheral vascular disease. One study showed that 32 per cent of the people afflicted with periph-eral vascular disease had abnormal homocysteine readings.[5]

Carotid artery stenosis, which mainstream medicine tries to correct with vascular surgery, also correlates strongly with high homocysteine, as does the vascular disease that often develops in people with diabetes.[6] Arteries aren't the only targets, either. Clots in leg veins also have been linked to the blood protein's presence,[7] as has sudden vision loss that may stem from a blockage of retinal blood vessels.[8]

Nor is the impact confined to the cardiovascular system. Homocysteine levels are also significantly higher in Alzheimer's patients[9] as well as in patients with multiple sclerosis,[10] menopause[11] and rheumatoid arthritis.[12] High readings also have been seen, not surprisingly, in women who have given birth to babies with neural tube defects.

Tragic as this tale may be, the treatment is cut-and-dried. We can predict a happy ending with virtual certainty. Proper doses of folic acid (along with vitamin B_6, the second most important nutrient in this regard, as well as with vitamin B_{12} and betaine) almost always render homocysteine's threat harmless.[13] I cannot recall even a single patient at the Atkins Center whose high homocysteine reading did not drop precipitously once treated with this nutrient combination.

Oestrogen Replacement I very often prescribe high doses of folic acid for conditions that are not yet associated with the nutrient in published research. I've discovered them largely on my own, and they've withstood the test of time with thousands of my own patients. Dr Carlton Fredericks taught me that high doses (between 40 and 60 mg) have a powerful, oestrogenlike effect. Mega-folic therapy, as I call it, proved to be a godsend for women who cannot tolerate the side effects of oestrogen replacement. The prescription hormone, in many instances, will worsen diabetes, low blood sugar, high blood pressure and high triglycerides. Folic acid will not.

Mega-folic therapy, along with the mineral boron, can delay menopause or relieve its symptoms, allowing women to halt oestrogen replacement therapy entirely or reduce their prescription dosages. It can revive a depressed libido, restore menstrual regularity and adjust hormonal imbalances. In adolescent girls it can coax delayed puberty back on track. It also helps to slow the bone loss that leads to osteoporosis, perhaps by decreasing homocysteine.

Intestinal Disorders Cells in the digestive tract require folic acid to replicate and heal. Ironically, the medications that are dispensed to treat Crohn's disease, colitis and other painful inflammatory bowel disorders, such as sulfasalazine, drain the body of folic acid and impede absorption. People with Crohn's disease already have a lower than average level of folic acid in their bodies, probably because of the disorder's own malabsorption problems, so an already painful problem becomes worse. A folic acid deficiency simply delays healing and prolongs the agony.[14]

Mega-folic therapy, I've discovered, tames these afflictions. Again, dosages of 40–60 mg work best, along with pantethine, the essential fatty acids, and a sugar-restricted diet. My staff and I have treated hundreds of people with this formula, chalking up a very gratifying success rate of about 85 per cent. The vitamin also dramatically relieves various forms of short-term and chronic diarrhoea,[15] providing an added advantage to colitis cases in which the frequency of bowel movements must be decreased.

Brain Disorders Cerebrospinal fluid contains – or should contain – a strong concentration of folic acid, because the nutrient is essential to the brain's health. In older people a below par level can contribute to dementia, while supplementation, conversely, can greatly improve their mental processes. Deficiencies have been found in people who have epilepsy as well as such psychiatric disorders as depression, mania and schizophrenia.[16]

Depression Many chemicals responsible for the brain's health and emotional balance are dependent on folic acid, but what's sufficient for one person may not be enough for someone else. People who become depressed, for instance, may have a higher need for the nutrient than do nondepressed, otherwise healthy people. It is known that depressed patients with low folate levels respond poorly to antidepressant drugs.[17] Once the greater need is satisfied, mental disposition can improve as markedly as it does with drugs. A 50 mg dose of folic acid (in the form of methyl folate) can, according to one study, treat depression as effectively as the drug amitriptyline.[18]

Peripheral Neuropathy This numbing, tingling pain in the legs and arms is often the result of a lower than normal supply of folic acid. I and other practitioners administer the nutrient intramuscularly to treat the disorder.

Cancer Folic acid alone can reverse cervical dysplasia, the abnormal cellular changes that cause positive Pap smears and portend the development of cervical cancer. Dosages of 10 mg per day, one study found, eliminated the precancerous cells and averted the need for surgery in just two months.[19] Larger dosages are completely safe and, I believe, possibly more effective. For my cervical dysplasia patients, I typically prescribe 30–60 mg a day, along with vitamin C, vitamin B_{12} and vitamin A. There is one precautionary note, however. Birth control pills should not be taken during treatment for cervical dysplasia, because they drain the body of folic acid.

Other malignancies are also vulnerable to folic acid. Low folic acid readings are also associated with cancer of the throat and colorectal cancer. Fortunately the supplement therapy news is encouraging. A year-long course of the nutrient (10–20 mg a day, plus 750 mcg of vitamin B_{12}) reversed dysplasia in smokers' lungs and, in a separate study, in the colon.[20] Supplements also cut in half the percentage of people in whom colitis leads to cancer.

Skin Problems Folic acid deficiencies are common among people with psoriasis, and folic acid is the nutrient behind the success of our psoriasis treatment at the Atkins Center. Along with vitamin B_{12}, the vitamin contributes to evening out the loss of skin pigmentation caused by vitiligo, and it helps clear up acne outbreaks.

Other Diseases Believe it or not, I still haven't reached the end of the list. A glance at the published research shows that folic acid (in a 6.4 mg daily dose, plus a little vitamin B_{12}) can match the pain relief of nonsteroidal anti-inflammatory drugs for people with arthritis.[21] It's proved beneficial for people with restless leg syndrome, chronic fatigue and HIV infection. And as a mouthwash, it helps fight periodontal disease.

SUPPLEMENT SUGGESTIONS

Folic acid combats so many health problems so successfully because an optimum amount is so frequently absent from our bodies. Only 11 per cent of all Americans, and a similarly low percentage of Britons, eat enough of the nutrient's chief dietary sources – liver, kidney, broccoli, beef, kale, turnip greens, beets and corn – to obtain even the minimally required daily amount. Cooking can destroy as much as 90 per cent of a food's folic acid. Regular alcohol consumption depletes our bodies of it, as do many anticonvulsant medications.

'Enriching' foods with an extra pinch of folic acid, as the FDA has ordered in America, won't make an appreciable difference to our everyday health. The amount falls far below our need, and the nutrient won't reach the bloodstream as surely as it would by taking supplements. Consider two crystal-clear illustrations:

1. When seventeen women took 200 mcg of folic acid per day, an amount slightly more than the RDA, they were not able to maintain an adequate blood level of the nutrient. Even worse, the dosage did not prevent homocysteine levels from rising.[22]
2. Eating 400 mcg worth of folic acid solely from food does not raise the bloodstream's concentration of the nutrient anywhere near the point attained by swallowing a supplement of the same amount.[23] What a blow to the generation of dietitians who have insisted that we don't need vitamin pills and can meet all of our nutritional needs exclusively from food!

For these reasons and others, I simply do not subscribe to the recommended daily allowance of folic acid and cannot applaud even a small step towards greater fortification of the diet. Everyone, I believe, needs to take at least 3–8 mg a day. People whose homocysteine levels are elevated or who have a high risk for heart disease should take 10–20 mg daily. For cancer, menopausal symptoms, postpartum depression, serious cases of colitis or any other condition linked to the nutrient,

I'll administer 20–60 mg per day. To enhance the body's absorption, take a bifidobacteria supplement. These helpful intestinal flora manufacture additional folic acid in our large intestines.

Folic acid is one of our safest supplements. The theoretical possibility of masking a vitamin B_{12} deficiency is easily averted completely just by making sure your diet and supplements contain a sufficient amount of B_{12}. Occasional unexplained, idiosyncratic reactions are rare. But the reactions to the *lack* of folic acid are not rare at all.

VITAMIN B_{12} (COBALAMIN): *The vitality shot*

Millions of people regularly go to their doctors for shots of vitamin B_{12}, and they leave the surgery knowing that the nutrient will make them feel better. Although doctors normally oblige their patients by giving the injections, many worry that their colleagues would frown on the practice. After all, they may think any improvement would just be in the patient's head.

Their concern is well founded. In the past, doctors have lost their medical licences after administering the vitamin for reasons other than those authorized by the arbiters of medical correctness. Why the vindictive reaction? At one time, only doctors could dispense vitamins or nutrients. Doctors were (and still are) steeped in the tradition of finding only one officially recognized cause of any given disease, and they followed the officially sanctioned treatment. To them, vitamin B_{12} was the treatment for pernicious anemia – nothing more, nothing less. If the results of a patient's laboratory tests didn't reflect the disease, he or she didn't need the vitamin. And doctors shouldn't administer it.

These narrow-minded rules are still on the books, even though the scientific reality is quite different. Research now proves that vitamin B_{12} influences our health in myriad ways beyond the prevention of pernicious anemia. It metabolizes food, guards against stroke and heart disease, fine-tunes the nervous system and contributes to relief from asthma, bursitis, depression, low blood pressure, multiple sclerosis and a variety of mental disorders. The millions of people who get B_{12} shots and take supplements, it turns out, were right. They feel better because they *are* better.

A DEFICIENCY IN DISGUISE

Although cobalamin, as vitamin B_{12} is technically termed, appears in all animal foods and can be manufactured by beneficial bacteria in the gastrointestinal tract, a deficiency and its health consequences are never very far away. Standard measurements of B_{12} status can be deceptive, and even sufficient intake doesn't assure that the body will absorb it properly. The repercussions of inadequate B_{12} consumption are bad enough, but even a blood level that's just moderately below optimum can inflict considerable damage to the brain and nervous system.[1]

Vegetarians and older adults are particularly susceptible, as are smokers, people with AIDS and anyone who has a long-term diarrhoea problem. A high percentage of people with sickle cell anemia[2] or thalassemia, two other inherited forms of anemia, also risk a deficiency. Pregnancy, too, increases a woman's dietary need; a mother-to-be who eats very little animal protein could expose her baby to B_{12}-related neurological problems. Also, certain medications interfere with the body's use of the vitamin.

Absorption depends entirely on a healthy intestinal supply of 'intrinsic factor', a substance made in the stomach that latches on to B_{12} and draws it into the bloodstream. With age, we generate less and less intrinsic factor, one of the reasons anyone older than fifty is vulnerable to a deficiency.[3] One out of every three people who have undergone stomach surgery is also deficient because of the lack of intrinsic factor.[4] Also, those taking popular anti-ulcer drugs have impaired B_{12} absorption.[5] While this situation is serious, the problem is easily overcome by taking high doses (at least 1,000 mcg a day) of B_{12}. Amounts closer to the RDA won't do the job.

Lower dosages also can't overcome B_{12}'s certified deficiency disease, pernicious anemia. Perhaps this condition no longer deserves its name now that B_{12} injections are known to work so well, but a subclinical form, which occurs when blood readings fall in the low end of the 'normal' range, may be just as pernicious – and considerably more common. Long before a blood test can detect official B_{12}-related anemia, symptoms will surface. Doctors can easily misdiagnose them, but if the true cause is not identified and addressed, the brain or nervous system could suffer permanent damage.

At first you may feel tired all the time or notice a little indigestion. A woman might miss her period. Other early signals include slower thinking, confusion, memory lapses and depression. Because the nutrient is required for the body to make myelin, the membrane that covers nerves, you may also notice a numbness or burning sensation in the feet. Many diagnoses of Alzheimer's disease, multiple sclerosis, peripheral neuropathy and Lou Gehrig's disease (amyotrophic lateral sclerosis) have turned out to be cases of vitamin B_{12} deficiency.

PERNICIOUS PRESCRIPTIONS

If, as with anemia, medicine properly labelled all of the illnesses related to a B_{12} deficit, health textbooks would teem with references to 'pernicious' variants of numerous diseases – pernicious insomnia or asthma, or pain syndrome, to name but a few. The failure to acknowledge the nutrient's full impact is, itself, pernicious. The evidence of B_{12}'s influence is readily available.

Mental Function A broad range of emotional and cognitive abilities rely on an optimal amount of B_{12}. In cognition tests of elderly people, for instance, those who had the poorest scores had the lowest blood measurements of cobalamin.[6] People diagnosed with depression had low plasma levels of cobalt, the mineral that forms the centre of the B_{12} molecule.[7] Restoring a healthier blood concentration relieves symptoms of dementia and confusion for many older people. It also contributes to deterring the mental deterioration that occurs in AIDS. People infected with the HIV virus frequently have too little B_{12} in their bodies.[8]

Heart Disease Cobalamin is part of the nutrient trio (the others are folic acid and vitamin B_6) that overcomes the threat posed by homocysteine, a blood chemical that in high amounts magnifies the risks of heart disease and stroke.

Multiple Sclerosis A higher than average homocysteine level also generally coincides with multiple sclerosis. People with this demyelinating disease don't metabolize B_{12} properly, which leaves them more vulnerable to nerve damage. A daily 60 mg supplement of a B_{12} preparation called methylcobalamin helps. Vision and hearing improved by 30 per cent, one experiment concluded, after a group of people afflicted with MS started to take the vitamin.[9]

Sleep Disorders On its own, B_{12} appears to help overcome insomnia. A 3,000 mcg dose, according to one study, enables people with sleep problems to drift off more easily and to remain asleep for a longer period.[10] Equally significant, large doses apparently help us adjust to changes in our sleeping and waking habits. The nutrient contributes to the manufacture of melatonin, the hormone actually responsible for resetting our biological clock's rhythm whenever we adapt to a new time zone or a major change in work schedule.[11] The age-related decline in B_{12} absorption probably accounts for the fall in melatonin secretion that occurs as we grow older.

Asthma and Allergy I'm not the only doctor who uses B_{12} to treat allergies and asthma. In one study, a 30 mg dose, administered intramuscularly for two weeks, completely relieved asthmatic breathing problems for ten out of twelve study participants.[12] Other research documents the vitamin's value in clearing up hives and chronic dermatitis.

Nerve Pain Science has established conclusively that aggressive cobalamin therapy eases pain from the nerve damage of diabetic neuropathy.[13] Discomfort from shingles or peripheral neuropathy also abates after B_{12} injections.

Low Blood Pressure Have you ever felt dizzy upon standing up suddenly? Take some vitamin B_{12}. It helps to correct the low blood pressure that causes those abrupt bouts of light-headedness.

Viral Infections A cobalamin deficiency impairs the immune system's ability to fight off germs and other microbes. This is one reason that supplements have been used for years to treat viral hepatitis. Low serum B_{12} levels doubled the rate of disease progression in AIDS patients.[14]

Hearing Disorders Tinnitus, a persistent ringing in the ears, often coincides with poor B_{12} intake. A deficiency, one study reported, was detected in 47 per cent of people who had chronic tinnitus and noise-induced hearing loss.[15] Among a similar group of people with no hearing problems, only 19 per cent had a deficiency.

Infertility Cobalamin is one of many nutrients essential for the reproductive health of both men and women. On its own, one study shows, the nutrient can raise a low sperm count.[16]

Cancer Before outright cancer develops, cells undergo a premalignant transformation called dysplasia. After a one-year supplement programme featuring 750 mcg of B_{12} and 10–20 mg of folic acid, the precancerous changes noted in smokers' lung cells had disappeared.[17]

SUPPLEMENT SUGGESTIONS

We all could use more B_{12} in our bodies. For a more clinically accurate assessment, you'll need a lab test. However, the measurement most commonly used, serum B_{12}, is inadequate. It won't reveal if your intake is great enough for the body to absorb and use the nutrient. A far better gauge is a blood test for methylmalonic acid, a nerve-damaging toxic compound responsible for many misdiagnosed cases of Alzheimer's disease. Higher methylmalonic acid readings mean that the body isn't absorbing or receiving enough B_{12}. As more of the vitamin is ingested and absorbed, methylmalonic acid declines.

Determining your body's need might be the easiest aspect of tending to your B_{12} health. From here, you have several options for how much to take, how to take it, and what form to use. Here are some treatment tips:

Dosage Individual circumstances will differ, of course, but all of us would be better off by taking at least 100 mcg every day. If you're forty years old, take 200 mcg; if you're older than sixty, take 400 mcg. For any other deficiency-related conditions, you'll need at least 1 mg (1,000 mcg) per day, as part of a comprehensive nutrient programme. The upper limit may be 'the sky'. I've prescribed 60 mg a day to some of my MS patients with no adverse impact.

Safety The nutrient is extraordinarily safe even in high amounts. No toxicity has ever been noted. My only precaution is the rule of B-complex balance: don't take supplements of B_{12} alone. Accompany them with a good balance of the other B vitamins. Folic acid is of special concern, because it works in tandem with B_{12}. Always take at least 1 mg with any amount of cobalamin.

Shots vs Tablets How should you get your B_{12}? Many of us in complementary medicine have long pondered the relative benefits of injections and pills. Both can be effective. Intramuscular injections are the speediest, most direct way to get the vitamin into your system. For any condition that demands quick relief – including asthma, a pain syndrome, diabetic neuropathy and acute viral hepatitis – go to the doctor and ask for an injection.

Shots also compensate for a lack of intrinsic factor, but then so, too, do high doses in pill form. Any amount above 1 mg will overcome the absorption impediment, working quite well against the ailments I've just listed. Chewing tablets or swallowing drops of liquid B_{12} also enhances absorption – by as much as fivefold, according to some experiments. I usually tell people to take sublingual lozenges. Dissolving these specially prepared pills under the tongue bypasses the digestive tract, permitting the nutrient to enter the bloodstream directly.

Oral Options Supplements come in many forms. Hydroxy-cobalamin and cyanocobalamin are fine for generally healthy people who want an optimal intake. Both correct deficiencies and reverse pernicious anemia. Hydroxycobalamin is the longer acting and raises blood levels higher. I prefer it to cyanocobalamin. On the other hand, the two so-called coenzyme forms, methylcobalamin and adenosylcobalamin, may have a therapeutic edge. Food contains the coenzyme form of B_{12}, and logic suggests that it might work when the other forms are ineffective.

I cannot end a discussion of 'the red vitamin', as it has been dubbed, without recalling the life's work of H. L. Newbold, MD, a doctor who, like me, practised complementary medicine in New York City. He developed a unique programme for treating most of his patients who complained of chronic metabolic fatigue, depression and brain fog. Besides a meat-based diet, he recommended a daily hydroxycobalamin injection in a dosage of 1–10 mg. I've had many occasions to see people he treated over the years, and their dedication to maxi-megadoses of B_{12} was profound. They were convinced that it turned their lives around. Their devotion – and their patient records from Dr Newbold – has nearly convinced me that the nutrient might have even more remarkable power when given in higher doses.

CHOLINE AND LECITHIN (PHOSPHATIDYLCHOLINE): *Nerve rebuilder*

In the name of good health, our fat-fearing society often does things that harm more than help. By renouncing eggs, for example, we scramble the body's ability to metabolize fat and deprive ourselves of nutrients that are fundamental to avoiding disease, including the heart problems that a low-fat diet ostensibly prevents.

Eggs are one of our only food sources (along with soyabeans) of phosphatidylcholine, known otherwise as lecithin.

Phosphatidylcholine (PC) is an essential protector of every cell, especially those of our nervous system, and it also serves as the main source of choline, which in turn is essential to the formation of acetylcholine, one of our most important neurotransmitters. Conversely, choline is essential for our bodies to manufacture our own lecithin. Some confusion may arise from recognizing that the product we purchase in the health food store as lecithin is not PC, but a natural concentrate containing PC plus a mixture of other similar compounds, called phospholipids. Because choline, PC, and lecithin supplements all will build up the blood levels of choline, we shall consider them together.

NERVE NUTRITION

Choline is found in breast milk, a usually sure indication that it is indispensable to health. Without it, infants would develop severe neural abnormalities, for the nutrient contributes to the production of myelin, the protective casing that surrounds nerves and brain cells. In treating adults, I have found that doses of 9–18 grams reduced the trembling, involuntary movements and slurred speech of tardive dyskinesia, a condition caused by antischizophrenic medications.[1] Choline and PC both seem to help ease the jerky, involuntary movements and spasms that characterize Huntington's disease and Tourette's syndrome.[2]

Alzheimer's Disease There is no scientific agreement on the nutrient's impact on this memory-stealing disorder. However, memory enhancement from choline supplements is more apparent in people without the disease. Ten grams of choline chloride, taken daily, one study demonstrated, considerably improved the short-term recall ability of healthy adults.[3]

Heart Disease The choline/PC/lecithin team fights heart disease in several different, though complementary, ways. A study of these mechanisms reveals why low-fat diet advice can be so counterproductive for keeping the heart healthy. For example, even though PC produces only a moderate reduction of total cholesterol, it improves the ratio between good and bad cholesterol.[4] Almost every time a heart patient of mine stopped taking lecithin or PC supplements, I soon found a worsening in that ratio, the amount of beneficial HDL cholesterol to the amount of total cholesterol. After my patient resumed lecithin supplements, the cholesterol ratio just as consistently began to improve

again. Why? Lecithin lowers harmful LDL cholesterol somewhat while simultaneously raising HDL modestly.[5] The extra
HDL further reduces LDL. Lecithin is also an emulsifier,
breaking down fats for better digestion and helping both cholesterol and triglycerides to remain fluid and less likely to build
up along artery walls. Also, PC preserves the blood levels of
carnitine, one of the body's most essential heart nutrients.[6]

Choline plays a part in helping to lower blood pressure by
causing blood vessels to relax and thus allow better flow of
blood.

Liver Disorders A low-choline diet impedes the liver's ability
to process fats, resulting in another ironic consequence of an
egg-free, fat-free diet – weight gain.[7] A deficiency, if extreme,
may lead to a liver disease or even liver cancer.[8] As abnormal
fat metabolism continues, cholesterol and triglycerides accumulate in the liver, eventually leading to fatty liver disease,
which, if untreated, is fatal.

Happily, though, choline supplements will clear the fat log
jam, and the liver can reverse the disease entirely. In one small
study, several people with fatty liver disease took between 1 and
4 grams of choline chloride every day for six weeks. As CAT
scans verified at the end of the study, the condition had cleared
up completely.[9]

Oestrogen-Based Disorders. Lecithin may heighten the overall
effectiveness of nutritional therapies for a whole spectrum of
women's health problems, including uterine fibroids, fibrocystic
breast syndrome, endometriosis and breast and endometrial
cancer. Dr Carlton Fredericks taught me that choline, along with
inositol and methionine, should always be part of the treatment
for these afflictions. They're the most effective nutrients for
enabling the liver to convert oestradiol, the form of oestrogen
with the greatest cancer-causing potential, into oestriol, a safer,
less carcinogenic form of the hormone.

SUPPLEMENT SUGGESTIONS

Eggs are our best dietary sources of phosphatidylcholine. Other good choline-containing foods are organ meats, dandelion greens, nuts, seeds and soyabeans. For the amounts needed to address health problems, supplements are certainly necessary. Lecithin granules are my favourite. They're a tasty addition to recipes and a great salad garnish. But though some people may warn you that, over time, lecithin granules may turn rancid and leave a bad taste in your mouth and have no nutritional benefit, this is precisely why I recommend them. Supplements can oxidize, too, but because you swallow them as capsules, you'd never know it. With granules, your taste buds warn that they've gone bad.

Phosphatidylcholine supplements are another good way to get choline nutrition; they are well tolerated and have been used safely in doses as high as 35 grams a day. Concentrated lecithin, a thick liquid, is another option. It typically contains 55 per cent phosphatidylcholine and releases choline slowly over time. For the concentrated form, the basic preventive dosage is 1/4 teaspoon daily. For neurological problems and memory enhancement, take between 1 and 4 teaspoons a day.

To round out the list, choline chloride and choline bitartrate are two other acceptable forms, but in the doses often required, you may notice an annoying but innocuous fishlike odour.

A minor precaution: high doses of supplemental lecithin and choline should be accompanied by additional vitamin C and calcium. Vitamin C serves to protect us from the nitrosamines that can be generated during choline metabolism, and calcium is required to tie up the extra phosphorus that lecithin contains.

INOSITOL: *Nature's sleeping pills*

Inositol was among the very first nutrients I used for pharmaceutical purposes. Dr Carl Pfeiffer taught me that this relative of the B-complex family relaxes nervous tension and encourages sounder sleep. Some ten thousand inositol-taking patients later, this old supplemental friend remains one of the most clearcut examples of a safe, natural vita-nutrient that virtually eliminates the need for a whole category of potentially harmful drugs: tranquillizers and sleeping pills.

Aye, but there's a rub. Before you have a chance to dream of a world without drugs, you need to be informed of the alternatives. And since inositol's seemingly self-evident action had never been subjected to an official scientific experiment, its virtues had to be described by word of mouth by the relatively few doctors in the know.

Only in the past few years have researchers begun to examine inositol's calming influence, with several studies using doses far bigger than I've used to treat severe cases of depression, anxiety and obsessive-compulsive disorder.

THE BRAIN AND BEYOND

Depression Inositol levels are often lower than average in people hospitalized for depression. To make a bad nutritional deficit even worse, lithium, commonly prescribed for manic-depressive disorder, further decreases the brain's inositol concentration. Resupplying the nutrient naturally can frequently lift spirits. Dosages of 6–12 grams a day for four weeks, two studies agreed, significantly alleviated a number of depressive symptoms.[1]

Anxiety Inositol's treatment power matches that of stronger psychotropic drugs in alleviating the most severe example of anxiety, panic disorder. It should be taken routinely for this almost paralyzing sense of dread, whose symptoms can resemble those of a heart attack. People with less severe cases of anxiety respond well, too, as can people with agoraphobia, the fear of being in public. Among the few differences research has noted between inositol, again in a dosage of 6–12 grams, and drugs was the nutrient's lack of side effects.[2] A dose of 18 grams daily proved safe and effective in treating obsessive-compulsive disorder.[3]

Alzheimer's Disease Inositol in doses of 6 grams daily helped the language and orientation of a group of Alzheimer's patients;[4] perhaps a longer-term study will prove its value.

Diabetic Neuropathy Inositol's other uses are better documented. For example, inositol escapes easily from the nerve cells of people with diabetes. The loss, experts believe, is at least partly responsible for diabetic neuropathy, the painful destruction of nerves in the arms and legs that occurs after years of poor blood sugar control. I've used inositol in my diabetes treatment ever since reading an impressive 1978 study in which a daily 1 gram dose eased pain and improved nerve function for a group of people with neuropathy.[5] Vitamin C is an important addition, for it may head off the inositol loss in the first place.

Obesity Inositol, choline and methionine are integrally involved in how the liver handles fats, giving rise to their scientific nickname of lipotropic, or fat-burning, nutrients. For a number of overweight people whose biggest obstacle to weight loss is a reluctant metabolism, supplements of the nutrient trio can trigger their bodies to burn off the excess fat. Note that this same trio of nutrients helps weaken oestrogen effects, as I described in the previous chapter.

Infant Health Breast milk is one of our richest natural sources of inositol, a fact that should have prompted manufacturers to include the nutrient in infant formulas. At first they didn't give it a second thought, but these days, thankfully, most infant formulas do contain it. Be sure to check the label, however.

Newborns need inositol critically for healthy growth. For premature babies, it increases survival rates, prevents vision loss from retinopathy and prevents respiratory distress.[6]

SUPPLEMENT SUGGESTIONS

By eating a lot of fresh produce, whole grains, meat and milk, we might be able to supply ourselves with as much as 1 gram of inositol daily. However, a substantial proportion would be in the form of fibre and thus not absorbed very well. Therefore supplements are necessary for most of our basic needs. For most everyday uses, such as temporary or full-blown insomnia, take 500–1,500 mg at bedtime. For moderate anxiety, I will give 1–2 grams a day. Clinical depression and panic and obsessive-compulsive disorders demand far higher doses, such as the 6–18 grams used in the research studies. Note that inositol is a chemical isomer (it has a slightly different configuration) of glucose, and these higher doses might inhibit weight loss.

PANTETHINE/PANTOTHENIC ACID:

Better than cholesterol drugs

One of the very first nutritional principles I learned was that our adrenal glands need pantothenic acid to manufacture their disease-modifying anti-inflammatory hormones. Applying the lesson in a little experiment gave me one of my first hints that a nutrient could in fact replace a drug. Eventually pantothenic acid would prove to be a powerful natural treatment for several rather disparate health plagues, arthritis, colitis, allergy and heart disease.

If pantothenic acid was so essential to the adrenals, I reasoned, supplements of this B-complex nutrient might enable the adrenal cortex to secrete an extra amount of its principal hormones, called glucocorticoids, perhaps enough to help ease the symptoms of arthritis, colitis or another inflammatory ailment. At the time, the only treatment for these conditions was prednisone, a drug whose horrible side effects include everything from water retention and facial bloating to weight gain, osteoporosis, diabetes and immune system failure. My modest hope was that the nutrient might let me reduce some prednisone users' medication dosages.

Pantothenic acid's impact far exceeded both my and my patients' expectations. I went on to help thousands of people not only lower prednisone dosages, but free themselves entirely from a lifelong need to take anti-inflammatory drugs. As a surprising side effect, the nutrient also decreased high cholesterol.

BIRTH OF A SUPPLEMENT

As the years went on, we learned the secret behind most of pantothenic acid's success. Once in the body, it forms a substance called pantethine, which is converted into an all-important enzyme called 'coenzyme A'. Coenzyme A is one of the few substances in the body directly involved in the metabolism of all three main food components – protein, fat and carbohydrates. It's also the basis for our production of hemoglobin, bile, sex and adrenal steroids, cholesterol and a few brain chemicals. While pantothenic acid supplementation does ultimately lead to the creation of coenzyme A, pantethine creates at least twice as much.

Once discovered, pantethine was researched extensively in Europe, especially in Italy and Spain, where it was marketed as a registered pharmaceutical. Wanting to obtain it closer to home, I found an American vitamin company that solved the technical problem of keeping pantethine stable in tablet form. Overcoming this obstacle gave birth to perhaps the single best substance on the planet for reestablishing optimal levels of cholesterol, triglycerides and other fats in the blood.

Pantethine is more powerful than any other side effect-causing medication used to reduce cholesterol. Dozens of solid medical studies from Europe and Japan attest to its efficacy and safety. Thousands more people are living proof. But it is certainly the most underappreciated vita-nutrient you will read about in this book.

PANTETHINE: THE POTENT PERFORMER

Pantethine's results aren't just good. They're spectacular. I use it and pantothenic acid together, making them the number one single or dual nutrient used in my practice. Because most of the therapeutic action comes from coenzyme A, pantethine is potentially the more valuable of the two, although for a few other illnesses, pantothenic acid retains its full value. Therefore let's consider them separately, starting with pantethine.

Autoimmune Disorders Soothing inflamed tissues doesn't apply only to arthritis. Whether for allergies, asthma, lupus or psoriasis, anyone who now takes prednisone or another steroid medication stands to benefit. At the very least, you can expect less need for the drug. Your doctor probably will have to reduce the dosage and may be able to wean you off the prescription entirely – two things I now do routinely for my patients. The less the dosage, the less your chance of suffering the drug's side effects.

Besides allowing the adrenal glands to generate more cortisone, pantethine also helps to increase omega-3 fatty acids in the body (EPA, DHA and the other essential oils).[1] These omega-3 fatty acids also exert a powerful anti-inflammatory action. And their only side effects are good ones, making pantethine indirectly responsible for cutting the risk of heart and artery diseases.

Cardiovascular Disease The escalation of our two most dangerous blood fats, low-density lipoprotein and triglycerides, stops dead in its tracks when confronted by pantethine. In one published account that's typical of the results I and dozens of other doctors achieve, a daily 900 mg dose of pantethine led to a 32 per cent drop in triglycerides, a 19 per cent drop in total cholesterol, and a 21 per cent drop in LDL. At the same time, the 'good' cholesterol, high-density lipoprotein (HDL), rose by 23 per cent.[2]

Without even trying, I found more than a half dozen similar accounts in the medical literature. All of them documented dramatic improvements in supplement takers' blood fats, even when the lipid abnormality was due to other illnesses.[3] Not a single paper failed to show reductions, and not a single paper reported side effects. Compare that to the well-established life-shortening consequences of most cholesterol-lowering drugs. Statin drugs create a shortage of the vital heart nutrient co-enzyme Q_{10}, and all the other drugs were associated with death rates from noncardiac causes that were higher than the control subjects. Pantethine outperforms these two-edged swords in every way.

Ironically, pantethine's effectiveness at cholesterol lowering has helped cause considerable incredulity among my patients as I tell them, with the confidence built on over twenty thousand cases, that they can eat steak, eggs and butter and, as long as they take their pantethine and other nutrients and stay away from carbohydrates (the Atkins Center's time-tested programme), their lipid profile, especially LDL and triglycerides, will improve dramatically. But those happy results take place over 90 per cent of the time.

Pantethine protects the heart and arteries in other ways. It encourages the production of enzymes that help break down blood fats and contributes to vitamin E's action against cholesterol buildup.[4] Pantethine is one of the few nutrients that increases the amount of clot-busting omega-3 fatty acids and reduces clot-promoting fats in cell membranes. By generating more coenzyme A, it enhances metabolism in the heart muscle, strengthens the force of its contractions, and slows the rate at which it beats. It can also improve a certain form of dilated cardiomyopathy and ease angina pectoris (cardiac chest pain). In short, pantethine helps the heart in so many different ways that no heart patient should be without it.

Colitis and Crohn's Disease Merely maintaining an average blood concentration of pantothenic acid won't raise the body's coenzyme A level enough to relieve the discomfort from the two major inflammatory bowel problems, colitis and Crohn's disease. A 'normal' concentration of the nutrient, one study of colitis sufferers demonstrated, didn't get the enzyme to where it was needed, the mucous membranes that line the colon.[5]

Pantethine reversed all of that. A daily 900 mg dose, matched by an equal amount of pantothenic acid, dramatically improved the vast majority of my Crohn's and colitis patients – and within just a week, something that I had never before witnessed. By helping beneficial bacteria to grow in the intestines, pantethine also controls the yeast infections found in the majority of our colitis patients.

Yeast and Chemical Sensitivities Candidiasis plagues a very large number of people even in the absence of colitis. Pantethine, as a natural detoxifier, helps the body get rid of yeast overgrowths and accumulations of other noxious substances, such as formaldehyde. It also supports the liver in breaking down such chemical by-products as acetaldehyde. Both alcohol consumption and yeast infections generate this toxin, which is responsible for the 'brain fog' associated with candidiasis.[6] Some research indicates that pantethine may even work against the desire to drink alcohol.[7]

Many of us received our first doses of pantethine from mother's milk. The nutrient, once in the intestinal tract, stimulates the growth of bifidobacteria, *Lactobacillus bulgaricus*, and other friendly flora. The more we maintain an intestinal balance weighted in favour of these good bacteria, the better protected we are against harmful microbes. Antibiotics present an imminent threat to this balance, because they destroy all bacteria, both friend and foe. While these drugs are a necessary evil in many instances, pantethine supplements, according to one study, greatly minimize their inherent risks.[8]

PANTOTHENIC ACID: WE STILL NEED IT

Don't conclude that pantothenic acid must play second fiddle to its virtuoso offspring. Pantethine's parent remains a therapeutic player in its own right, especially for healthy skin. Unusually high doses (as much as 10 grams a day) can alleviate acne, although six months or more may pass before the megadoses pay off.[9] Once the complexion begins to improve, the dosage can be cut to a maintenance level of a mere 1–5 mg a day. Besides clearing up pimples, a topical cream that contains a 20 per cent concentration of pantothenic acid will also shrink enlarged pores and make the skin feel smoother. The B-complex nutrient appears to promote skin health in general. A recent study found that 900 mg of pantothenic acid daily will improve wound healing and surgical recovery.[10]

Gout We've used calcium pantothenate for years as a gout remedy. Taking 200 mg four times a day pretty reliably breaks down the excess uric acid that leads to the condition's arthritic leg pain.[11]

Inflammation Symptoms of the so-called burning-foot syndrome are also relieved with pantothenic acid supplements, as is the burning feeling of an ulcer. Add pantothenate to the list of natural alternatives for arthritis relief. The often used nonsteroidal anti-inflammatory drugs carry a substantial risk of causing ulcers.

Obesity Because my low-carbohydrate diet is so effective for losing weight, I haven't delved into some relatively new research that suggests a hefty amount of pantothenic acid (10 grams a day, taken in several divided doses) helps people shed excess weight.[12] It certainly makes sense, however, because the body's production of coenzyme A drops when we try to lose weight. We should not let that happen, because coenzyme A, when present in sufficient amounts, decreases appetite, burns long-chain fatty acids and restores energy.

But I certainly cannot condone the use of drugs to lose weight – or to relieve inflammation or ulcer pain or to control cholesterol. For general health, take between 100 and 200 mg of either pantothenic acid or pantethine every day. To stabilize cholesterol and triglycerides or to tame inflammation, allergies or an autoimmune condition, you'll need 600–900 mg a day of both pantethine and pantothenic acid.

PABA (PARA-AMINOBENZOIC ACID):
Energizer, stiffness fighter

Whether you're bothered by menopausal symptoms or are struggling with a far more serious disease like scleroderma, you might find a friend in PABA. People unwittingly treat themselves with this nutrient every summer. Because it absorbs ultraviolet light, PABA is the active ingredient in many topical sunscreens. Few people realize that you don't have to ladle on the lotion to get the sun shield. An oral supplement of 1–2 grams, taken before going out into the sun, will also protect your skin. As a bonus, you might be shielding yourself from feeling tired. The nutrient is high on my list of fatigue-fighting remedies, although it doesn't help everyone.

While not an official member of the family, para-aminobenzoic acid, as PABA is formally called, is typically included in B-complex supplements because it's required to synthesize folic acid in our gastrointestinal tract. This fact probably explains, in part, why PABA often proves helpful in treating hot flushes, irritability and other menopausal maladies. The folic acid it helps to create is integral to keeping a good balance of female hormones.

Tough Approach to Tough Skin

Medicinally, PABA is one of the handful of nutrients capable of substantially swaying the course of two diseases that are otherwise very difficult to treat, as well as a few other skin-related conditions somewhat more serious than a summertime sunburn.

Scleroderma In this disorder of the immune system, hard, fibrous tissue grows throughout the skin and blocks blood flow to internal organs. Usually the condition is ultimately fatal. PABA, however, offers some hope. When treated with the nutrient, 76.6 per cent of the people in one study survived longer than ten years, about double that of the usual expectation for the illness. Almost all PABA users with the disease will at least notice softer skin and an improvement in other symptoms.[1]

Peyronie's Disease Conventional urologists may unwittingly practice a bit of nutritional medicine when they prescribe Potaba, the pharmaceutical version of PABA, to treat this disease in which fibrous tissue grows inside the penis. The condition usually isn't otherwise serious, but the hardened skin doesn't permit erectile tissue in the penis to expand uniformly, resulting in an inconvenient, occasionally painful curved erection. PABA, in high doses, is the best nonsurgical therapy available.[2]

Joint Disorders It's worth anyone's while to try PABA for a possible remedial effect against two other conditions caused by the growth of fibrous tissue: posttraumatic contractures and Dupuytren's contracture. In the former, hardened scar tissue forms near the site of an injury and limits joint flexibility; in the latter, a tendon, usually the fourth flexor, tightens in the palm, making it difficult to straighten the affected finger. In my practice, PABA is frequently helpful in relieving all sorts of connective tissue problems, including arthritis.

Skin Discoloration More than fifty years ago doctors used PABA to treat vitiligo, the loss of pigmentation that leaves blotches on the skin.[3] Even modest doses are very beneficial, with dramatic improvements possible after six months of regular supplementation.[4]

Other Ailments Probably because it soothes inflammation, PABA can influence other autoimmune disorders, including thyroiditis.[5] Additional research suggests it may be useful in treating chemical sensitivities and oxidative damage from ozone exposure.[6] For people allergic to gluten and its related proteins, found in such foods as wheat, oats, barley and rye, supplements can counteract stomach distress and other symptoms of gastro-intestinal damage.

In nutritional folklore, PABA purportedly can restore colour to greying hair. Unfortunately this claim may not be true. I've never seen it happen with any of my patients, and it's never been documented.

SUPPLEMENT SUGGESTIONS

Unless you're affected by a PABA-related condition or are planning to spend a lot of time beneath the summer sun, you won't need daily supplements. Most of us get what we need from food, with help from the beneficial bacteria in our intestines, where the nutrient is manufactured naturally.

People with vitiligo can take as little as 400 mg per day. The more serious health conditions require far greater dosages and a doctor's supervision. For example, in Peyronie's, between 6 and 12 grams a day are necessary, although as much as 20 grams has been used (prescription-only Potaba is the best way to get such high amounts). But 1 gram, taken in divided doses over the course of the day, may be effective in treating gluten allergy. Your stomach won't tolerate big dosages of over-the-counter PABA very well. Aside from the intestinal upset, however, the nutrient causes no serious adverse effects in dosages under 15 grams per day. The liver problems that one study associated with a large amount are quite rare; I've never encountered them.

Some people experience an allergic reaction to topical applications of PABA. If this has occurred, don't assume that you also can't take it orally. You won't necessarily be sensitive to supplements.

BIOTIN: *Diabetes benefactor*

Like vitamin B$_2$, biotin is a team player, and team players are normally forgotten amid the fuss over the big-name attractions. Biotin could become a memorable member of the B-complex clan, however, if researchers played to its strengths. In amounts a hundred times the standard dose, this nutrient might reverse a crippling consequence of diabetes.

The typical B-complex capsule contains a paltry 100 or 200 mcg of biotin. Why? For one, the nutrient is quite costly. For another, outright deficiencies rarely occur, because the body, with the assistance of the intestines' beneficial bacteria, manufactures its own supply.[1] When a deficiency does occur, the patient is usually an infant, because a baby's gastrointestinal tract may not hold enough of the beneficial bacteria. People who are fed intravenously for a long time or who take a lengthy course of antibiotics might run a small risk of a biotin shortage. So can someone who drinks alcohol regularly or who must take anticonvulsant medications. Consuming a number of raw egg whites every day might also increase your need.

RESTORING NERVES TO NORMAL

The standard biotin dosage probably ensures that your skin and hair remain healthy, but when the amount is multiplied by a factor of 100, exciting therapeutic changes can occur. If further research confirms the results from some small studies, we may have a genuinely incredible treatment for anyone with Type I or Type II diabetes. In dosages of 15 mg and higher, lab experiments have demonstrated, biotin aids in managing blood sugar.

It accomplishes this by enhancing the effect of enzymes involved in processing glucose.[2]

In one small study, megadoses also were able to halt or even reverse diabetic neuropathy, a degenerative nerve condition caused by elevated sugar levels. Subjects were given 10 mg of biotin by intramuscular injections three times a week for six weeks. After that they took 5 mg a day orally. Within four to eight weeks neuropathy symptoms improved markedly. Muscle cramps in their legs eased considerably, and symptoms of 'restless leg syndrome', the nagging discomfort relieved by movement that's felt deep inside the limbs, had all but disappeared. After a year of biotin therapy, each of the supplement takers could walk 300 metres without assistance – no small feat for someone afflicted with neuropathy. All in all, the study participants enjoyed a general increase in their ability to get around. Even better, the large nutrient dosages caused no side effects.[3]

The early success of this experimental therapy, although enormously encouraging, raises more questions than it answers. Can biotin, for instance, also influence such diabetes-related disorders as low blood sugar and obesity? Will it enhance the effects of chromium or zinc? To glean some answers, I've been giving high doses of the nutrient, between 5 and 15 mg a day, to some of my diabetes patients. They've been faring well, but because they receive other effective nutritional measures, it is difficult to discern the role played by biotin.

Skin Disorders Along with beneficial bacteria supplements, biotin can be useful in treating cradle cap in infants. Its impact is less dramatic against the adult version, seborrheic dermatitis. Adults require a more comprehensive approach that includes all of the B vitamins, as well as the essential fatty acids and such minerals as zinc. In large doses biotin can partially restore weak or brittle nails. One study documented a difference using a daily dose of 2.5 mg.[4]

Hair Problems Because it optimizes the body's use of fatty acids and makes the scalp less oily, biotin can improve the hair's general texture and appearance. Even though claims that it stimulates hair growth are not backed by any published papers, I prescribe it routinely for my patients in the same dose I give to diabetics. Supplements will surely stop hair loss caused by a biotin deficiency, but hormonally caused male pattern baldness is a different story. Judging from my patients' results, a significant number of balding patients improve with biotin supplements.

Supplement Suggestions

Unless you want to explore its ability to curb diabetes, daily biotin supplements aren't necessary. To compensate for a possible low level, make sure your meals include healthy portions of such biotin-containing foods as cheese, organ meats, nuts, egg yolks, soyabeans, royal jelly and brewer's yeast. Take a general bifidobacteria supplement, too. For diabetes and to explore the possibility that hair loss will prove to be biotin-responsive, add 5–15 mg of biotin at meals, in divided doses, to your complete vita-nutrient program.

VITAMIN C: *The nutrient that does it all*

Vitamin C is so fundamental to our health that I am unable to think of an ailment that supplements do not in some way improve. In an attempt to focus this discussion, I asked myself, What do I commonly see in my practice, and how does C help? Almost every medical problem I could think of, be it colds, cancer, high blood pressure or asthma, has a vitamin C-based solution, each one documented by a plethora of scientific evidence.

Thus, you will note the encyclopedic nature of this section, which should serve as a rallying cry for one and all to get the right daily dose of this nutrient.

And with that we touch upon the key to vitamin C: the right amount. Here's a clue for how much that might be: It's not the RDA, or double the RDA, or even quadruple it. The RDA was set long ago at 60 mg, but science has learned far more since then. As has been demonstrated over and over, we need a full gram (1,000 mg, or almost seventeen times the RDA) for prevention of illness and probably much more for dealing with it.

Once the nutritional pioneers discovered that ascorbate was necessary to curing scurvy, the bleeding gums disease first noticed in our seafaring forebears, they quickly established a daily requirement based on the few milligrams required to prevent symptoms from reappearing. With the minimum requirement as a starting point, a consensus soon evolved among academic nutritionists that 300 mg would probably be the uppermost dosage bounds for safe, acceptable experimentation. Their conclusions may have been based on the assumption that a toxic dose must bear some relationship to the minimum requirement. As a result, higher doses were seldom studied; however, this assumption was false.

In recent years many enterprising investigators paid no heed to the arbitrary constraint, which had become, over the years, accepted and enforced almost as law by those who determine medicine's professional standards and guidelines. And as the research mavericks continued to demonstrate that dosages above 1,000 mg brought a variety of health advantages, political forces on medical consensus panels continued to endorse the RDA. Within the last couple of decades, however, the mavericks have become the majority in medical research, and 1,000 mg is now the popular, 'politically correct' starting point.[1] But the policy-setting old guard still hangs on stubbornly and stodgily to the status quo.

Notwithstanding the industry debate, contemporary studies show success after success, making vitamin C the featured performer in the drama to replace pharmaceuticals with nutrients. One simple experiment in comparative physiology (the study of other species), demonstrates that our true vitamin C requirements are far higher than officially recognized.[2]

Humans, along with primates, guinea pigs and a few other species, are the only beings that do not synthesize their own vitamin C. Most animals make about 30 mg per kilogram of body weight. For a person who weighs, say, 68 kilograms, that adds up to about 2 grams a day. Rats, mice and rabbits manufacture seven times that amount when under stress. Paleontologists have calculated that even before evolution cast off the mechanism to manufacture ascorbate, primitive humans ate between 400 mg and 2 grams every day. (If science ever conclusively establishes that 2 grams guards health better than 60 mg, you'll see how it all fits together.)

More specific research, particularly that done by Mark Levine, PhD, at the US National Institutes of Health, offered the first precise measurement of ascorbate's performance in real-world circumstances, as opposed to test tubes or the mainstream medical mind. His conclusive result: our metabolism requires at least three times the vitamin C that the RDA provides.[3]

Those who dismiss ascorbate and other nutrients as nothing more than the ingredients of expensive urine will be interested to learn that its presence in the urine in no way indicates whether or not the body has enough or too much vitamin C. Overconsumption is the least of our problems, even according to the outmoded RDA. A full 25 per cent of all Americans consume less than 39 mg a day[4], and the figure is unlikely to be very much better in the United Kingdom. Few people, especially children, eat enough of the fruits and vegetables that are our primary dietary sources. Heat, storage, cooking and biochemical processing all destroy much of the vitamin C we would otherwise consume. In the body even more is burned off by stress, cigarettes and other sources of cellular damage like exposure to smoke and smog. Commonly used medications like aspirin and oral contraceptives are big depleters of whatever vitamin C does manage to get into our bodies.

There is another lesson to be learned, however, from the early history of vitamin C research. Albert von Szent-Györgyi, the doctor who discovered vitamin C, had actually discovered an entire nutritional complex in ascorbate-containing foods. Milligram for milligram, this 'natural' vitamin C proved to be more effective than the source most of us use today, the one responsible for the impressive therapeutic accomplishments you'll read about momentarily.

The C complex's success, particularly against scurvy, can be attributed to the fact that the natural sources contain synergistic components, such as rutin and other bioflavonoids, a copper enzyme (tyrosinase), and other factors. None of these are found in standard-issue synthetic vitamin C, which has been in general use since 1934. The problem lies in getting a source of vitamin C complex per se. It's not commercially available in quantities close to what I believe are necessary to overcome illnesses other than scurvy. Were C complex generally available at a realistic cost, our dosage requirements could be scaled down considerably.

TOUCHING ALL THE BASES

Ascorbate is one of our chief antioxidant nutrients, killing free radical molecules and microbial invaders on its own and extending the lives of other antioxidants, including vitamin E and glutathione. Though it also works in other ways, the bottom line is that people who consume more vitamin C live longer than those who consume less. Let me count the ways:

Infections Everyone knows (don't we?) that vitamin C can knock out a cold or other infection. Though it does kill bacteria directly and aids in neutralizing bacterial toxins, the primary reason that C fights colds so well is that it boosts our natural defences. Almost all cells of the immune system receive some nutritional support, but the biggest beneficiaries are interferon, antibodies and white blood cells, which lose vitamin C during an illness.[5] A good illustration of the vitamin in action is the nutritional treatment of recurrent furunculosis, an ugly infection that forms numerous boils on the skin. In one study, a gram of vitamin C was given to twelve people who both harboured the infection and exhibited an impairment in the function of their neutrophils, the major type of white blood cell. Ten of those twelve cases cleared up completely, but the boils victims whose neutrophils were working normally did not benefit.[6]

At the Atkins Center and at a majority of complementary doctors' surgeries around the world, vitamin C is the mainstay of virus treatments. Its use has been championed more by word of mouth than by the reports and pronouncements of mainstream medicine, which still considers such infection-based diseases as chronic fatigue syndrome, recurrent hepatitis, the various herpes viruses and even AIDS almost untreatable. I am but one of thousands of doctors who finds vitamin C dramatically helpful in fighting these disorders.

The extent of our treatment success often depends on how much vitamin C the body can stand. Most complementary doctors rely on the 'bowel tolerance' system developed by Robert Cathcart, MD. Simply put, you take it until your bowels can't take it. Once the body receives more vitamin C than it can use, the bowels will loosen, causing a temporary case of diarrhoea. The more severe the illness, Cathcart discovered, the more ascorbate the body can tolerate – a fairly obvious sign of a greater need. In some severe cases of mononucleosis, hepatitis or AIDS, people can ingest more than 50 grams over the course of a day without provoking diarrhoea.[7]

When a doctor prescribes such a large amount of vitamin C, he or she will typically administer it intravenously. This circumvents the bowels, avoiding diarrhoea but fully saturating the body with this master nutrient.

High-dose intravenous administration, an innovation of Fred Klenner, MD, who used it to treat polio back in the 1940s,[8] offers particularly gratifying relief to people with AIDS. With this treatment they rarely develop the unpleasant opportunistic infections so commonly endured at the hands of conventional medicine and its pharmaceutical therapies. The injections are safe, reliable and, perhaps, therapeutic in ways we do not yet understand. Though by no means an AIDS treatment per se, vitamin C does deter viruses from reproducing in laboratory experiments involving cell cultures,[9] and it neutralizes a suppressant factor that further weakens the immune system. Topically applied, it can help treat the Kaposi's lesions so commonly developed by HIV patients. Daily oral doses of 100 grams or more have strengthened the immune systems of many people with AIDS; smaller doses are somewhat less effective.

The same immune response that fights viruses assists us in overcoming a bacterial infection – luckily for us, because of the difficulty in initially distinguishing between, for example, a viral and a bacterial pneumonia or bronchitis. If the immune system is operating at full strength when an acute infection first hits, it can prevail over either challenge.

This is the strategy we must mimic nutritionally at the first sign of some malady, whether it turns out to be a cold virus or a bacterial infection. At the onset, both are vulnerable to aggressive vitamin C therapy, along with infection-fighting partners like zinc, vitamin A and the bioflavonoids.

So we return to the original question: does vitamin C cure the common cold? Even advocates of alternative medicine don't agree fully, but evidence from more than twenty studies suggests that the nutrient will reduce the severity of cold symptoms. The body also fights nasty respiratory infections, such as bronchitis and pneumonia, more effectively when ascorbate is employed.[10] Marathon runners susceptible to postcompetition upper-respiratory infections can avoid most of these episodes with 1 gram of ascorbate daily.[11]

Therapeutic dosages that were tested in the early days are small by today's standards, but even 1 gram or more taken daily decreased the length of a cold by 20 per cent.[12] Amounts of up to 6 grams have been tested routinely in recent years, and the higher dosages prove to be somewhat more effective at minimizing the strength and duration of symptoms.

Asthma and Allergies Snuffing out sniffles becomes even more intriguing when you consider that vitamin C very capably combats allergies. With supplements of 1,000 mg or more a day, it acts as an antihistamine.[13] The benefits may not be seen for weeks, though, because the concentration within body tissue must first reach an adequate level.

Asthma is the best example. The risk for this inflammation of lung tissue rises when consumption of vitamin C is low. At least seven studies demonstrate that a daily vitamin C dosage of 1–2 mg can improve lung function and reduce the chance of an asthmatic attack.[14] The same amount, according to double-blind studies, can protect the bronchial airways and lungs from cold temperatures, hay fever and smog.[15] Finally, 2 daily grams of vitamin C eliminated exertional asthma, the exercise-induced form of the bronchial condition, in about half a group of children and young adults.[16]

CHALLENGING CANCER AND HEART DISEASE

The new generation of scientists is taking vitamin C to its farthest therapeutic reaches, attempting to harness its antioxidant power to tame heart disease and a variety of cancers. It's a logical extension. The subject of enormous research, vitamin C is the first line of our antioxidant defence system against cancer and is widely regarded as the most powerful anticarcinogenic nutrient known.[17]

One of the many ways C earns its reputation is by blocking the creation of nitrosamine, a carcinogen. Nitrosamine forms in the body from nitrates, which come from smoked and cured meats, tobacco and even natural gastric secretions. Vitamin C's interference here contributes to cancer prevention in the stomach and throughout the gastrointestinal tract.

Regardless of the mechanism, though, the evidence strongly suggests that a gram or more of ascorbate per day reduces the risk of both gastric cancer and precancerous lesions.[18] When consumed in optimal amounts throughout a woman's lifetime, vitamin C can ward off breast cancer,[19] cervical cancer and the precancerous cellular changes called cervical dysplasia. A low intake also greatly increases the risk of pancreatic cancer, while optimal supplementation reduces the danger.

Research offers evidence of vitamin C's preventive role against colon cancer, bladder cancer, endometrial cancer and oesophageal cancer. Eighty-eight population studies have demonstrated this protective effect.[20]

Why do complementary doctors use vitamin C to treat established cancer? Two reasons: we see that it works for our patients, and the published evidence supports our observations. For instance, one hundred people with terminal cancer survived up to four times longer than expected when they took 10 grams of the nutrient every day.[21] After just five days of supplementation, they said they felt better, stronger and more alert. Their appetites increased, too.

Other studies confirm that multigram doses can lengthen survival time and improve quality of life.[22] The nutrient may control tumour growth, some researchers suspect, by enveloping the malignancy in scar tissue, as well as by strengthening collagen tissue enough to limit the spread.

While not a cure, vitamin C does assist the body in controlling the disease – and in controlling the consequences of conventional cancer therapies (which, by the way, are rarely cures, either). Surgery, radiation and chemotherapy all greatly lower the body's ascorbate content. Some newer research suggests that the vitamin may augment the effectiveness of chemotherapy and, at 40 grams a day, can prevent the almost inevitable hair loss associated with the treatment.[23] From my clinical experience, I've found that it also augments the nontoxic natural therapies I employ as a first line of defence against the disease.

Though anyone with cancer can benefit from ascorbate, it certainly is more effective for people who have not been exposed to chemotherapeutic drugs. These medications damage not only the tumour, but the immune system, removing a primary mechanism through which vitamin C works. This explains the lack of a nutritional benefit shown in some studies, especially a Mayo Clinic experiment that seemed to be designed specifically to undermine the nutrient's worth. Nearly all of the patients involved in this study had been subjected to chemotherapy before starting ascorbate supplementation. Their demise was probably compounded by the abrupt discontinuation of the high doses of ascorbate that were being administered. Such a sudden withdrawal causes 'rebound scurvy', which can have deleterious effects on any disease.

Heart Disease A low tissue concentration of vitamin C, many researchers now agree, should be considered a bona fide risk factor for heart disease.[24] The nutrient's stellar performance in protecting blood fats from turning into atherosclerotic plaque makes it one of our best tools against what is still the number one killer in many Western, industrialized nations, including the UK.[25]

Ascorbate rescues low-density lipoprotein from oxidation, the dangerous process through which this 'bad' type of cholesterol builds up on the insides of arteries. A controlled study of smokers who took 1 gram daily showed a significant reduction in LDL oxidation.[26] Another study demonstrated that the wall thickness of the neck's carotid arteries, another measure of atherosclerosis, was greatest in people who consumed the lowest amounts of the nutrient, as well as the lowest amounts of vitamin E and carotenoids.[27] The two co-partners are undoubtedly important to the body's overall antioxidant defence system. But while vitamin E and beta-carotene slow LDL oxidation once it has begun, only vitamin C – when present in an adequate quantity, of course – can prevent it completely.

A gram of vitamin C has more than twice the antioxidant potential of a glass of red wine, highly touted as a substance that prevents LDL from oxidizing. Vitamin C does not share alcohol's mineral-depleting or liver-irritating properties.

Vitamin C is indispensable to the heart in ways other than as an antioxidant. A high intake raises the body's HDL, the artery-protecting form of cholesterol.[28] Less cholesterol in general is absorbed from food when vitamin C is present, and when administered a dosage of 2 grams per day, heart patients experience a decrease in abnormal arterial spasms or constrictions.[29] Another role of vitamin C, its ability to form collagen, is theorized by Mathias Rath, MD, to protect the heart's blood from attracting sticky particles. Hundreds of case histories attest to the success of his treatment protocol.[30]

But Does It Work? To answer that question, Japanese cardiologists gave 119 patients that had undergone angioplasty a daily dose of 500 mg of vitamin C. Normally, because of the reblockage of arteries, one out of three patients must have the angioplastic procedure redone. Only 14 per cent of the patients who had the modest dose of vitamin C supplements had to repeat the procedure.[31] Yes, vitamin C works.

The principal consequence of Type II diabetes (the high-insulin type) is atherosclerosis. Here, vitamin C is almost as important as well-controlled blood sugar. Besides helping to avert cholesterol buildup, it safeguards the body from the damage wrought by high blood sugar. The more vitamin C a diabetic ingests, the greater the reduction in glycation, which is the name given for harmful effects of sugar upon our tissues. This is not to say that vitamin C does not help control blood sugar in diabetes: a study using 2 grams daily shows that it does.[32]

Hypertension, another big risk factor for heart disease, also appears to depend in part on an individual's vitamin C status. Among sixty-nine adults participating in one study, those with the highest blood levels of the nutrient had significantly lower blood pressure readings. A 1-gram-a-day dosage proved to lower blood pressure effectively.[33] Diastolic pressure, the bottom number in the blood pressure reading, was higher among people with lower ascorbate concentrations, according to another study.[34]

Stress Coping successfully with the emotional and physical toll of stress may depend more on vitamin C than on any other single nutrient. The adrenal glands, which secrete the hormones we need to function during stressful situations, contain more ascorbate than any other part of the body. Vitamin C both assists in the manufacture of these stress hormones and protects the body from toxins created as the hormones are metabolized. Schizophrenia and a variety of other mental disorders may stem, in part, from such toxic by-products of stress.

Obesity Weight loss without a calorie cutback? That's certainly possible on the Atkins diet, but one research effort claims the same can be accomplished with a daily supplement of 1–3 grams of vitamin C.[35] While I am not convinced that the nutrient adds to the weight loss, it does make the process healthier by ridding the body of toxic compounds that are released whenever fat is metabolized. Finally, vitamin C helps the liver withstand the greater free radical stress that weight loss imposes.

Gout Supplements relieve gout's discomfort, but again, the secret is in the dose. Only a daily dose of more than 8 grams will effectively reduce uric acid, according to lab tests.[36] Gout sufferers should not, however, immediately begin to take such a large amount. Start with 1 gram a day and raise the dosage slowly.

Gallstones Vitamin C, 2 grams daily, has been shown to delay the process of stone formation by 350 per cent.[37] One could logically assume that gallstone formers would benefit by staying on C supplements.

Vision Disorders Like certain carotenoids, vitamin C bathes the eyes in antioxidant protection that, according to the US Department of Agriculture's Human Research Center, can prevent cataracts and slow their growth. A minimum of 800 mg per day is required, taken in conjunction with vitamin E and beta-carotene. Ascorbate also eases pressure within the eye, thus decreasing the risk of glaucoma, which occurs more often when Vitamin C is low.[38] As little as 500 mg a day will suffice, some researchers assert. A larger amount, administered intravenously, also lowers intraocular pressure more rapidly.

Drug Addiction Especially when combined with a high-protein diet and B-complex supplements, megagram doses of vitamin C (as much as 50 grams a day) have eliminated withdrawal symptoms in people recovering from heroin addiction. Smaller doses can keep current users from craving the drug. In this regard, vitamin C has proven to be safer and more effective than methadone therapy, which merely replaces one addiction with another.[39]

SUPPLEMENT SUGGESTIONS

For general health, all of us need to consume at least 500 mg of ascorbate every day, along with an equal amount of the bioflavonoids, nutrients found in natural sources of vitamin C that enhance its effectiveness. Milligram for milligram, natural C complex is more potent than the usual synthetic versions of the vitamin, but it's unavailable commercially in sufficient quantity or at a reasonable price.

However, bioflavonoid supplements will help to compensate. Include at least a gram of bioflavonoids whenever your ascorbate dosage exceeds a gram. To further ensure that you obtain C-complex factors, at least 75 mg of your total ascorbate intake should come from food. There's a trade-off here, for almost all food sources, especially fruits, are high in sugars and carbohydrates (therefore you should choose wisely if you have diabetes or another insulin-related condition). Dark green vegetables, lemon juice, red peppers and tomatoes are smart selections, as are cabbage, broccoli, citrus fruits, strawberries, cantaloupe, paprika, mustard and horseradish. Even when their ascorbic acid content is negligible, foods contribute cofactors of C that will make your supplements more effective.

Taking enormous dosages of vitamin C is remarkably, unequivocally safe. Charges to the contrary have long since been discredited. Even in amounts of 10 grams a day (which a lot of nutrient advocates take routinely), vitamin C will not increase the risk of kidney stones or destroy body stores of vitamin B_{12}, as some have alleged.

Concerns about quantity aside, you can follow several other suggestions to help saturate your every cell with this healthful antioxidant.

• *Divide the dose* Consuming a large amount at any given point is fine, but the body uses vitamin C quickly after receiving it. You need to maintain a consistently high concentration, which is easily achieved by dividing your daily total into several smaller doses taken over the course of the day. Slow-release formulations accomplish the same thing, and some research suggests that they ultimately yield a higher blood level.

• *Build up and taper off* Don't shock your body by suddenly introducing a large quantity of vitamin C, and don't abruptly discontinue regular supplementation. Begin with no more than 1 gram per day and gradually up the amount over the course of a week. When you end high-dose therapy, wean yourself by decrementally cutting back on the daily amount. A sudden halt of ascorbate supplements can aggravate the condition for which they were taken, a side effect known as 'rebound scurvy'.

• *Add some enzymes* Digestive enzymes also contribute to a better blood concentration of vitamin C, which is why the nutrient should be taken with meals. A digestive enzyme supplement will help.

• *Mix it with minerals* For general health and nutritional support against illnesses, the widely available ascorbic acid form of vitamin C is just fine. Mineral ascorbates, though, are more bioavailable and thus preferred. They're buffered, too. Based on my clinical experience, magnesium ascorbate seems to allow maximum absorption. The mineral also targets many of the same health problems for which vitamin C is used. Despite some scattered claims to the contrary, calcium ascorbate offers no advantage over any other form, including plain old ascorbic acid. A patented product called Ester-C is touted as providing better blood levels, but this claim has been challenged. I like to prescribe it simply because it is very well tolerated, and it is not acidic, as are most vitamin C preparations.

BIOFLAVONOIDS: *The first family of antioxidants*

As science learned its nutritional ABCs in the 1930s, we briefly had a vitamin P. Once it was reclassified as nonessential, however, the dietary alphabet lost an integral member. We simply can't spell health as well without it.

Vitamin P was the collective name given to the bioflavonoids, an abundant group of pigments, some four thousand strong, that colour many of the plant world's flowers, leaves and stems. Their nutritional demotion was hasty and premature. Because of a wellspring of solid basic science during the last few years, these mighty little antioxidants will be vindicated one day. They're destined to become a routine part of treating cancer, heart disease and inflammation.

MORE THAN C'S SIDEKICKS

In supplement formulas the bioflavonoids often keep company with vitamin C – and for good reason. Nature teamed them with the vitamin in our food to form a C-complex family of nutrients that is somewhat like the B-complex vitamins. Ascorbate allows the bioflavonoids to flex their varied medicinal muscles by protecting them from destruction. In return they empower vitamin C with therapeutic abilities it otherwise would not have. On their own, to use one small study as an example, vitamin C and the citrus flavonoid hesperidin have no effect on menopausal symptoms. Together, however, they eliminated hot flushes for a majority of the study's ninety-four participants.[1]

Citrus contains only some of nature's bioflavonoids. Other plants have other kinds, each with specific health-improving properties. The bioflavonoids in *Ginkgo biloba,* for example, bring oxygen and energy into the brain, while those in hawthorn help the heart. Bilberry's flavonoids improve sight at night. Genistein, the chemical most researchers cite to explain a high-soya diet's link to cancer protection, is a flavonoid, as are the ingredients that account for green tea's antitumour shield. Red wine, too, owes a good deal of its reputation as a heart tonic to flavonoids. Alone or together, the C-complex components also *ward off allergies, ease asthmatic airways, cool inflammation and reinforce collagen and connective tissue.*

Science upholds the use of many individual bioflavonoids, including catechin, epicatechin, resveratrol and the anthocyanosides. Some of them are better known by the plants from which they come, such as *Ginkgo biloba* and bilberry, so I'll explain them in the chapter devoted to herbs. But two bioflavonoids have earned their reputations individually.

QUERCETIN

Because of its versatility as a preventive and curative nutrient, quercetin deserves the title of 'king of the flavonoids'. At the Atkins Center it's a royal member, along with vitamin C, pantethine and the essential oils, of our 'Big Four' allergy treatment, but we also rely on it to help treat heart disease and cancer.

Allergies and Inflammation You'd be hard-pressed to find an antihistamine better than quercetin. I've prescribed it for years, along with the citrus bioflavonoids, to relieve hay fever and other allergies. Quercetin also interferes with pain-promoting inflammatory substances that are generated in the body by such diverse ailments as rheumatoid arthritis and colitis. Newer research done at Cornell, my alma mater, points to another way quercetin may snuff out sneezing and cool inflamed tissues. Flavonoids from grapefruit juice, this study showed, fight off an enzyme that neutralizes cortisone, a natural anti-inflammatory produced by the body's own painkilling machinery.[2]

Heart Disease The flavonoids in general, but quercetin in particular, may be more potent than vitamin E for disarming cholesterol's potential threat to the heart. A high intake of the nutrient corresponds to a significantly lower risk of cardiovascular disease and stroke, according to several large studies (including one that involved elderly people from seven countries).[3,4] As the most effective antioxidant among the flavonoids, quercetin safeguards LDL cholesterol from oxidation, making it less likely to turn rancid and build up inside artery walls. This shield covers blood vessels and cells throughout the body. Quercetin also keeps blood from thickening and more readily forming clots.

Cancer As both a preventive and therapeutic nutrient, quercetin may allow medicine to make significant inroads against cancer. Besides reinforcing the immune system, it accelerates the production of certain natural detoxifying enzymes that rid the body of potential carcinogens. By alleviating inflammation, it works against yet another process that might contribute to malignant growths.

High-dose quercetin therapy slows the advance of many different types of cancer, according to animal studies.[5] In people it stops the growth of leukaemia cells and impedes the development of breast cancer cells.[6] Other work suggests it may also be useful to prevent or treat colon cancer,[7] ovarian cancer and endometrial cancer, among others.

SUPPLEMENT SUGGESTIONS

You could drink more unfermented green tea and red wine to get more quercetin. Apples, onions, green peppers, tomatoes and broccoli are good quercetin-containing foods. Because a large amount is required, however, the best source is the supplement.

To combat allergies, arthritis or other inflammatory ailments, I normally advise a patient to take, in divided doses over the course of the day, between 600 and 1,200 mg on an empty stomach. To guard against heart disease or cancer, 300–600 mg per day will serve you quite well. As part of an aggressive cancer treatment, a minimum therapeutic dosage starts at 1,500 mg a day.

PYCNOGENOL AND GRAPE SEED EXTRACT

I hold these extraordinary antioxidants and anti-inflammatories close to my heart, for I had been recommending them before my colleagues had had a chance to confirm their therapeutic potential. Their active bioflavonoids, called proanthocyanidins (PCOs), neutralize an even wider range of free radical forces than does vitamin E. By no means does this imply that they can replace E, but their presence certainly magnifies the overall effectiveness of your antioxidant programme.

A considerable body of research attests to proanthocyanidins' contribution to the strength of our capillaries, making them especially valuable for circulatory disorders of all kinds, including varicose veins, hardening of the arteries and impaired blood flow to the brain.[8] PCOs seem to be the bioflavonoids that best speed the healing of bleeding gums, protect the skin of people who bruise easily and curb heavy menstrual flows.

In Scandinavian countries doctors often prescribe pycnogenol, the pine bark extract that I worked with initially, as an allergy treatment.[9] Little support for this remedial role exists in scientific journals, but then none is necessary. Complementary doctors and supplement takers can see and feel the results with their own eyes.

Pycnogenol was the first PCO supplement in the United States, and its 85 per cent bioflavonoid concentration became the gold standard for all other PCO supplements. We later discovered, however, that grape seed extract's concentration is a little higher, between 92 and 95 per cent. Because it also contains some flavonoids not found in pine bark, grape seed extract now probably holds a slight qualitative edge. It's also generally less expensive.

Supplement Suggestions

For all practical purposes, the differences are slight, and dosages remain about the same for either pycnogenol or grape seed extract. For allergies and most other afflictions, I normally dispense between 50 and 300 mg per day. Circulatory and capillary problems require more. To limit a heavy menstrual flow or stop bleeding gums, I'll tell a patient to take 1,000 mg three times per day. At that dosage a therapeutic change can come about in as little as a month. For instance, by the time of her cycle, a woman accustomed to a heavy seven-day menstrual flow might finish within three or four days.

VITAMIN D: *Bone benefactor*

Vitamin D is unique in several ways. It is the only nutritional necessity (therefore a vitamin) that actually functions as a hormone. But then, it is not a *nutritional* necessity because skin will manufacture the vitamin if it gets a little sunlight.

Independent of diet, our skin manufactures vitamin D (from cholesterol, by the way) after a little exposure to the sun – direct exposure, that is. Sitting behind a closed window won't help at all, because glass blocks the ultraviolet rays that trigger the process. During the autumn and winter, elderly people who live in the Northern Hemisphere lose a greater degree of bone mass, the most notable consequence of a vitamin D insufficiency, because of their restricted time outside. Night-shift workers and anyone else who burns the midnight oil, along with people who are bedridden or chronically ill, face a very real danger from a lack of sunshine.

Those of African descent living in the Northern Hemisphere are among the other people who need to monitor their nutrient status, for the darker the skin, the less vitamin D will be produced in response to sunlight. Vegetarians and followers of a low-fat diet share the risk, because the nutrient requires some dietary fat for absorption. In addition, the antiseizure drug phenytoin is a notorious depleter of vitamin D.

Skeletal problems, particularly osteoporosis, are the most

notable repercussions of not keeping your body fully supplied with the nutrient, but they're not the only consequences. The immune system's vitality rises and falls directly with vitamin D's concentration in the body. A vitamin D measurement is one of the factors that doctors use to predict the length of survival for someone with AIDS.[1]

BONING UP

Researchers classified the sunshine supplement as a vitamin after discovering that it prevented rickets, the abnormal skeletal growth seen in children. We've learned only recently, however, that the nutrient, once converted inside the body to its active form, vitamin D_3, is actually a hormone. In addition to making the gastrointestinal tract more receptive to absorbing calcium, vitamin D_3 mobilizes the minerals from other places in the body and directs them to the bones. How well we use magnesium, zinc, iron and other minerals also depends on the nutrient/hormone, as does our susceptibility to skin disorders, heart problems and cancer.

Bone Disorders With the spotlight shining brightly on hormone replacement therapy, vitamin D's enormous effect in combating bone thinning and osteoporosis has been left in the shadows. As we age, our skin loses its ability to synthesize vitamin D_3 from sunlight. The intestines, too, are less able to absorb the nutrient. Supplements thus become imperative. When a group of older people began to take 800 IU of vitamin D_3, along with some additional calcium, every day, one study found, the number of hip fractures they suffered dropped 43 per cent.[2] Women would lose less bone mass during the winter, other research found, if they took 500 IU of the vitamin and 377 mg of calcium.[3]

Psoriasis Clinical studies endorse what many health practitioners have known for some time – natural vitamin D_3 creams cut down on the characteristic skin flakiness of psoriasis.[4] Although pharmaceutical companies have synthesized a D_3

derivative to sell as a psoriasis drug, the real thing – 1.25 dihy-droxy vitamin D – works no less effectively.

Bowel Ailments A lack of vitamin D is one of the most frequently encountered deficiencies among people with Crohn's disease and ulcerative colitis. Supplementation helps eliminate some of the unpleasant symptoms that these intestinal illnesses cause.

Multiple Sclerosis Women afflicted with this degenerative nerve disease frequently have a low blood concentration of the sunshine vitamin. Supplementation reinforces the overall effec-tiveness of MS therapy, although we're not quite sure why. Some nutrient experts think that a better absorption of calcium and magnesium improves the body's reconstruction of the protec-tive membranes that surround nerves.[5]

Diabetes There is considerable evidence that vitamin D improves sugar tolerance in animals. A recent Dutch study found that elderly men with the lowest levels of vitamin D[6] had the greatest impairment in sugar and insulin metabolism. Studies are under way to see if D supplements will help diabetics.

High Blood Pressure Healthier levels of active vitamin D_3 corre-spond with lower blood pressure readings. According to one study, the incidence of pregnancy-related hypertension, called preeclampsia, fell by more than 40 per cent once the 666 parti-cipants began to take vitamin D and calcium supplements.[7]

Arthritis Progressive osteoarthritis, especially in the knees, may partially stem from a lack of vitamin D. This relationship could explain the vitamin's success in a tiny study of five people whose leg and arm pain was not relieved by a whole panoply of drugs. They were deficient in vitamin D, though, and the pain disap-peared along with supplementation.[8]

Cancer Nutritional oncologists question vitamin D's impact only against colon malignancies. Otherwise the nutrient emerges with flying colours from a rigorous review of its anticancer qualifications:

- The rate of breast cancer declines as women consume more vitamin D or receive more exposure to sunlight. A similar relationship exists with the incidence of ovarian cancer. Taking calcium supplements enhances the vitamin's modest protective effect against the two malignancies.[9]
- Cancerous prostate cells are vulnerable to vitamin D_3, making the nutrient good for both prevention and treatment. The only downside in this respect is that rather large amounts are necessary, which may raise the body's calcium level precipitously.[10]
- The vitamin stops tumour cells from spreading, according to laboratory experiments, and has reduced cancerous growths by more than 50 per cent.[11]
- In lab cultures the nutrient inhibits the growth of glioblastoma, the most common type of brain tumour. It also checks the growth of leukaemia cells.

SUPPLEMENT SUGGESTIONS

As with any other hormone, there is an optimal dosage for vitamin D. If exceeded, problems can occur. Knowing that D_3 increases the amount of calcium in the blood, it's logical to expect that too much D_3 leads to an excess concentration of calcium. Should that occur, the mineral may seep into the walls of our blood vessels and other soft tissues, which could speed the formation of artery-blocking plaque.

That's one of the ways we sow the seeds of heart disease, especially if magnesium is in short supply. Plaque can start to accumulate inside arteries even in childhood. Rather than fear vitamin D, I'd prefer to address the lack of magnesium, a more widespread health threat and therefore a solution to a variety of diet-related disorders.

In any event, I don't advocate high-dose vitamin D therapy, although consuming an amount several times higher than the 400 IU RDA represents no danger, at least in the short run. Exposing your face or arms to outdoor sunlight twenty minutes a day for four months out of the year should meet almost anyone's requirement. Supplemental sunning isn't always possible or practical, however, so other sources are nee

But contrary to popular beliefs, milk isn't a good bet. For one thing, the various forms of milk typically contain too much simple sugar, which can send blood sugar skyrocketing. For another, milk does not always live up to its reputation as a source of the nutrient (some 20 per cent of milk products that claimed to provide vitamin D, according to one analysis, actually contained none). Finally, milk is very high in phosphorus, which interferes with the metabolism of both vitamin D_3 and calcium. To be sure, colas and similar beverages carry an even greater risk of phosphorus-related vitamin D problems.

Elderly people, women, shift workers, low-fat dieters, vegetarians, those of African descent and other dark-complexioned people, those who suffer seizure disorder, carbonated beverage drinkers, people who stay indoors – all those at risk for a vitamin D deficiency or a D-related health problem should protect themselves by taking between 400 and 800 IU of vitamin D_3 per day. If you intentionally avoid the sun or shield every exposed inch of skin with sunscreen, chances are you will probably need more of the vitamin.

VITAMIN E: *The chief executive antioxidant*

Vitamin E, for many years derided in mainstream medical circles as 'a vitamin in search of a disease', has recently received such enormous media attention that it would certainly win the 'Most Valuable Nutrient' award, if one existed. Why? Vitamin E controls the number one killer in the Western world, coronary heart disease. A spate of recent research has also established that in addition to the vitamin's deficiency-related impact on blood and muscle function and on reproduction, it also influences tissue inflammation, menopause, cataracts, cancer and bronchial disease. And when 1997 research established the vitamin's ability to benefit Alzheimer's and diabetes, as well as improve our immune function, the remaining sceptics should have been blown away.

THE HEART OF THE MATTER

Suppose your doctor announced that the results of your cholesterol tests were not very good. What would you do? Based on the traditional recommendations, you might stop eating eggs and steak, filling up instead on rice, pasta, skimmed milk and bananas. After a few months a new round of cholesterol tests will show, in all likelihood, that your dietary efforts were not successful, and the doctor probably will convince you to begin taking a cholesterol-lowering drug. After the medication did all that it could do, your risk of dying from a heart attack would decrease by no more than 0–10 per cent, according to medicine's own analyses. If, on the other hand, you had taken a daily 400 IU capsule of vitamin E, the risk would have dropped by more than 40 per cent.

The staggering superiority of vitamin E therapy over the most concerted drug efforts was most convincingly demonstrated by conventional medicine, based on the findings of two Harvard studies: one of 40,000 male doctors, the other involving more than 100,000 female nurses. Dozens of other studies concur. The more vitamin E consumed, the lower the rate of cardiovascular disease.[1] Another study of 2,002 people with heart disease showed that the nutrient, in a dosage of 400 and 800 IU per day, slashed the occurrence of heart attacks by 77 per cent and the death rate from heart disease by 47 per cent.[2]

Several things happen when you take vitamin E regularly. The most important comes from the nutrient's antioxidant shield, which prevents LDL cholesterol from sticking to artery walls and, once enough builds up, blocking the flow of blood. At the same time, vitamin E reduces the amount of LDL cholesterol in the bloodstream, works to eliminate triglycerides (another dangerous blood fat), and increases the amount of artery-cleansing HDL cholesterol. In addition, it lowers insulin and spares the heart from damage caused by a magnesium deficiency or a lack of oxygen. Vitamin E greatly improves the biochemical changes caused by stress in patients suffering congestive heart failure.[3]

Helping to rid the blood of harmful fats improves circulation throughout the body, but vitamin E goes a little further by naturally 'thinning' the blood. The latter term is really a misnomer; actually, blood tends to form clots through the process of platelet clumping. A clot that lodges in an artery can impede blood flow, causing a heart attack or, if the brain is affected, a stroke. When volunteers in a 1996 study took 400 IU of vitamin E daily along with an aspirin, they suffered far fewer transient ischemic attacks (TIAs). These 'ministrokes' interrupt blood flow to the brain only briefly but often portend a more serious stroke.[4] Compared to Coumadin and similarly risky pharmaceutical blood thinners, vitamin E stands as a worthy, and far safer, alternative.

Diabetes People with diabetes are particularly susceptible to blood clots. Their blood platelets, lab analyses show, contain less vitamin E than the platelets of their nondiabetic peers. The anticlotting action is only one way in which the nutrient improves the health of people with diabetes. When vitamin E levels are low, the risk of acquiring Type II diabetes rises by a ratio of nearly four to one.[5] Besides improving sugar metabolism, taking a daily supplement diminishes the severity of several diabetic complications. In a recent study, providing Type I diabetics with 100 IU of vitamin E daily for three months significantly reduced the tissue damage from high blood sugar, a process called 'glycation', as well as the accumulation of triglycerides, the diabetes-related heart disease risk factor.[6]

E'S EFFORTS ELSEWHERE

Vitamin E achieves many, but not all, of its cardiovascular feats as a fat-soluble antioxidant. By safeguarding our cells from marauding free radicals, it rescues us from a number of other health threats.

Cancer Hundreds of studies have examined the relationship between vitamin E and various kinds of cancer, and many reach the same, almost inevitable, conclusion: The higher the nutrient intake, the less likely the cancer.[7] The converse is true, too. As illustrated by an eight-year-long study of more than thirty-six thousand adults, the people with the lowest levels of vitamin E had a greater risk for developing cancers of all kinds.[8] Scientists have found specific correlations with colon cancer, cervical dysplasia and cervical cancer, breast cancer, lung cancer and oropharyngeal cancer.[9]

However, this conclusion is not unanimous. And the reasons touch on the very nature of antioxidant nutrition. Vitamin E's role is preventive. It cannot reverse already existing damage. In some of the research that finds no anticancer benefits from vitamin E, the participants have smoked for years or have not minded their nutritional health. Neither a drug nor a nutrient can reverse tissue destruction caused by decades of unhealthy living. For instance, a daily vitamin E dosage of 400 IU can prevent nitrites (certain compounds found in smoked and pickled foods) from converting to carcinogenic nitrosamines; it will not, however, turn back the reaction, reverting nitrosamines into nitrites.

In addition, the presence of other antioxidant nutrients magnifies vitamin E's potency. Vitamin C, the carotenoids and selenium are notable partners that enhance the anticancer shield. Studies with disappointing results often test vitamin E all by itself. Finally, to touch on one of the main refrains of this book: It's the dosage that does it. The amount of vitamin E derived from food will not guard against smoking-induced cell destruction, nor will the 30 IU commonly found in multivitamin supplements. Protective dosages, research shows consistently, begin at 400 IU.[10]

Neural Impairments Vitamin E's role in protecting the health and function of the nervous system make it a routine prescription at the Atkins Center for those vulnerable to neural impairments. In a dosage of 3,200 IU per day, coupled with 3 grams of vitamin C, it slowed the progression of Parkinson's disease.[11] The antioxidant serves a second purpose for people with Parkinson's by fighting off the free radicals generated by L-dopa, the major drug therapy for the disease. It also plays a vital role in the treatment of tardive dyskinesia, a neurological side effect from taking antischizophrenia medications. Vitamin E's benefit for the heretofore untreatable brain-robbing Alzheimer's disease was published in the prestigious *New England Journal of*

Medicine and widely covered in the media. The vitamin, 2,000 IU daily, prevented deterioration significantly, and as well as Selegiline, the leading drug for this purpose.[12]

Lung Disease In a large group of older people with respiratory symptoms, the measurements of pulmonary function improved proportionately to the amount of vitamin E in the daily diet.[13]

Arthritis Joint pain eases markedly when people with arthritis take vitamin E supplements. Eighty-one per cent of the participants in one study felt a dramatic improvement in joint discomfort after taking 2,500 IU per day.[14]

Vision Loss Though others may produce more impressive results, any antioxidant will help combat the free radical damage behind certain eye diseases. A low level of vitamin E is associated with an increased risk of cataracts, while a healthy blood reading coincides with a smaller risk of macular degeneration, one of the primary causes of blindness.

Menopausal Symptoms Daily doses of 400–1,200 IU can trigger the release of a little oestrogen from fat cells, thereby serving as a natural version of oestrogen replacement therapy. Vitamin E can also cool off hot flushes.

Blood Disorders Without enough vitamin E, red blood cells die sooner than they should, causing vitamin-deficiency anemia and its considerable reduction in energy level.

Immune Weakness Supplements of 1,200 IU a day, according to a small study of thirty-two men and women older than sixty, will enhance certain markers of a healthy immune system. The ability to resist infections and illnesses wanes with age, making the nutrient all the more important as we get older.[15] Another well-publicized recent study showed that the immune system benefits might be optimal for elderly people with doses of just 200 IU. It produced a sixfold increase in antibody response and a striking increase in skin test measurements. Both higher (800 IU) and lower (60 IU) doses were less effective.

SUPPLEMENT SUGGESTIONS

To tap vitamin E's power, taking supplements is a must. Most people don't consume even the terribly inadequate RDA, probably because few foods contain the nutrient. The best sources are vegetable oils and fats. Oddly, though, consuming a greater amount of these oils is counterproductive, for they increase the rate at which the body metabolizes the nutrient. The more vegetable fats and oils we use, then, the more vitamin E we need. The daily amount necessary to cut the risk of heart-related death is impossible to get just through food.

I rarely see a patient for whom I would recommend less than 400–1,200 IU per day, to be taken along with a meal that contains some fat for the best absorption. For severe cases of heart disease, I typically prescribe more than 1,200 IU. Smokers require even higher dosages, as do regular exercisers (strenuous aerobic activity stimulates free radical oxidation). You'll also need more if your supplement programme includes healthy amounts of vitamin A or fish oil.

Doses of vitamin E up to 3,200 IU per day are very safe. Despite a smattering of reports to the contrary, adverse reactions are uncommon. Sometimes, however, the nutrient will prompt a slight increase in blood pressure in people who already have hypertension, especially if they don't build up gradually to the higher amounts. My only other precaution is a common-sense reminder related to one of the nutrient's main therapeutic actions. Because vitamin E prevents clotting, don't take supplements before any scheduled surgery.

Several forms of vitamin E exist. Generally, the natural form, d-alpha- tocopherol, is more potent than its synthetic counterpart, dl-tocopheryl acetate. Tocopherol is absorbed more effectively than tocopheryl and better stimulates the immune system. Don't sell the synthetic version too short, though. Some studies suggest that vitamin E succinate possesses the most anticarcinogenic potential of all other forms.

Natural mixed tocopherols (including alpha-tocopherol, beta-tocopherol, gamma-tocopherol and delta-tocopherol) more closely reproduce how the vitamin appears in nature. Taking alpha-tocopherol to the exclusion of the others, research indicates, will increase the need for gamma-tocopherol. Smokers and anyone exposed to secondhand smoke need gamma-tocopherol's protection more than most of us.

Water-soluble, or micellized, preparations of vitamin E are absorbed easily and needn't be ingested with fat. This form is excellent for joint inflammation and acute infections, particularly when taken with micellized vitamin A.

TOCOTRIENOLS: *The undiscovered antioxidants*

These members of vitamin E's extended family once were considered of minor significance to our health. We should have known better than to second-guess nature's nutritional master plan. The four tocotrienols, now starting to attract the scientific attention they deserve, are making big waves in stroke and heart disease research.

THE BETTER ANTIOXIDANT

These new kids on the nutritional block reduce inflammation and cancer risk, too, and they might be as much as forty to sixty times stronger than vitamin E in stopping oxidative damage to our cells.[1] If further research verifies the results of one very small clinical experiment, the tocotrienols may have opened the skies for reversing disease far beyond our highest ambitions. This creates a curious parody – nutrients that are not classified as vitamins, yet are more effective than the vitamins they emulate.

The study that raises this possibility examined fifty people with plaque buildup inside the main artery that supplies blood to the brain. The condition, called 'arteriosclerotic narrowing of the carotid artery', can be an ominous prelude to an eventual stroke. Each subject was given 40 mg each of alpha-tocotrienol and gamma-tocotrienol. After eighteen months, fifteen of the twenty-five tocotrienol takers appeared to benefit from the programme. For seven of them, the cholesterol accumulation decreased, opening the artery to a greater flow of blood and decreasing the risk of stroke.[2]

I have seen no other single treatment – no drug, no nutrient, no other special therapy – work quite that well. Such a remarkable reversal of disease risk could, if shown to work for other people, change the way we prescribe nutrients.

In other promising research, taking 200 mg of gamma-tocotrienol for a month reduced blood readings of cholesterol by a whopping 30 per cent.[3] Thromboxane, a component of blood that encourages clotting and inflammation, also fell, by more than 20 per cent.

SUPPLEMENT SUGGESTIONS

Mainstream nutrition theory deprives us of the tocotrienols in two ways – first by ruining one of our best dietary sources, then by advising us to avoid it. Palm oil, a saturated fat, contains an abundance of tocotrienols, along with some vitamin E, carotenoids, and a few other nutrients. In cultures where palm oil is a dietary staple, the incidence of heart disease is low. In our food-refining and maligning culture, the oil is processed and hydrogenated, which strips it of nutrients and transforms it into a decidedly unhealthy fat. Dietitians who recommend avoiding partially or completely hydrogenated palm oil are absolutely right, but for the wrong reason: they cite its classification as a saturated fat.

Barley and rice bran are other good food sources of the tocotrienols, but no food provides the amount necessary to influence your health. Everyone who can afford this very expensive nutrient, therefore, should take 100–300 mg of a palm-based supplement. Make sure the product you pick contains all four tocotrienols, not just gamma-tocotrienol. Even though research thus far shows gamma-tocotrienol has more of a health-promoting ability than its brethren, we need the complete tocotrienol clan.

VITAMIN K: *The key to bone health*

One of the least known of all nutrients, vitamin K will rarely, if ever, appear along with its nutritional colleagues on a food label. The average health food store may very well not carry it as part of the regular stock, and even people with more than a passing interest in supplements are likely to be unfamiliar with it.

Because it is mentioned so infrequently, you may conclude that a vitamin K deficiency is improbable or inconsequential. Not true at all. A lack of the nutrient – very often but not always a result of anticoagulant therapy – is widespread and probably represents our most underappreciated cause of osteoporosis. As many as one out of every three women unknowingly has a deficiency.

BONING UP ON OSTEOPOROSIS

The K stands for 'koagulation', the Danish spelling of the blood-clotting process that can't occur without the nutrient. Though intestinal bacteria can manufacture vitamin K for us, the fat-soluble nutrient nevertheless was designated as essential when it was discovered in 1929. Our intake, primarily from leafy green vegetables, varies widely, and the low rate of clotting disorders that doctors see doesn't correspond to a low rate of deficiencies. Many of us might be able to get by with a less than ideal amount, although people worried about the health of their bones should pay a little more attention.

Without enough vitamin K, we can't form osteocalcin, the structural framework inside bones around which calcium crystallizes. The mineral then passes through the body, usually through urine, and the risk of bone fractures rises correspondingly.[1] Women with osteoporosis have, on average, only 25 per cent of the vitamin K found in their otherwise healthy counterparts.

Replenishing the supply improves the prognosis enormously. Osteocalcin production resumes, calcium excretion slows and bone begins to form again. A study of postmenopausal women showed that supplementation elevates a test marker that measures how much bone the body makes.[2]

Research into the nutrient's other functions has been woefully inadequate, but a few studies hint that it might contribute to cancer prevention. It may selectively kill cancer cells.[3]

Laboratory experiments show that supplements, in conjunction with vitamin C, can inhibit the growth of cancer cells in the breast and the endometrium.[4] Another study demonstrated that daily 5 mg doses, in a form called menadione, can, again with vitamin C, alleviate pregnancy-related nausea and vomiting.[5] Expectant mothers can also use vitamin K to prevent a bleeding disorder in their newborns known as late hemorrhagic disease and in the UK, mothers are given the option of having their babies injected with vitamin K soon after birth.

HIDDEN HEALTH ROBBERS

Insufficient intake only partly explains why people might easily suffer from a lack of vitamin K. One of the worst offenders is that bottle of anticoagulant pills in the medicine cabinets of so many people with heart disease. Part of consensus medicine's cardiovascular therapy often calls for warfarin (Coumadin) and similar 'blood-thinning' drugs to destroy any vitamin K that circulates in the body.

Are people with heart disease told that their bodies' natural clotting mechanism presents a greater peril than does a vitamin K deficiency? Would you trade the risk of one disease for the risk of another? The irony is that this unfortunate dilemma need not be faced because the two aren't mutually exclusive. The pharmaceutical approach, heavy with side effects, may not be the best answer. A daily handful of certain nutrients – fish oils, vitamin E, and bromelain among them – by preventing platelets from aggregating, can safely prevent clots without creating a deficiency of vitamin K. And the other effects of these nutrients is a further benefit.

Well-intentioned heart therapy isn't the only medical threat to our vitamin K status. Chemotherapy can also lead to a deficiency, as can the use of antibiotics and most antiseizure medications.[6] Gastrointestinal maladies also may be responsible. Because most of the body's supply of the nutrient comes from our beneficial intestinal bacteria, deficiencies often exist in people afflicted with chronic diarrhoea, Crohn's disease, or colitis.[7]

Supplement Suggestions

Despite the risks a deficiency presents, if you are being treated with prescription blood thinners, do not begin to take vitamin K supplements or dramatically increase intake of your foods high in the nutrient. Supplements will counteract the medication and raise the chances of developing the very blood clot your doctor is trying to prevent. Instead talk to your doctor, explaining your desire to forgo drug therapy in favour of a safer, more natural approach.

Virtually everyone else should eat more kale, parsley and other green leafy vegetables. Eggs also contain the nutrient. Even people who are undernourished in vitamin K usually have normal blood clotting, so supplements probably aren't necessary unless you fall into one of the groups at high risk for osteoporosis. Some researchers suggest that women, in particular, should take a daily 100 mcg supplement (provided, of course, that they are not undergoing anticoagulant therapy). The relationship with bone strength also seems to call for an adjustment in the current RDA for the vitamin, now set at just 65 mcg for women and 80 mcg for men. A daily dose of up to 500 mcg is perfectly safe.

CHAPTER 4

MINERALS

CALCIUM: *Bone builder*

After protein, fat and carbohydrates, calcium is the body's most abundantly stored dietary component. Required in a comparatively enormous amount, it carries the highest RDA of any nutrient. Without it we would literally be mush, because we wouldn't have bones or teeth. Nevertheless, multiple vitamin and mineral tablets often fail to provide the full daily requirements (which are measured in grams, not milligrams). This is not an oversight; it is a practical expediency. Still, there is a solution. Calcium is present in many more foods than people are aware of, making it an ideal nutrient for which we should seek dietary sources.

IS MILK THE ONLY ANSWER?

In the diluted version of nutrition underwritten by the dairy industry, calcium supplementation is a sacred cow. A decades-long public relations blitz has convinced millions that calcium bestows perfect health upon women and growing children, especially if they use milk products. As a consequence, many people take calcium to the exclusion of all other supplements. In so doing, these well-intentioned bearers of a milk moustache miss out on many of calcium's benefits, for the mineral works best with other nutrients. But the real secret is calcium's significance beyond our bones, teeth and nails. In fact, it is crucial in treating a host of disorders, in fields as varied as obstetrics, cardiology and oncology.

It's in Our Bones

No evidence has ever clearly demonstrated that high doses of calcium, taken long-term, can prevent osteoporosis. We do know with more certainty that consuming less than 500 mg a day greatly multiplies the chance of bone deterioration. Although some studies conclude that simply taking calcium tablets (1,500 mg per day is an often mentioned dosage) contributes to bone strength and is a good hedge against postmenopausal bone loss (one reviewer concluded it slows menopausal bone loss by 30–50 per cent),[1] other equally authoritative research asserts that supplements reinforce bone density only if combined with regular weight-bearing exercise.[2]

Neither conclusion can be correct in a vacuum, however, for bone sturdiness depends upon a sufficient supply of other nutrients – vitamin D, magnesium, copper, zinc, manganese, boron and vitamin C. Because academic scientists frown on experimenting with combination therapy (it makes identifying a single substance more difficult), the ideal programme has never been strictly tested. One study, though, did find a quite dramatic benefit with a daily regimen that included 1 gram of calcium and small amounts of zinc, manganese and copper.[3] Adding boron, magnesium, folic acid and vitamin D to the mix, I believe, would provide conclusive evidence for osteoporosis prevention.

Of all skeleton-supporting factors, the calcium-magnesium ratio is pivotal. When the amount of magnesium in the bloodstream falls, the kidneys readjust the balance by holding on to less calcium. When magnesium's concentration rises, the kidneys excrete less calcium. Because blood levels of magnesium respond better to supplementation, the more magnesium we ingest, the more calcium our bodies automatically keep.

What we eat also determines the extent of bone deterioration. In this regard, many of our menu selections could hardly be worse. A diet high in sugars, grains and other carbohydrates weakens bones. For example, when a group of women between the ages of nineteen and twenty-one began to eat foods higher in carbohydrates, they lost bone density.[4] Why? Sugar acidifies the blood, forcing calcium out of the body. The phosphorus in grains and soft drinks drains an additional amount. The content of milk sugar (lactose) is why milk is not as ideal a source of the mineral as is cheese (all the lactose has been fermented away).

And to bury another medical myth, a high-protein diet does not contribute to either osteoporosis or calcium loss. That misconception sprang from a series of short-term experiments showing that eating a lot of protein increased the amount of calcium excreted in urine. Newer studies invalidated this previous work, showing that the additional excretion doesn't persist in the long run.[5]

CALCIUM'S OTHER VIRTUES

Calcium is vital to other parts of the body besides the bones. As a therapeutic nutrient, the mineral has basked in quite a bit of scientific attention.

Hypertension Cardiologists and obstetricians are both fascinated with calcium's association with blood pressure. In a review of twenty-five clinical trials involving hypertensives, twelve showed that the mineral could cut the risk of high blood pressure, and twelve did not. The chance of preeclampsia, the pregnancy-related hypertension disorder, was similarly reduced.[6] However, a more panoramic view of the medical literature shows that the blood pressure benefit is actually slight and unimpressive. I tend not to incorporate calcium into the Atkins Center's programme for normalizing high blood pressure, simply because I find magnesium to be the more important element for doing so. The effect of magnesium, I believe, determines the degree to which calcium influences blood pressure readings.

High Cholesterol Supplements may also contribute to heart health by helping to lower cholesterol and triglycerides, other research indicates. A higher amount of the mineral in the blood, one study of more than ten thousand people shows, corresponds to a higher amount of the 'good' HDL cholesterol. Alas, total cholesterol was elevated, too, meaning that the unhealthy LDL cholesterol also remained high.[7]

Pregnancy Complications Women have fewer preterm deliveries, incidents of spontaneous labour and low-birth-weight babies when they take 1,200 mg of calcium every day. Still, in this case supplements may be a double-edged sword, for dosages of more than 1,500 mg can impede the body's absorption of zinc, iron and magnesium.

Cancer Finally, supplements may guard against cancers of the endometrium, pancreas and colon.[8] With a daily 1,250 mg dose of calcium carbonate, the proliferation of colonic epithelial cells decreases. Another study of 1,900 men found that 1,200 mg per day reduced the incidence of colon cancer by 75 per cent.[9]

Insomnia One of the reasons I am most likely to prescribe calcium is that it is a very potent sleep inducer. That's why it has become a major constituent of my nutritional insomnia therapy and why taking supplements at bedtime may produce a bonus benefit for a better night's sleep.

SUPPLEMENT SUGGESTIONS

Many of my patients are concerned when their targeted supplement programme contains less than the RDA of calcium. This actually occurs because an adequate amount of calcium tends to crowd out other nutrients in a multiple formula and because not everyone's digestive tract can tolerate calcium pills taken alone (although two calcium carbonate tablets, 500 mg each, is not too hard to swallow). Fortunately I can also count on the fact that most of us consume many foods, other than milk, that provide us with more calcium than a pill would.

Some good nondairy sources of the bone-building mineral are sardines, sesame seeds, pink salmon with bones, almonds, Brazil nuts, kale, Swiss chard, cooked spinach, bok choy, mustard greens and pinto beans. The best example of a high-calcium, low-carbohydrate diary product is cheese. So unless your diet is quite limited, it should provide what you need.

In certain circumstances, supplements will be necessary. By all means, take them if

- you have osteoporosis or another bone disorder or are at risk for the same.
- you face a high risk of colon cancer or other disease that calcium may benefit.
- you want a guaranteed source of mineral nutrition and don't mind swallowing extra pills.

I've found that calcium hydroxyapatite and calcium citrate are the most readily absorbed supplemental forms of calcium, even though the hard-to-find calcium orotate may have a special affinity for bone, as European researchers claim.

Whatever you choose, make sure your calcium pill is packed loosely enough so that it dissolves easily. A home test to determine this involves placing your tablet in 175 ml of vinegar. It should disintegrate into fine particles within half an hour. Depending upon the health objectives, both men and women will need to take between 800 mg and 1,500 mg per day.

MAGNESIUM: *The heart's most important mineral*

Magnesium is scientifically established as the heart's most important mineral. More than three hundred different enzymes in the body depend on the mineral, yet some 80 per cent of those on a typical Western diet fail to consume as much as they need. Even worse, few cardiologists bother to prescribe it routinely. No wonder heart disease is so rampant.

ELEMENTAL MEDICINE

We face threats to rob us of magnesium no matter where we turn. The mineral is all but absent from the sugary junk foods that now constitute more than 35 per cent of the average person's diet. Crops are grown in soil that steadily becomes more deficient in the mineral. The body expends much of its meagre supply to cleanse itself of smog, pesticides and so many other toxins. Perspiration and stress drain off what's left, as do diuretics and other drugs. For most of us, a deficiency seems unavoidable. Age brings it even closer to reality. As we get older, we absorb less of many nutrients, including magnesium, from food. Because of dental problems, we may avoid nuts, seeds and other good dietary sources, and we will probably be taking more nutrient-depleting medications.

Magnesium touches almost every aspect of our health, but because it's one of the strongest explanations for the presence or absence of cardiac problems, the heart is a good place to start.

Cardiovascular Disease As a cardiologist, I see more people for heart-related ailments than for any other problem. About 98 per cent, I'd guess, need magnesium, and all of them benefit from it.[1] Yet only a handful of them were ever instructed by their previous doctors to take it. The following summary of what's possible with regular supplement use reads more like a wish list for any person with heart disorders.

- Irregular heart rhythms become more stable.[2]
- High blood pressure improves.[3]
- The body keeps a better balance of potassium, another important cardiovascular mineral.
- The heart pumps a larger volume of blood with no extra demand for oxygen.[4]
- Constricted blood vessels relax, allowing blood to flow more freely.
- The chest pains of angina pectoris strike less frequently.
- By not allowing platelets to clump together, the blood becomes less likely to form artery-blocking clots.[5]
- HDL cholesterol rises and LDL cholesterol falls.[6]

Acute Heart Attacks Hospital cardiologists are quite interested in what magnesium can do when a patient is first admitted to a coronary care unit, because half a dozen studies showed it to be effective in preventing complications.[7] This led to a larger study, which failed to demonstrate benefit. Dr Mildred Seelig, the magnesium guru, feels that the mineral's benefits could be maintained with the individualization of treatment and a flexible dosage system.[8] Magnesium, when given by the vein, as in these studies, can stabilize or destabilize the heart.

Blood Sugar Disorders How well the body metabolizes sugar is tightly linked to magnesium, making the mineral essential to anyone with diabetes or insulin resistance. In and of itself, poor sugar control raises the risk of a magnesium deficiency, which in turn further impairs sugar metabolism. Supplements allow people with Type II diabetes to regulate blood sugar more easily. As a result, their need for oral diabetes drugs usually diminishes and could disappear altogether.[9] People susceptible to bouts of hypoglycemia, too, can stabilize the roller-coaster rise and fall of their blood sugar. Although the mineral doesn't affect Type I diabetes as dramatically, it is nevertheless a benefactor that shouldn't be neglected.

High Blood Pressure Following our nutritional approach, about 80 per cent of the Atkins Center's hypertension patients reduce or eliminate their need for diuretics and other blood pressure medications. All of the ingredients we use contribute to that success, but magnesium is largely responsible. A person with high blood pressure typically will have a lower level of the mineral compared with somebody who has a healthier blood pressure reading.[10] Supplements work like a natural calcium channel blocker, another standard antihypertension drug, but without ill effects.[11] Excess insulin in the blood, low potassium levels, constricted blood vessels – the nutrient addresses all of the condition's primary causes simultaneously.

Pregnancy Complications For expectant mothers and their babies, magnesium supplements can frequently overcome several serious blood pressure disorders that may arise. As medicine has known for more than fifty years, the mineral is a choice treatment for preeclampsia, a relatively common complication seen in the latter part of pregnancy that raises blood pressure and causes water retention, among other problems. In extreme cases of preeclampsia, a woman may suffer convulsions or lapse into a coma. Again, magnesium is a very effective treatment. Some 60 per cent of all such hypertension-related complications could be avoided, researchers estimate, if pregnant women were to take supplements.[12]

By administering magnesium instead of drugs, doctors also might be able to rescue certain babies whose lives are endangered by high blood pressure. As described in a medical journal article, doctors gave the nutrient to seven infants after all other medications failed to help them. The babies were expected to die, but injections of magnesium sulfate brought down their blood pressure and saved their lives.[13]

Mitral Valve Prolapse This condition, which involves a weakness of a valve in the heart, increases magnesium excretion. Resupplying the mineral helps to correct low blood sugar, one of the main problems linked to mitral valve prolapse, and counteracts fatigue, which is probably the most frequently encountered symptom.

Asthma By diminishing wheezing and encouraging bronchial muscles to relax, magnesium reinforces my better-breathing programmes for bronchitis, emphysema and other chronic lung disorders. When given intravenously, it stops an asthma attack cold.[14] Safe and consistently effective, this 'IV push', as we call it, is also a great on-the-spot treatment for allergic flare-ups.

Migraines The IV push significantly relieves migraine headaches, too. In most cases it'll stave off a recurrence for more than twenty-four hours. Not surprisingly, people who enjoy the most prolonged relief usually have the lowest blood levels of the mineral.[15] Regular migraine sufferers need not anticipate a future of daily visits to the doctor's surgery if they want sustained relief; taking magnesium orally is a good preventive.

Fibromyalgia For anyone who copes with the muscle and joint pains of this rheumatic ailment, magnesium is a valuable part of an effective treatment. I also use it, in a dosage of 300–600 mg, for a related condition, chronic fatigue syndrome. It's especially powerful when combined with 1–2 grams of malic acid.[16]

Brain Function Magnesium readings are markedly lower than average in people who have multiple sclerosis, Parkinson's and Alzheimer's or other types of dementia.[17] Many of them have an unusually high amount of aluminum in their brains, and the metal is known to interfere with magnesium. Institutionalized psychiatric patients also have reduced blood levels of the mineral. An outright deficiency can aggravate psychiatric symptoms, some research suggests, and cause the brain to age prematurely.

Osteoporosis For preventing and perhaps reversing osteoporosis, magnesium might be more important than calcium. Although constituting only a fraction of bone matter, the mineral plays a disproportionately important role, balancing the body's calcium supply and keeping it from being excreted. Some scientists go so far as to say that how much magnesium we eat is a stronger predictor of bone density than calcium consumption.[18] Without enough magnesium and the other trace minerals, any additional calcium we ingest will be deposited not around our bones, but elsewhere, perhaps in the walls of our arteries.[19]

Strength Training Muscle growth and strength, especially from a weight-training programme, depends on magnesium. Supplements attracted a good deal of interest from competitors in the 1988 Olympics, especially athletes involved in rowing, weight lifting and other power sports.

Premenstrual Tension Supplements have decreased the number of mood swings that may occur as menstruation nears. They also help tame premenstrual migraines and yeast infections.[20]

Cancer Scientists haven't studied humans directly for a link between magnesium and cancer, but other evidence suggests a strong relationship. For instance, tumours can develop in animals that eat a low-magnesium diet, and higher rates of the disease seem to exist where the local water and soil contain low concentrations. Cancer drugs and radiation therapy, in addition, deplete the body of magnesium.

Other Conditions Magnesium should be a part of any nutrient program for better sleep. Besides encouraging a more restful slumber, it works against bruxism, an involuntary grinding of the teeth while asleep. Its wide range of actions helps against chemical sensitivities, bacterial and viral infections, leg cramps, kidney stones and intermittent claudication, an impairment in blood flow to the legs that causes pain upon exertion.

SUPPLEMENT SUGGESTIONS

Giving the cells in your body the optimal amount of magnesium isn't as easy as swallowing a supplement or two every day. Quantity alone is no guarantee, and an overload could be harmful. For a nutrient like vitamin C, to give an example, you can dose yourself into a case of diarrhoea, but that's about the only side effect you'll suffer. Big doses of magnesium, particularly magnesium oxide, also cause diarrhoea, which makes it a good short-term treatment for chronic constipation, but diarrhoea is not a benign consequence. Taking too much could be dangerous, especially if your blood's concentration already is high, as can happen when certain kidney problems prevent the mineral from being excreted. No one with seriously diminished kidney function should take magnesium supplements without careful medical supervision.

Blood tests are the best way to determine your true need and track the effectiveness of supplements. Don't rely on standard blood serum measurements. They can be misleading and will often fail to detect a deficiency. A much better gauge is the mineral's concentration within red blood cells. I've found that the optimum dosage for magnesium-related health problems typically brings the red blood cell reading to a point slightly above the middle of the 'normal' range. For most people this usually translates into a daily dosage of 400–1,000 mg.

To reach the ideal point, some formulations work better than others. Magnesium oxide, the type most frequently found in mineral supplements, does easily raise the standard blood serum level, but other forms deliver the nutrient to tissue cells more successfully. My favourite is magnesium orotate, which, although once difficult to find, is now beginning to be found in health food stores. Other good forms are magnesium taurate, magnesium chloride, magnesium glycinate and magnesium aspartate.

As an alternative, go soak your feet – and the rest of your body. Epsom salts are known chemically as magnesium sulfate, and your skin will absorb as much of the mineral as you need. Drawing a bath and pouring in some Epsom salts can be as nourishing as it is relaxing.

POTASSIUM: *Our most valuable electrolyte*

The essential mineral potassium is vital to life and to the functioning of every living cell. Understanding its role is crucial to practising medicine. Potassium, sodium, chloride and bicarbonate are called electrolytes. They are responsible for the acid-base balance and osmotic pressure in the body; excessively high or low levels are life-threatening. In the case of potassium, abnormal levels are usually caused by a medical condition – either the illness or, all too often, the treatment – rather than by a dietary deficiency.

Potassium's main role is maintaining the proper function of our cell walls. This is accomplished when in harmony with sodium. Potassium stays within the cells; sodium stays outside. Its second chief duty is to support the concentration and activities of magnesium, a major heart nutrient; if the blood level of one is low, the other is likely to be low, too.

Promoting the cellular equilibrium through an emphasis on potassium is one of the most important strategies we can adopt against heart disease and cancer. Getting enough potassium is more important than limiting salt intake for regulating blood pressure. Potassium is also critical for optimum energy, nerve health, muscle contraction, athletic performance and a range of other functions.

Drugs That Threaten Potassium

I have never seen a case of hypokalaemia – the name given to low blood potassium – caused by poor nutrition. Illness is a much more likely cause. Vomiting, diarrhoea, or perspiration can, if severe or recurrent, drain off enough potassium to induce dangerously low levels. Trauma also causes a precipitous drop (between 50 and 68 per cent of trauma patients have low levels).[1] But the main reason hypokalaemia is becoming increasingly prevalent is the widespread use of diuretics, usually prescribed for high blood pressure or heart failure. An estimated 20 per cent of all people who take 'water pills', as these drugs are known, are hypokalemic.[2] Two other common antihypertension drug types, ACE inhibitors and beta-blockers, also impair blood potassium levels. This is precisely the opposite of what people with hypertension and heart disease need most.

A potassium-poor diet might contribute to this trend by failing to help restore its depleted levels. Processing and chemical-based farming methods can both rob food of the mineral. Manufacturers exacerbate the problem by adding sodium to their products – and increased sodium leads to a potassium shortage. More than one-third of the body's energy, in fact, is expended maintaining the potassium and sodium balance within cells. In cultures with food supplies that are more natural and richer in potassium, rates of heart disease and cancer are far lower. These people often have potassium-to-sodium dietary ratios one hundred times greater than most of those living in Western industrialized nations.

You don't have to be a heart patient to risk a potassium deficiency, although this condition would certainly increase your risk. Cardiovascular health is closely linked to the mineral, making it an appropriate beginning for a review of potassium's therapeutic uses.

Heart Disease The interdependency with magnesium probably accounts for potassium's cardiovascular significance. When potassium is low, there is greater risk of life-threatening arrhythmias, heart failure and stroke. So intimate is its cardiac relationship that potassium readings can be used with a great degree of accuracy to predict an individual's risk for heart rhythm abnormalities.[3] A single daily serving of a potassium-rich food, one study found, can cut nearly in half the risk of death from a stroke.[4] Yet cardiologists would rather use high-risk medications to treat these heart problems. Even when the goal is to help the body retain potassium and magnesium, heart doctors prefer to use drugs rather than the safer option, therapeutic amounts of the depleted minerals.

Blood Pressure I find it curious that conventional medicine dwells so intensely on the sodium side of the sodium-potassium balance to treat high blood pressure. Scientific literature demonstrates that potassium may be more important in both treatment and prevention.[5] What I've seen in my practice convinces me that potassium is far more important, so I'm not too obsessed with salt. Inordinately high intake, of course, is unhealthy, and restricting the seasoning's use is appropriate for anyone with heart failure or tissue swelling. But the rest of us can satisfy our salty tooth within reasonable limits with little risk of hypertension. Ensuring a high intake of potassium, many population studies show, is more effective at preventing the onset of the 'silent killer'.[6]

Research that measured the actual magnitude of salt's impact showed that cutting back intake reduced blood pressure only by an average of two or three points.[7] In contrast, a high-potassium diet proves to be very effective, especially when combined with a sugar-free diet and supplements of magnesium and taurine. Even a high-potassium, high-magnesium salt substitute was judged to be effective. However, the longer potassium is used, the less effective an antihypertensive agent it becomes.[8] More than thirty controlled studies attest to the success of potassium as a blood pressure control agent.[9]

Weaning patients off their potassium-wasting diuretics is a major treatment goal of mine. The drugs don't resolve anything; their use not only compounds the hypertensive threat by further depleting the body of both potassium and magnesium (very possibly to dangerously low levels), it also induces the body to make an increased amount of its normal blood pressure–raising biochemicals.

Muscle Weakness and Fatigue Fatigue or weakness may be the most common indicators of a need for more potassium. Leg cramps, particularly the ones that awaken you at night, may also stem from low levels of the mineral (as well as of magnesium and calcium). I've observed many patients, people who, because of their low blood concentration of the electrolyte, couldn't even climb a flight of stairs without tiring. Low-calorie dieters and heavy-duty exercisers are especially prone to a potassium-related loss of energy. So are older people. An inadequate amount of potassium and magnesium may contribute to the onset of chronic fatigue syndrome.

Replenishing the body's supply, using 250–500 mg each of potassium aspartate and magnesium aspartate, can often single-handedly restore muscle tone, promote a higher energy level and boost endurance.[10] The reversal often can occur within a week. If the nutrient duo doesn't work on its own, it still may prove a valuable adjunct to treating other kinds of fatigue.

Supplement Suggestions

The best way to get potassium is from food, not supplements. Whole, organically grown, unrefined foods contain higher amounts than do chemically grown foods.[11] My favourite sources are parsley and sunflower seeds. Other good potassium foods are almonds and other nuts; certain meats and fish, especially halibut, cod, turkey, chicken breast and sirloin; some vegetables, including mushrooms, chard and spinach; and a few fruits, such as cantaloupe and avocado.

Yes, you should have no bananas. Though encouraged routinely by many doctors, probably by hand-me-down misinformation, bananas have only a moderate potassium content. So does orange juice. Both, unfortunately, are quite high in sugars, which can disturb blood sugar stability.

The best way to get your potassium is to go to the supermarket and buy a salt substitute such as Losalt or Solo made from potassium chloride. Sprinkle it liberally on foods as a seasoning. Don't waste your effort getting over-the-counter pills from a health food store, since they will contain more than 99 mg, which is not a very meaningful amount (it takes fifteen of them to equal two prescription potassium pills). In addition, some pills may irritate your stomach. If you are truly experiencing a potassium deficiency, you probably have a medical reason for it and you will need to learn why you have it, plus you will need prescription-strength dosages of 3,600 mg or more, which must be taken under a physician's care. Almost all doctors are knowledgeable about prescribing the mineral, and they should be able to determine why your level is low.

IRON: *The double-edged sword*

Iron is the long-standing remedy for 'tired blood', essential to the blood-borne haemoglobin that carries oxygen to every cell in the body. Many of this century's earliest health tonics may have worked because they contained iron, and the mineral may also explain the occasional effectiveness of two other antiquated treatments: bloodletting and the laying on of leeches. Iron is a double-edged sword in nutrition, and one of the edges is toxic and rusty – a possible contributor to hardening of the arteries, heart disease and cancer. We must therefore wield the sword with precision.

Whether or not to take iron supplements should be one of our most carefully considered nutritional decisions. Deficiencies are clearly a more imminent threat to health (nutritional anaemia is a major global problem, especially in the third world). To a surprising extent, Western industrialized nations such as the US and the UK face a similar, if less immediate, hazard because of the concerted effort to discourage people from eating red meat, perhaps the safest, single best source of the mineral. Most of us can satisfy our body's iron requirements just by eating red meat. The widespread hawking of supplemental tonics and pills, especially those made from overload-prone forms of the mineral, has caused the medical powers-that-be to ignore the cost of taking too much.

DEFICIENCY DANGERS

Anaemia may be the best-known repercussion of an iron

deficiency, but it's not the only one. Even a minor shortage leads to learning disabilities, fatigue, a weakened immune system, lower body temperature, impaired physical performance and a reduced output of thyroid hormone. Stomach cancer also is associated with low iron stores. Women may be tipped off to iron depletion by a persistent inability to lose weight, a consequence of the lower thyroid output. In one study, women who took iron supplements responded with an increase in thyroid function.[1] And when a group of teenage girls took supplements to correct slight, nonanaemic deficiencies, they increased their ability to learn, as demonstrated by their better scores on memory and learning tests.[2]

Children, women in their menstruating years and older people face the greatest likelihood of an iron deficiency. The growth demands of pregnancy, childhood and adolescence increase the body's need, and as we age, we're less able to absorb the mineral. Any kind of blood loss or internal bleeding also poses a risk. For example, during a typical menstrual period, a woman can lose as much as 30 mg of iron.

Eating a meatless high-carbohydrate or high-fibre diet contributes to an iron deficiency. Drinking tea or coffee with meals also reduces your absorption, as can eating high-calcium and iron-rich foods during the same meal. Women absorb about 30–50 per cent more iron from a meal if the calcium content is low.

Finally, taking aspirin or other nonsteroidal anti-inflammatory medications may provoke or compound an iron loss by encouraging internal bleeding that often goes undiagnosed. As many as 52 per cent of the people with rheumatoid arthritis, one study found, have low iron reserves.[3] I believe the treatment may account for more of the deficiency than the arthritis.

IRON OVERLOAD: NO WAY OUT

As we all know, too much of a good thing can be detrimental. There are several reasons. The fact is that once iron enters the body, it has no way out. Most of it is recycled, not excreted or otherwise consumed. Except during growth stages, pregnancy, menstruation or another cause of blood loss, we eliminate only a minute amount, principally through urine, sweat, certain illnesses and the turnover of skin cells.

Here's the second catch. You may remember from your school chemistry class that iron (like copper) converts readily between the ferrous (with two electrons) and the ferric (three electrons) forms. This makes it a player in oxidation-reduction reactions, useful for transmitting oxygen via our red blood cells, but also capable of acting like a free radical and oxidizing tissues, thereby damaging them.

This means whatever amount of the mineral that isn't affixed to the haemoglobin in our blood or to other proteins for other uses roams around in the body as unbound 'free iron' and is vulnerable to the rustlike process of free radical oxidation. Once transformed into free radicals themselves, oxidized iron molecules go on to similarly damage whatever other tissue cells they touch. Finnish heart researcher Jukka Salonen, MD, blew open the medical profession's understanding of cardiology by revealing the true impact of cholesterol and iron on hardening of the arteries. His research established that LDL cholesterol becomes an artery-blocking danger only when it oxidizes and that men with high a concentration of iron (or copper) in their bodies are at a particularly grave risk.[4]

Thus it turns out that iron, not oestrogen, explains the low risk of coronary heart disease among women in their child-bearing years and why the threat magnifies after menopause or a hysterectomy. The compelling evidence is that even when the ovaries are not removed after a simple hysterectomy and continue to produce oestrogen, the woman's heart disease risk begins to escalate – very similarly to those women whose ovaries *were* removed. Menstruation ensures that excess iron is excreted, not left to become an oxidizing menace. The regular blood loss keeps a woman's overall iron level low, if not deficient. Oestrogen contributes to cardiovascular protection mainly to the extent that it enables ovulation and a monthly period. This fact alone undermines one of the usual rationalizations for hormone replacement therapy.

Excess iron is implicated in other diseases, too. It could accumulate to a toxic extent in our organs and tissues, including the joints, the liver, the gonads and the heart. It could feed the growth of harmful bacteria and malignant tumour cells, as well as stimulate additional cancer-promoting free radical activity.[5] One of the reasons that fibre protects us from colon cancer could be that it binds to iron, which prevents the mineral from sparking oxidation damage. By burning off excess iron, exercise may work in a similar way. Remember, though, that a lack of the mineral can also lead to cancer. As I mentioned, maintaining an optimal balance is tricky.

High amounts of iron have been found in the brains of people afflicted with Parkinson's disease,[6] and it could disrupt the central nervous system enough to aggravate, if not cause, mental disorders. When seven psychiatric patients in one small study were treated for excess iron, their disturbed behaviour patterns diminished significantly. In the months following treatment, their symptoms did not return.[7]

THE BOTTOM LINE

If both low and high levels of iron can be bad, then which is worse? Well, by the time you've reached your seventies the answer is high iron is better, according to a 1997 US government survey of nearly four thousand seniors. Men and women with the highest serum level had 38 per cent and 28 per cent lower all-cause death rates, respectively.[8]

GOOD IRON AND BAD IRON

Believe it or not, our bodies were designed to circumvent the iron dilemma entirely. Orthodox medicine and popular dietary practices, though, seem designed to circumvent nature. Two forms of iron exist. Knowing which to use and where each is found is fundamental to protecting your body from the mineral's potential harm. The two kinds are:

1. *Heme iron* The natural, organic, biologically available form cannot build up to excess and is not vulnerable to free radical oxidation. Only 2 mg of heme iron, which comes from red meat, chicken and fish, can be absorbed

by the body during any single meal, so no surplus accumulates.[9]

2. *Non-heme iron* This synthetic, inorganic form is the kind we need to avoid, yet it's the predominant type found in most iron supplements and fortified foods, including those made with 'enriched' flour. It usually appears on labels as ferrous gluconate, ferrous sulfate or ferrous fumarate. The body can absorb as much as 20 mg of non-heme iron at any one time, possibly leading to a higher level of accumulation that would, in turn, increase the heart disease and cancer risk.

In Belgium, Germany, France, Italy and the Netherlands, food processors are forbidden to add iron to their flours, and it is not a common practice in the UK. And Swedish research confirms that iron-fortified flour can more than triple the incidence of primary liver cancer[10] and multiply by more than ten times the incidence of haemochromatosis, in which the intestines absorb more iron than the body needs. But ironically enough, inorganic iron-fortified flour is celebrated by the US government's food pyramid, which demands that Americans consume at least six servings of it daily.

SUPPLEMENT SUGGESTIONS

Almost any of us could be a candidate for iron supplementation, but with this good/bad mineral, generalizations are difficult to make. Usually women who have heavy, prolonged menstrual flows could need a supplemental source, as could heavy-duty exercisers.[11] People who probably should not take extra iron include

- *older people who do not suffer from anaemia* The risk of cancer increases with age, so the elderly need to avoid iron supplements and food fortified with the mineral.
- *people with a gastrointestinal infection* Iron supplements should be shelved for the duration of the infection, because disease-causing microorganisms in the gastrointestinal tract feed on the mineral.

- *breast-fed infants* Contrary to earlier pediatric research, the iron in mother's milk is well absorbed and not readily available to gastrointestinal germs. Additional iron can often cause or worsen a baby's gastrointestinal infections.

To be safe, don't take any kind of iron supplement, tablet or tonic without first going to a doctor for a blood check. Not any old blood test will do, however. The ordinary haemoglobin and haematocrit counts will let you know if you're anaemic, but they don't accurately gauge an iron deficiency. Plasma iron tests are almost meaningless, too.

The best answer is a serum ferritin test, which measures how much of the mineral is stored in the body. It will be low if you're deficient, high if you have an overload. Serum iron will also be low if you have a deficiency, while serum transferrin (an iron carrier molecule) will be elevated or normal. The upper range for 'normal' ferritin is about 250 µg/L in women and 450 µg/L in men. If your ferritin reading is above 750 µg/L, ask your doctor to check you for haemochromatosis. Iron overload is more common than mainstream medicine now recognizes, and it's frequently overlooked.

Should testing reveal a deficiency, the therapy of choice is both easy and delicious: additional servings of red meat, at least 900 grams a week. Chicken and fish also are suitable. Animal meat, as I mentioned, contains heme iron, which, unlike synthetic supplements, will not accumulate in the body. Nor will it lead to an increase in free radicals, a process linked to colon cancer.

As an alternative to eating meat more frequently, search health food stores for supplements of heme iron. Newly available over the last few years, they are sold as ferritin capsules. The only drawback may be cost. The per-capsule dosage is limited to 5 mg, and ten or more pills daily may be needed to overcome anaemia. Liquid liver extract is another source of safe, natural iron. But do your utmost to avoid synthetic supplements of non-heme iron, except when the anaemia requires immediate treatment.

To enhance iron absorption, consider taking a little extra vitamin A (about 20,000 IU) and vitamin C. Vitamin A can help increase the level of iron in the blood, which may be of particular concern to someone with an underactive thyroid, a condition that impairs the ability to convert beta-carotene into vitamin A. When tested for iron status, people with low thyroid function should make sure their need for vitamin A also is measured.

Vitamin C, whether from fruits, vegetables or regular 500 mg supplements, helps the body derive more heme iron from food. High doses pose no risk of excess iron absorption.

ZINC: *Immune booster, wound healer*

Zinc is critical to the healthy functioning of every cell in our bodies. Insufficient consumption the world over threatens to emerge as a veritable public health crisis. As we continue to deplete our soil of zinc and forsake animal protein, some experts believe that large-scale supplementation or food fortification will become necessary.[1]

Meeting the body's optimum need for the mineral has revolutionized nutritional medicine's control of an incredibly wide scope of deficiency-related consequences – a list of afflictions that includes schizophrenia and other psychiatric disorders, diabetes, prostate enlargement, cataracts, heart disease, brain and nervous system deterioration, immune malfunctions, inadequate digestion, ulcers, food allergies, toxic metal accumulation, poor wound healing, colds, osteoporosis, skin problems, fatigue, lack of appetite, hearing impairments, eating disorders and the many symptoms of a blood sugar imbalance.

Though a person's zinc status is an important health measure, until recently nutritional medicine never had a good way to gauge how much of the mineral is actually inside the body's cells. Typical blood measurements have never given us an accurate assessment. But a simple taste test that anyone can perform at home can prove to be a crucial part of determining the adequacy of your supply of this mineral.

The test works because our sense of taste depends on zinc. Simply take a swig of zinc sulfate heptahydrate, a widely available liquid supplement, and swish it around in your mouth. If you immediately notice its bitter taste, you don't have a deficiency. If, however, you taste nothing or have a delayed recognition of the taste, you need to replenish your body's zinc supply.

My guess is that you won't instantly taste the mineral. Our land is becoming increasingly barren in zinc content, and high-carbohydrate diets are leaving us with even less. Calcium supplements and high-calcium diets can reduce our zinc absorption up to 50 per cent.[2] The mineral is quickly expelled from the body by stress (whether physical, emotional or chemical) as well as exposure to toxic metals, pollutants and pesticides. Growing old gives us an inborn disadvantage, because we don't secrete the amount of stomach acid necessary for absorption. Based on the high incidence of zinc deficiency among the sick elderly, zinc supplements should probably be mandatory for all older adults.[3]

Neurological Illnesses As part of my introduction to nutritional medicine, Dr Carl Pfeiffer taught me that zinc (along with its supporting mineral, manganese) is the essential treatment for such serious psychiatric disorders as schizophrenia and clinical depression. He saw schizophrenia as a 'dysperception syndrome' caused by biochemical imbalances. Hearing voices, for example, was simply a flawed perception that often could be eliminated by giving zinc, manganese and B vitamins.

A zinc deficiency, we now recognize, can be implicated in a whole range of neurological and neuropsychiatric disorders – epilepsy, multiple sclerosis, Huntington's disease, dyslexia, acute psychosis, dementia, anorexia nervosa, attention deficit disorder and depression.

Zinc supplements may help to prevent Alzheimer's disease. The presence of the zinc-dependent thymus hormone, thymulin, is almost undetectable in people with Alzheimer's, implying that a zinc deficiency plays a role in the disease's onset.

Immune System Strength Like vitamin C, zinc knocks out cold viruses, if you catch them early enough.[4] Sucking on lozenges works better than swallowing tablets. A Cleveland Clinic study found that using zinc lozenges cut down cold symptoms from an average of about seven days to four days.[5]

People with AIDS are almost universally deficient in zinc, which contributes significantly to the continued decline of their already damaged immune systems. Restoring their supply, in doses of up to about 100 mg every day, has been found to be one of the most important strategies for stabilizing their immune function and reducing complications of the disease.[6]

Cancer forms more easily when zinc levels are low. People who are stricken with a malignancy dramatically increase their excretion of the mineral, implying, according to Czech researchers, that the body utilized its zinc reserves at the early inflammatory stages of cancer development.[7] Supplementation stimulates the manufacture of white blood cells, one of the immune system's tumour-fighting components, and more generally supports the activities of our neutrophils, T lymphocytes, and our natural tumour-fighting (NK) cells.[8] It also is required for producing thymulin, the major thymus hormone.[9]

Diabetes In the long run, zinc's most valuable medical contribution may be its ability to balance blood sugar.[10] The mineral assists the pancreas in manufacturing insulin and may protect the receptor sites on all cell membranes that allow the hormone to enter.[11] In people who have diabetes, zinc also helps lower high cholesterol.[12]

Skin Health Just about all skin disorders improve if you build up your zinc stores. In doses of 100 mg or more, it's especially helpful in treating acne, thought by some researchers to be a zinc and essential fatty acid deficiency disease.[13] Supplementation won't work immediately. Weeks or months may pass before you notice its effect on your skin.

Sexual Health Although it has a reputation as a male nutrient, zinc is fundamental to the sexual and reproductive health of both genders. All of us require it for fertility, and I'll usually recommend it whenever a patient, male or female, needs a libido boost. It's also integral for more gender-specific problems:

• *Men* Benign prostate enlargement, now reaching almost epidemic proportions among men older than fifty years of age, is strongly tied to a lifetime of inadequate zinc intake. The frequent urge to urinate and other symptoms of an enlarged prostate diminish very reliably with the mineral, especially when combined with saw palmetto extract, the essential fatty acids and several amino acids, including glycine, alanine and glutamic acid. A lack of the nutrient can also impair sperm formation and testosterone production, whereas giving zinc glutamate supplements to a group of men in their sixties actually *doubled* their serum testosterone levels.[14]

• *Women* Zinc deficiency can lead to a host of pregnancy-related problems, including spontaneous abortion, toxaemia, growth retardation and delivery problems. Even the modest 22 mg daily supplement tested in one study enabled women to give birth to babies significantly larger in birth weight.[15] Doses of 10–60 mg per day are very safe to take when you're pregnant.

Zinc levels generally are lower in women who experience premenstrual tension. A deficiency may decrease progesterone production, which in turn may lead to a craving for sweet and salty foods.16

Wound Healing As a first-aid treatment for almost any wound or skin irritation, people have long reached for the bottle of calamine lotion. Its healing power comes from its rich zinc content, which promotes protein synthesis. That's why I tell my patients to take extra doses of the mineral both before and after an operation.

Applied directly, a zinc oxide paste improves the healing of leg ulcers by 83 per cent, according to the research. People who get these wounds typically have a lower than normal level of the mineral.[17] Zinc liquid is also an effective topical treatment for canker sores.[18] Zinc supplementation is a 'must' before and after any surgical procedure.

Ulcers If you're taking anti-inflammatory drugs or antihistamines that reduce stomach acids, you'll need zinc to help heal any ulcers that may result. If you're on an acid-reducing medication, you run the risk of a deficiency, because zinc absorption depends on the stomach's hydrochloric acid.[19]

Eating Disorders All the people I've treated for anorexia, bulimia or another eating disorder have been helped profoundly by a liquid supplement of zinc sulfate heptahydrate. It's truly a remarkable preparation.

Poor dietary habits already predispose teenagers to many mineral deficiencies, and insufficient zinc stores are associated with both anorexia and bulimia. Supplementation goes a long way towards helping them regain a healthier body weight. In one controlled study, the sixteen anorexic young women who received zinc supplements gained double the amount of body weight than did the placebo group.[20]

Eye Health Antioxidants are crucial to maintaining sight and protecting our delicate eye tissues. But they don't work alone. A zinc deficiency may contribute to one of the most common causes of blindness, macular degeneration. Taking supplements in doses of 100–200 mg can slow the progressive retinal deterioration that causes this condition.[21] The mineral is also helpful in treating and preventing cataracts.[22]

Gastrointestinal Problems Forty per cent of the people who have Crohn's disease are deficient in zinc, and replenishing their bodies' supply is critical to overcoming this common digestive disorder. In developing nations, giving supplements to zinc-deficient children cuts down the number of cases of dysentery and diarrhoea.[23]

Rheumatoid Arthritis People with this inflammatory joint disease are generally quite depleted in zinc. If you plan to take zinc supplements, make sure you are also given copper, an extremely valuable treatment. The zinc/copper ratio should be roughly eight to one.

Other Uses We become more vulnerable to the toxic influence of environmental pollutants when our zinc levels fall out of the optimum range. In one study of two hundred randomly chosen people with a chemical sensitivity, 54 per cent were low in zinc.[24]

Sickle Cell Anaemia This blood disorder increases the risk of zinc depletion, making supplements especially important.

SUPPLEMENT SUGGESTIONS

For preventive care, most of us can get by with a daily dose of 15–25 mg of zinc. Let the zinc taste test (ZTT) be your guide. If you have difficulty tasting it, increase the dosage to a maximum of 150 mg or until you can taste it. Liquid zinc sulfate heptahydrate is itself highly absorbable and a great way to take a supplement. In capsule form, I prefer to prescribe zinc monomethionine, although zinc picolinate, zinc aspartate, zinc orotate and zinc chelate are quite effective. Common zinc sulfate works well, too.

Taking zinc is very safe, although you should be aware of a few caveats. Zinc competes for absorption with other minerals, especially copper, manganese and iron. Taking more than 200 mg per day may contribute to deficiencies in these other minerals or even to their associated forms of anaemia. One recent report suggests that excess zinc may lead to weight gain.[25] If you have one of the conditions just mentioned that requires nutritional treatment and your ZTT is still showing a deficiency, you may need to take high doses. Do so only under the guidance of a health care practitioner, and unless you are treating a high copper problem such as depression or schizophrenia, make sure that your supplements keep zinc and copper in a ten-to-one ratio.

I hope you can see why so many nutrition doctors live by the motto 'Thinc zinc'.

COPPER: *Rheumatoid arthritis reliever*

Copper is a powerful mineral. Not only is it essential to helping the heart to function correctly, but it also controls cholesterol, sugar and uric acid levels. In addition, it increases bone strength, enhances development of red and white blood cells, maintains immune function, contributes to infant growth and is a major treatment for rheumatoid arthritis.[1] But as with iron, maintaining the correct balance is vital. Both shortages and excesses can increase free radical activity, thereby increasing the risk of heart disease and other chronic degenerative illnesses. A doctor and lab tests can determine whether your copper levels are too high or too low.

Many people living in Western industrialized nations such as the US and UK are more prone to suffer copper shortages than surpluses. Recent surveys show that only 25 per cent of Americans consume enough copper and it is estimated that a similar number are deficient in the UK. Most are getting only 50–60 per cent of the recommended daily amount[2], which is only 2 mg per day. Vegetarians also risk shortages, and our ever-increasing consumption of high-fructose corn sweeteners, which can deplete copper levels, increases deficiencies. Finally, copper shortages are widespread among nursing home residents.

COPPER AND THE HEART: FRIEND OR FOE?

Copper is essential in maintaining the heart's pumping ability, preventing aneurysms and ensuring the growth of strong arterial connective tissue that won't rupture. The heart muscle's own connective tissue relies on copper as well to prevent a nutritional form of cardiomyopathy.[3] When we limit copper, we lose an enzyme called ceruloplasmin, a vital antioxidant that protects us from the threat of free iron.

Copper deficiency has been implicated as a possible major contributor to coronary heart disease.[4] But more is not always better; high serum copper levels can be risky as well. An overload encourages cholesterol to stick to the interior wall of blood vessels, thereby increasing the risk of a heart attack. At normal levels, copper would prevent this occurrence.[5] Finnish heart researcher Jukka Salonen found that men with high copper levels were much more prone to having high levels of oxidized LDL cholesterol, and his colleagues confirmed that high copper (and low zinc) levels were strongly associated with increased likelihood for coronary heart disease.[6] That's why it is important to supervise copper with blood tests to monitor our copper status.

Bone Health Because it's needed to manufacture collagen in bone, copper is a key supplement for healing. Deficiency of this nutrient is frequently found in older women who develop leg fractures. Supplementation could reduce the frequency of these injuries.[7]

Rheumatoid Arthritis The use of copper to treat rheumatoid arthritis provides one of the best examples of how a nutrient can be superior to mainstream drug therapies. I have used it regularly to benefit thousands of my patients, following my reading of a landmark scientific paper by researchers Walter Hangarter and John R. Sorenson. They gave 1,140 people with rheumatoid arthritis intravenous doses of a copper salicylate compound. For 89 per cent of them, joint swelling decreased and joint mobility increased. Fevers and other signs of rheumatic activity went into remission for an average of three years.[8] In another Sorenson study, copper salicylate left some 168 of 280 people free of leg pain and all other symptoms of their sciatic neuritis.

Copper helps the body produce superoxide dismutase (SOD), its most therapeutic intracellular anti-inflammatory enzyme. Sorenson's key to success was finding the right copper compound; copper salicylate and copper aspirinate were the most effective. Because they help heal peptic ulcers as well, they are polar opposites of the ulcer-provoking nonsteroidal anti-inflammatory drugs (NSAID) typically prescribed for arthritis.

These copper compounds have never had the sponsorship to undergo testing; therefore, for all practical purposes, they do not exist. The best supplemental alternative available to us is copper sebacate, which mimics SOD's anti-inflammatory influence and is far more beneficial than any of the other compounds, such as copper gluconate, copper sulfate and copper acetate. Animal research shows that it's very difficult to ingest a toxic dose of copper sebacate. It's a compound that is absorbed well by the body and, as part of a mineral complex, it will not bind to proteins (as can simple copper compounds). In contrast, copper gluconate, the compound most commonly found in run-of-the-mill multivitamins, may not effectively raise concentrations of the mineral in blood, urine or hair samples.

Yeast Infections Copper is important to the bacterial balance that wards off candida, but an excessive amount counterproductively strengthens the yeast's own pathogenic nature.[9] The copper complexes, such as copper sebacate, show direct antifungal and bactericidal effects.

Other Conditions Further research and clinical experience will help doctors to fully flush out copper's treatment uses. Copper sebacate, for example, appears to offer some help against diabetes, radiation damage, cancer and convulsions. It may also improve wound healing. A deficiency of the mineral will weaken the immune system.[10] Restoring an optimal level will revive its strength.

WHEN YOU TAKE TOO MUCH

Let's examine the other side of the penny and learn more about the risks of excessive copper. The risk actually depends more on form than on quantity; it's a question of organic vs inorganic. For example, people who drink tap water that comes through copper-lined pipes are more vulnerable to overdose than those who ingest generous amounts of biological copper.

Copper's relationship with zinc is fundamental to understanding its effects on us. Part of the toxic potential of a high copper intake is the corresponding reduction of zinc. Dr Carl Pfeiffer taught an entire generation of nutritionally oriented psychiatrists that high copper causes many cases of schizophrenia, depression and anxiety. In his sophisticated laboratory tests, he found a copper surplus in more than 20 per cent of his psychiatric patients. He treated the overload with a programme that included supplements of zinc, manganese, molybdenum and vitamin B_6.

That same high copper-to-zinc ratio has been blamed for triggering migraine headaches, although some researchers theorize that copper is responsible because it allows the accumulation of compounds that constrict blood vessels. An excess has been seen in people who have the retinal disease macular degeneration, and animal studies verify that an elevated amount can damage the eyes.[11]

Women's greater susceptibility to excess copper is probably connected to the mineral's relationship with oestrogen as well as with zinc. Premenstrual tension and use of birth control pills, for example, are associated with high copper in the blood. So is preeclampsia,[12] breast cancer,[13] lymphoma and chronic leukaemia.[14]

SUPPLEMENT SUGGESTIONS

Until I've run blood tests to check for serum copper, zinc and sometimes manganese, I will not recommend copper supplements to women. If a man does not have a family history of heart disease and does not harbour any psychological problems, I'll forgo the blood tests and allow a cautious supplement programme of perhaps 2–3 mg per day, balanced by 30 mg of zinc. However, in treating rheumatoid arthritis or some similar condition, I will use between two and four pills of copper sebacate per day.

Once supplementation begins, I'll be on the lookout for any greater susceptibility to infection, mental and physical fatigue, a decrease in memory, insomnia or feelings of depression. In some people these reactions are possible even with standard supplement doses.

Better food sources for the mineral include nuts, seeds, organ meats and soya products. You can keep tabs on your copper status by paying attention to what might help deplete the body of the mineral. Anything fortified with iron, for instance, will reduce copper absorption by 50 per cent. If you're anaemic or if you regularly take iron supplements, have your doctor gauge the amount of copper in your red blood cells. You'll also need to be careful if you take vitamin C, especially in high doses.

MANGANESE: *The cell protector*

The name 'manganese' comes from the Greek word for magic, because the ancient Athenians believed the element had magical properties. But while manganese is special in certain ways, it's typical of many trace minerals: though only a small amount is needed, all too often an even smaller amount is available in our diets.

A lot of people don't have as much manganese as they should, according to my patients' trace mineral analyses, which can be done on hair samples. That can be bad news, because manganese is essential for growth, reproduction, wound healing, peak brain function and proper metabolism of sugars, insulin and cholesterol. Without an optimal level, we raise the odds for getting rheumatoid arthritis, osteoporosis, cataracts, multiple sclerosis and seizure disorders.

Our rapidly increasing consumption of refined flours and sugars is the most prominent reason low manganese levels are becoming more common. Lack of the mineral in soil translates into a lack of the mineral in food, while grain milling removes nearly all of what's left. Further, iron and calcium supplements can also have an antagonistic effect.

Here's a look at just some of the ailments that manganese can help to treat:

Diabetes Natural diabetes remedies from around the world often feature manganese-rich herbs. The mineral is an integral part of the Atkins Center's treatments for all variations of sugar and insulin disorders. People with diabetes typically have only half of what's considered a 'normal' manganese level, and the deficiency contributes to their bodies' inability to process sugars. With the nutrient, research shows, they are better able to manage blood glucose.[1]

Cell Damage An important antioxidant, manganese is one of the minerals required to form SOD (superoxide dismutase), one of the 'bodyguard' enzymes that protects us against unstable, cell-damaging free radicals.[2] Manganese can protect against the injurious effects of excess iron, which also generates a tremendous amount of free radicals.[3]

Heart Disease People with heart disease have far less manganese in their heart muscle than do their healthy counterparts. The mineral also strengthens arterial tissues, making them more resistant to plaque formation. Another main reason we use it to treat Atkins Center cardiovascular patients is its relationship with cholesterol. In good supply, manganese can help lower high triglycerides and high cholesterol, with a particular effect on stabilizing LDL and decreasing its atherogenic potential to create blockages. But with experimental manganese deficiency, cholesterol falls to an unusually low point. This condition is linked to an increased likelihood of cancer and a tendency toward suicidal behaviour.

Birth Defects Although potential fathers need manganese for sperm motility,[4] complications seem more problematic when women lack the nutrient. There is a risk of foetal malformations, including increases in neural tube defects, when the mother doesn't have an adequate amount of manganese.

Bone, Joint Health Manganese is just as important as calcium for preventing and treating bone problems. Bone cartilage can't grow or repair itself adequately without it. It's an essential part of glucosamine, a spongy, sugarlike compound that is a major benefactor for our joints. When glucosamine is in short supply, various forms of arthritis tend to arise, eventually leading to severe joint deterioration. Though manganese deficiencies are more common in women with osteoporosis, men should also be aware of this problem. A well-known professional athlete was sidelined with repeated foot fractures that were traced, in part, to his manganese-deficient vegetarian diet. After taking manganese and other mineral supplements, his bones healed, and he was able to resume his athletic career.

Neurological Disorders Early on in my practice, I made manganese supplementation a must for treating a seizure disorder. By now, six different studies confirm that people with epilepsy have lower manganese levels than others. The discrepancy is not caused by their anticonvulsant medications or by the seizures themselves. Research repeatedly demonstrates that a manganese deficiency increases the likelihood that an animal will go into convulsions. Therefore it seems safe to conclude the greater the deficiency, the more frequently seizures occur.[5] My personal conclusion is that manganese supplements will lessen seizure activity and should be routinely prescribed for such patients.

Other Conditions A little more research could broaden manganese's therapeutic horizons. We do know that when it's combined with calcium, it can help relieve premenstrual tension. Manganese helped thousands of schizophrenics treated by Carl Pfeiffer, MD, and his many followers. In doses of 5–20 mg per day, the mineral has alleviated symptoms of tardive dyskinesia. It also might be involved in helping asthmatics breathe more easily; people with asthma often have only one-quarter the amount found in their asthma-free peers.[6]

SUPPLEMENT SUGGESTIONS

You can't set manganese dosages in a vacuum. They have to be determined in relation to zinc and copper, two competing minerals that can affect each other's concentration in the bloodstream. Manganese should be taken whenever you use zinc supplements for any length of time; you should use manganese with two to five times the amount of zinc. A typical dose then might be 35 mg of manganese along with 100 mg of zinc.

A manganese overload, usually from air pollution, is toxic and can damage brain cells. But possible excess rarely comes from food or nutrient supplements (in fact, most of us need to go out of our way to provide our bodies with enough). We can enhance our absorption with supplements of zinc and vitamin C and by eating more animal and soya protein.

IODINE: *Thyroid fuel*

Unlike an estimated one billion people throughout the rest of the world, Americans have remained largely free of iodine's deficiency-related consequences ever since its inclusion in the national salt shaker back in 1924. In the UK, it is possible to buy iodized table salt, but its inclusion is by no means universal. Even in America the shield isn't as secure as it once was. Public health officials harangue people to avoid salt, while touting the benefits of low-sodium foods, thus bypassing the supplementation strategy and posing a very real risk of creating iodine deficiencies.

Contrary to conventional medical advice, salt has little effect on blood pressure in most people. Iodine's impact throughout the body is far greater. By avoiding salt, Americans face throwing the baby out with the bathwater. And there is more to iodine deficiency than thyroid weakness. Our immune systems, our brain function and our hormonal balance all require optimal iodine.

A Pain in the Neck and Elsewhere

The thyroid gland, whose hormones regulate metabolism and the growth of nearly all body tissues, is always the first victim of an iodine shortage. Lack of sufficient nourishment by the mineral causes the gland to malfunction, forcing it either to pump out an overload of thyroid hormone or, most often, to slow production almost to a halt.

Replacing the missing iodine won't heal an underactive gland; at best it may renew hormone production, but only if an actual deficiency exists. In all other cases, iodine supplementation offers no benefit and in fact could be hazardous. Since iodine is toxic in large amounts, it should be used only under a doctor's supervision. Some people mistakenly believe that even if the gland is healthy, supplements will accelerate weight loss by triggering the release of additional thyroid hormone. Not true.

Iodine, then, is a preventive nutrient, not a therapeutic one. Big doses won't bring better health benefits. But this fact doesn't detract from the mineral's enormous impact on human health. While the thyroid's effect is far-reaching, an iodine deficiency has other repercussions.

Birth Defects Throughout pregnancy, especially during the first two trimesters, iodine is critical, and ensuring an adequate intake is imperative. When a woman lacks the mineral, she threatens her foetus with the mental, neurological and physical abnormalities of cretinism.[1]

Learning Impairments Children whose diets are low in iodine usually display little intellectual motivation and will likely develop learning disabilities. Testing the thyroid isn't always an accurate gauge of the potential risk.[2] Even when the gland's output falls within an acceptably 'normal' range, a low-iodine diet may lead to a decrease in IQ and a loss of eye coordination. Researchers in China have associated a general decline in national IQ scores with a dearth of iodine in the Chinese diet. Because the mineral has been studied only as a preventive, scientists don't know if iodine supplements can reverse the learning disabilities or improve scores on intelligence tests.[3]

Immune Weakness Experimentally, high doses of iodine have been used to treat polio, viral diseases and some disorders of the central nervous system. Here, the mineral affects the overall health of the immune system through its relationship with the thyroid.[4]

Female Hormonal Diseases Fibrocystic breasts, endometriosis and uterine fibroids are a few of the specific women's health conditions that iodine supplementation may relieve.[5] The requisite high dosages of molecular iodine used in these studies can be toxic, however, and must be taken only under medical supervision.[6] The mineral accomplishes this by helping to convert oestradiol, a more potent and possibly carcinogenic form of oestrogen, into oestriol, a safer, less bioactive form.

Cancer Throughout the world, where the soil's concentration of iodine is lowest, cancer rates generally are higher. Researchers don't understand the precise mechanism, but they do suspect that, at least for women, it involves the mineral's regulation of the oestradiol–oestriol balance. The ratio between the two forms of oestrogen can accurately predict a woman's risk of cancer.[7]

SUPPLEMENT SUGGESTIONS

Because of its toxic potential, don't take iodine supplements in a cavalier manner, especially in high amounts. Eating seafood and seaweed such as kelp gives the body a rich, safe supply.

And don't deprive yourself of salt. The seasoning can be used moderately by almost everyone with no risk of raising blood pressure.

At the very most, a daily multimineral supplement that contains 100 mcg of iodine will cover most people's needs. Larger doses, to repeat, should be supervised by a doctor. The Japanese consume up to 3 mg of iodine a day, and they have far fewer thyroid problems than do Americans or Britons. If they have found the optimal dose, the reasons why are apparent.

CHROMIUM: *Blood sugar balancer*

Uncontrolled blood sugar and disturbances of the insulin process account for most of our chronic diseases. One of the primary reasons so many of my patients fare better than their drug-taking counterparts in this regard is that I have corrected their insulin resistance. While years of experience show that restricting carbohydrate consumption is the easiest, most certain overall therapy to bypass the disorder, the number one nutrient treatment is chromium.

Taken regularly, this trace mineral throws considerable therapeutic weight against the entire roster of problems caused or worsened by insulin resistance – including obesity, hypoglycaemia (unstable blood sugar), stroke, high blood pressure, Crohn's disease and colitis, ulcers, gastritis, multiple sclerosis, Ménière's disease, migraines, premenstrual tension, seizure disorders and a host of psychiatric disturbances.

THE METAL'S METTLE

Chromium is far and away the most pivotal nutrient involved in sugar metabolism. More than 90 per cent of all Americans are deficient, as are a similarly high percentage of Britons, and sadly, those who are most lacking are the ones who need it the most. Chromium deficiencies are self-perpetuating. When your body exhibits low levels of the trace mineral, your craving for sugars grows. But the more sugar you eat, the more you deplete your chromium stores. With the average American now consuming about 68 kilograms of sugar and corn syrup every year, it's no wonder that insulin-resistance problems and chromium deficiency are so pervasive.[1]

Except for supplements, there is no good way to rebuild the body's stockpile of chromium. True, mushrooms, barley and whole grains contain the trace mineral, but only if they're grown in chromium-rich soil. Seafood and meat are also supposed to be good dietary sources, but again, the animals must have first consumed a chromium-rich diet. The only 'food' truly rich in the mineral is brewer's yeast. Unfortunately, the large number of people who are sensitive to this substance or are susceptible to yeast infections would not be wise to avail themselves of this source.

Science got a glimpse of chromium's importance with the discovery of 'glucose tolerance factor', a molecule built around the mineral. From there, researchers developed chromium compounds that are more easily absorbed and utilized in the body (picolinate and polynicotinate, for example). Once these compounds hit the supplement market, a spate of research took place, providing solid proof of the nutrient's role in insulin metabolism and other aspects of health.

Diabetes Chromium is indispensable for controlling noninsulin-dependent (Type II) diabetes, the vastly more common and complex disease variant. It may also benefit people who have the insulin-dependent (Type I) form of the condition.

Type II, also known as adult-onset diabetes, is the embodiment of insulin resistance. Although family history is a strong predisposing factor, it develops almost exclusively from years of eating refined carbohydrates. If you have Type II diabetes, your body doesn't metabolize the chromium in food, which is why you need supplements. Once an optimum amount is circulating in your bloodstream, you may very well find your blood sugar completely under control. At the very least, chromium supplements could permit a doctor to reduce your requirements for diabetic drugs or insulin injections.[2]

The mineral has been hailed as 'spectacular' by a team of scientists headed by Richard Anderson, PhD, from the US Department of Agriculture's Agriculture Research Service. Using

180 people from Beijing, China, who had Type II diabetes, Anderson and his colleagues proved that a daily 1,000 mcg (1 mg) dose of chromium picolinate could stabilize blood sugar in just two months, something that medications couldn't achieve. After four months of supplementation, they gained even stronger control of their blood glucose, insulin and cholesterol.[3]

Obesity If you are overweight, you are very likely to be insulin-resistant. Weight gain is both a cause and a consequence of the disorder. Besides going on a low-carbohydrate diet, taking chromium supplements is your best bet for losing unwanted fat. According to the research, chromium works on several fronts:

- By reducing sugar cravings, chromium makes it easier to stick to the Atkins diet or another low-carbohydrate eating programme.
- Even without dieting, the mineral can increase your total lean body mass, which in turn speeds up your metabolism and burns additional fat.[4]
- Chromium helps to prevent the loss of lean muscle tissue if you do intentionally cut back on calories.[5]
- The mineral enhances the calorie-burning results of exercise, making weight loss even easier.[6] Working out also increases your excretion of chromium, compounding your need to use supplements.

Heart Disease Insulin disorders and obesity are major risk factors for heart disease. A deficiency of chromium has also been associated with a higher chance of developing heart problems, but not just because it helps to foster better sugar control and weight loss. As I see almost daily in my surgery, adding the mineral to my nutrient prescription helps raise the blood's concentration of artery-clearing HDL cholesterol and, at the same time, decreases LDL cholesterol and triglyceride levels. Total cholesterol also declines. The reduction is even more impressive, researchers report, when a little niacin accompanies the chromium.[7]

High Blood Pressure Why ban the salt shaker when more than 60 per cent of all hypertension cases are now recognized as the consequence of hyperinsulinemia and insulin resistance? It would be a better world if food labels boasted of a rich chromium content and low number of carbohydrates. The repeated rise and fall of blood sugar apparently stimulates the body's sympathetic nervous system, which helps regulate blood pressure. If we ever hope to master the 'silent killer', we need to correct these sins of neglect.

Aging We would certainly find the gold at the end of the rainbow if we could discover a substance that could truly slow the aging process. The bucket of gold may be within our grasp – but it may be filled with chromium.

In the search to discover why we grow old, scientists are focusing on a process called 'glycation'. It's a form of cell damage and death caused by high blood sugar, and it appears to be a major factor in aging. There's no better manager of blood sugar than chromium. What's more, another related mechanism also comes into play: when circulation diminishes to any part of the body, tissue in that area becomes starved for oxygen and other nutrients. Of the many supplements that contribute to the health of the arteries, chromium is one of the most important.

Other Ailments Chromium's value in other areas isn't as solidly established as it is with diabetes, heart disease and high blood pressure, but it may extend in many other directions. For example, it may alleviate chronic headaches and contribute to the treatment of acne, which appears to be caused in part by disturbed insulin metabolism. Chromium makes bones strong by increasing DHEA levels, so it could figure into a treatment programme for osteoporosis.[8] And though we can't say it will prevent glaucoma, the mineral (along with vitamin C) may deter the buildup of pressure inside the eyes.

SUPPLEMENT SUGGESTIONS

Some people might notice a little insomnia or irritability after taking their first chromium supplement, but only occasionally.

My one caveat is for people with diabetes who are chained to a daily regimen of insulin injections or sugar-lowering drugs. Chromium supplements most likely will reduce your requirements for these medications. Safely adjusting the dosages requires medical judgment. Therefore you should refrain from taking chromium supplements until you have a knowledgeable doctor on your side.

As for which kind of chromium is best, there seem to be two good choices. I prescribe both the picolinate and polynicotinate forms; the differences between them are rarely noticeable. Both are beneficial and thoroughly safe, although I feel that the picolinate has a stronger effect. These forms also seem to be more effective than other forms of the mineral. To recruit chromium's help against obesity and other problems related to insulin resistance, I usually suggest taking 200–600 mcg every day. For full-blown diabetes or extreme obesity, I normally raise the amount to between 600 and 1,000 mcg per day.

VANADIUM: *Diabetes therapy*

The case for nutrients to replace pharmaceuticals is powerfully strengthened by the recent explosion of knowledge about a trace mineral that dramatically helps diabetics: vanadium.

DIABETES ON THE RISE

Diabetes is on a dramatic upsurge; there are 1.4 million confirmed cases in the UK, and another 1 million are thought to be unaware they are sufferers – that's about three in every hundred people. Symptoms include insulin resistance, excess insulin release, high triglycerides and high blood pressure. Plus, the majority of the overweight population has problems related to elevated insulin. Vanadium is on its way to being recognized as an essential nutrient for all who suffer from these insulin-related problems.[1]

Is Vanadium Essential?

A nutrient has to jump through many hoops before it can be considered essential. Such an examination is now taking place for vanadium. While a handful of studies have suggested that the mineral is essential for animals, its status for humans has yet to be proven. Though we do ingest 10–60 micrograms per day from food, there have not been any studies in humans that examine the effects of a vanadium-free diet. One thing, however, appears clear from animal studies: vanadium is vitally important in the treatment of diabetes.[2]

New Kid on the Block

Vanadium first grabbed the spotlight in 1985 when researchers found that it could control diabetes in animals. While nearly all the early research was done on animals, the results are hard to ignore: not only does vanadium lower fasting blood sugar in diabetic mice, it also lowers LDL cholesterol and triglyceride levels.[3,4] The mineral works by acting like insulin and thereby helping cells to absorb sugar more effectively. The drawbacks? Uncertainty about its toxicity potential and the fact that it is not absorbed well. As a result, one needs large doses to benefit, particularly when using the vanadyl sulfate form.

The human studies with vanadium executed so far are impressive: they show that it can greatly reduce the needs for insulin and hypoglycaemic medications. Vanadium also lowers blood sugar as well as the need for insulin.[5,6] Vanadyl sulfate has been found to benefit both Type I and Type II diabetes. In humans it appears to have the insulin-mimicking effect that Type I diabetics[7] need, as well as the ability to overcome the insulin resistance that is the defining abnormality in Type II diabetes.[8]

In Search of the Right Dose

I, other complementary doctors, and the scientific community are all in the process of discovering vanadium's significant effects on insulin and both types of diabetes. What remains to be discovered, however, is the *optimal dose*. I have used 25–50 mgs of vanadyl sulfate per day in my diabetic patients with good results. But three recent studies have suggested that the more optimal dose might be closer to 100 mg, so I occasionally use doses in this range. It is certainly possible to overdose on vanadium; for instance, multigram doses may cause kidney problems,[9] which certainly suggests that doses above 100 mg per day should be avoided until more is known about the long-term effects of such doses. Doses over 20 mgs should be taken only for existing diabetes and with a doctor's supervision. It also should not be taken with the monoamine oxidase (MAO) inhibitor drugs used to treat depression. Although I have found it thoroughly safe, I usually recommend that it be taken in moderation.

WHAT'S THE BEST FORM?

The most interesting vanadium research of the last decade has been the work of John McNeill, PhD. Though he first studied vanadyl sulfate, McNeill has recently been developing a new vanadium compound that may surpass vanadyl sulfate in importance,[10] effectiveness and safety. It's called BMOV, which stands for bis(maltolato)oxovanadium(IV). This compound appears to be better absorbed and metabolized than vanadyl sulfate, and it also prevents cataracts and cardiac dysfunction in diabetic rats. However, all the studies to date have been done on animals, so it remains to be seen whether BMOV is also the superior form of vanadium for humans.

Yet I feel BMOV may be the breakthrough on the horizon. It certainly can be used at lower doses than vanadyl sulfate and therefore has less theoretical potential for long-term toxicity. Some of my colleagues are using doses below 1 milligram and reporting benefits for their diabetic patients, but I have not seen BMOV work as well as the higher dose of vanadyl sulfate. As this book goes to press, I am using BMOV for long-term management of diabetics once their blood sugar has been lowered by vanadyl sulfate.

VANADIUM WON'T MAKE MUSCLES BIGGER

Because vanadium can act like insulin, an anabolic hormone

that helps increase muscle mass, some weight trainers have begun taking high doses of vanadium in hopes that it will turn them into another Mr Universe. However, the mineral does not affect insulin metabolism in healthy people, and numerous studies have clearly proved that vanadium has no muscle-building effects whatsoever. And it is potentially dangerous: as we've noted, very high intake of vanadium may cause health problems. The weight-lifting crowd has been known to exper-iment with such high doses, and I strongly warn against such experimentation. Vanadium's power appears limited specifically to people with diabetes; its insulin-enhancing effects are not seen in nondiabetics.[11]

BOLSTERING THE DIABETIC VITA-NUTRIENT ARSENAL

Vanadium contributes to the excitement engendered by chromium. I am hoping that traditional medicine will attempt to confirm what I have observed in my own patients: that vana-dium – combined with chromium, zinc, manganese, magnesium, biotin, CoQ_{10}, niacinamide and a sharply lowered carbohydrate intake – can just about do away with the need for Type II diabetes medicine. Not bad for a trace mineral not even consid-ered essential.

I have discussed the dosage range for vanadyl sulfate in diabetes, ranging from 20 to 100 mg daily, and I do not recom-mend it at present for someone who does not have an insulin/glucose disorder. It is too early for me to recommend a dosage range for BMOV.

SELENIUM: *Anticancer antioxidant*

A substance that can cut cancer occurrences by almost 40 per cent and decrease the cancer death rate by 50 per cent should be heralded as our greatest medical breakthrough and dispensed to every person in the world. If it's not harmful in any way, why would the medical profession urge the public to avoid it?

As 1996 came to a close, we learned that selenium supple-mentation had, in fact, achieved these earth-shattering results.

But publication of the research details in the prestigious *Journal of the American Medical Association* was, not surprisingly, accompanied by the now familiar editorial advisory: 'Don't jump to premature conclusions without more research.' Needless to say, drug studies aren't greeted with such hesitation so routinely.

Selenium's Role as an Antioxidant

This kind of reaction is particularly astonishing given selenium's impressive track record. The cancer study's impressive results simply confirm what we've already known: this nutrient is an immune-strengthening, cancer-deterring dynamo with a widespread effect on our health. No other trace mineral is so vital to our antioxidant defences. When we lack selenium, we also lack glutathione peroxidase, a powerful antioxidant enzyme. Its absence leaves a huge hole in our protection from, among other oxidation-related afflictions, hardening of the arteries, heart disease, rheumatoid arthritis and cataracts.

The mineral also reinforces the body's immune defences against viruses and other invading pathogens, with lab experiments showing measurable changes in such immune system elements as white blood cells, natural killer cells, antibodies, macrophages and interferon. Taking supplements preventively, some studies suggest, could prevent hepatitis, herpes and even infections from the ebola virus.

The following conditions respond well to selenium supplementation.

AIDS Doses of selenium might help keep the HIV virus dormant and prevent it from developing into full-blown AIDS. In people who are infected with HIV, a selenium deficiency is very common, and the lower it drops below normal, the more damage HIV can inflict on an immune-crippled body.[1] In fact, one of the theories of how AIDS becomes manifest is that HIV drains selenium from an infected cell until it reaches a critically low point. The cell then bursts and the virus replicates.

Maintaining an optimum level of selenium does more than replenish this loss and fortify the immune system. In fact, the mineral works much like a number of AIDS drugs, inhibiting a virus-related substance called reverse transcriptase. For all these reasons, the most knowledgeable selenium authority I know, Gerhard Schrauzer, PhD, asserts that the mineral may be the single most important nutrient for people infected with the deadly virus.[2] Because the full immune stimulation of a standard supplement programme may not be seen for as long as six months, Schrauzer suggests that doctors may coax a speedier response by prescribing a very brief initial course with daily dosages as high as 8,000 mcg.

Viruses depend on selenium to grow and replicate, yet a lack of the mineral makes viruses more virulent. Lab studies demonstrate that when deprived of selenium, a range of viruses, including those responsible for hepatitis B and the common cold, will mutate into more dangerous forms.[3] This is exactly what we don't want.

A Conqueror of Cancer? Any substance that empowers the immune system and wards off oxidation can be expected to defend us in the war against cancer. Selenium's association with cancer prevention is solidly documented; the study that found a 50 per cent decrease in cancer deaths, then, is no bolt out of the blue that should be greeted with scepticism.[4]

First, the epidemiology allows us to predict selenium's value. It is firmly established from the world population studies that wherever soil selenium levels are higher, there are significantly lower levels of cancers of the lung, rectum, bladder, oesophagus, cervix and uterus. Studies from Finland have shown that male cancer patients have lower levels of selenium in their blood than healthy persons, and selenium may be one of the most important protective nutrients against these forms of cancer.[5] Patients with lymphoma, a form of cancer that is increasing dramatically in prevalence, is much more common among people with low selenium levels.[6]

The first evidence heralding selenium's cancer reduction success came from a study in Lin Xian, China. It was the only study in which giving synthetic beta-carotene worked impressively, cutting the cancer rate among thirty thousand people. But only in Lin Xian did the subjects get selenium, 50 mcg daily for over five years.

On December 25, 1996, perhaps the most successful cancer prevention study ever executed was published.[7] It is a ten-year study conducted with the support of the US National Cancer Institute on 1,312 volunteers (75 per cent of them men). This time, 200 mcg of selenium (from yeast) was administered daily. The selenium users had a 49 per cent decrease in the death rate from the three most prevalent cancers (lung, prostate and colorectal). The data in the study should change the way the world views cancer prevention and nutritional supplementation. It certainly should teach us that to be optimally protected from cancer, we need more selenium than is provided by the diet. Supplements provide an excellent and inexpensive protection against this killer disease.

And It's Good for Your Heart, Too As an important antioxidant, selenium would be expected to play a role in the prevention of heart disease. Indeed, it has been found that those with low selenium levels have a 70 per cent greater risk of coronary heart disease than those with normal levels, and that low plasma levels of selenium have been found (in a Danish study) to be a significant risk factor for heart disease.[8] Many population studies have shown that selenium is a protective nutrient against the development of heart and artery disease.[9] Clinical observation has also shown that selenium is an important supplement for the management of cardiac arrhythmias and the prevention of sudden cardiac death.[10] Selenium protects the heart, not only through its role in producing glutathione peroxidase, which maintains antioxidant activity,[11] but by restricting the body's load of toxic metals such as cadmium, mercury and lead, which can damage heart tissue. Finally, the mineral protects the heart against low levels of oxygen, against the toxic effects of drugs like Adriamycin[12], and against Keshan disease.

Inflammatory Conditions Selenium levels are low in people with rheumatoid arthritis, and its anti-inflammatory properties have helped relieve arthritis symptoms, especially when combined with vitamin E and other antioxidants.[13] Osteoarthritics have also benefited from it.[14] However, the effects are not instantaneous; it may take six months for selenium's benefits to become apparent.[15]

Low selenium levels have also been found in asthmatics. In a study of New Zealanders, where soil selenium levels are low, those with low levels of the selenium-dependent enzyme, glutathione peroxidase, were six times as likely to have asthma.[16] Because glutathione peroxidase has anti-inflammatory properties, selenium is valuable in a wide range of other inflammatory conditions, such as colitis and psoriasis. (The best results with psoriasis take place with the direct application of selenium to the affected skin.[17]

Thyroid Disorders Selenium is important for thyroid function because the enzyme that activates the main thyroid hormone (T_4) depends on it. Without selenium, the benefits of thyroid replacement therapy may be incomplete; this means that selenium deficiency may lead to a sluggish metabolism or even obesity. Selenium does more than just activate thyroid hormone: it protects the thyroid gland from free radical damage that can lead to decreased thyroid function.[18] Selenium's supplementation appears to be particularly important in older adults with thyroid problems.[19]

Metal Poisoning A major unappreciated contribution to good health is selenium's ability to disarm the threat of toxic metals, such as lead, platinum and mercury. It binds with the metals, leaving them inert and harmless. A case in point is that of mercury workers in the former Yugoslavia. Although they are exposed to a high amount of the metal, their diets are nevertheless high enough in selenium to protect them, thanks to the richness of selenium in their soil. A clinical advantage recently demonstrated is its ability to reduce the toxicity of platinum-containing chemotherapeutic agents.[20]

A major cause of multiple sclerosis, I found, is a systemic accumulation of toxic metals. MS cases occur more frequently in areas that lack selenium. Low glutathione levels, a sign of selenium deficiency, are found in MS patients.[21]

Birth Defects Fertility in both men and women depends on an optimum selenium intake. So does a baby's good health. Along with folic acid and zinc, selenium is crucial to preventing the malformed spines seen in neural tube defects.[22] Mothers of newborns with this birth defect and the infants themselves generally have lower levels of the mineral than do their healthy counterparts. Pregnant women who don't get enough selenium are more likely to have a miscarriage, and newborns may suffer from muscle weakness. Babies who die from sudden infant death syndrome have shown several signs of a selenium deficiency, suggesting a possible preventive role for supplementation.[23]

Pancreatitis When sudden abdominal pain, nausea and vomiting signal the onset of an acute case of pancreatitis, selenium can be lifesaving. Doctors found that administering the mineral to patients reduced pancreas inflammation within twenty-four hours.[24]

No easy way exists to determine the selenium content of food. Two plots of land just a mile apart can differ a thousandfold in their mineral content. Overfarming, topsoil erosion and acid rain all contribute to the increasing depletion of selenium in soil and, ultimately, in what we eat.

The food tables purporting to list the nutrient content of various fruits and vegetables, therefore, should be taken with a proverbial grain of salt. Fruit and vegetables don't require it for growth; meat and other protein-containing products don't necessarily contain it, either. With this proviso, I can say that good sources are supposed to be nuts, eggs, meat and whole grains; Brazil nuts are a notably good source. And as a rule, organic produce contains a higher amount than produce treated with chemicals.

A low-protein diet compromises intake of the mineral, as does eating a lot of refined grains, which are stripped of whatever selenium they otherwise might have possessed. Use of fish oil and polyunsaturated vegetable oils – from sunflower seeds, corn and flax – can unfortunately increase the body's need for the mineral.

SUPPLEMENT SUGGESTIONS

To get the most we can from selenium's anticancer shield, all of us should be taking a 200 mcg supplement every day. For added insurance against inflammation, viral infections, immune weakness or heavy-metal contamination, 400 mcg is more appropriate and still very safe. A topical selenium solution works best against psoriasis.

Short-term dosages as high as 1,000 mcg (1 mg) are usually safe to take, but not for a sustained period. Selenium can be toxic. In certain parts of the world with selenium-rich soils, where the normal daily diet provides as much as 700 mcg a day, area residents display no side effects or indications of toxicity. But no matter what dosage you might be using, pair it with some vitamin E. The two antioxidants compensate for each other if one is in short supply.

Several forms of selenium are available. The best, I've found, are selenomethionine and sodium selenite. Yeast-derived selenium is beneficial, too, some studies report, but avoid it if you're susceptible to yeast infections.

MOLYBDENUM: *Detoxifier, purifier*

For a nutrient needed in such a small amount, molybdenum packs quite a health-promoting punch. Dosages well beyond the officially recommended 75 mcg a day alleviate ailments ranging from mental grogginess to arthritis. This trace mineral's primary contribution to our health is as a cell purifier.

THE PURIFIER

In this role, molybdenum cleanses the body of toxic compounds whose accumulation in our cells contributes to depression, pain, fatigue and liver malfunction, among other maladies. It's one of the most important nutritional weapons we have to combat sulfite allergies and chemical sensitivities.[1] By helping to rid the body of aldehydes, noxious by-products of a yeast (*Candida albicans*) infection, the mineral clears away the brain fog that often muddles the thinking of people afflicted with an over-growth of the yeast that normally resides in our large intestines.

MOLYBDENUM'S MANY MODALITIES

In addition, molybdenum performs several other important roles to preserve our health. It generates energy and helps us manu-facture haemoglobin, the oxygen-carrying protein in red blood cells. In daily amounts of 500 mcg, it can relieve a broad range of aches and pains, including arthritis.[2] Other research indicates it may relieve asthma, especially when given intravenously.[3] Molybdenum can also help to overcome seizures in newborns.[4] It lowers the risk of gastrointestinal cancer.[5] It contributes to preventing tooth decay. It also opposes toxic accumulations of copper, making it a useful treatment for Wilson's disease, an inherited disorder that involves copper metabolism, liver impair-ment and mental abnormalities.

SUPPLEMENT SUGGESTIONS

A daily dosage of 200–500 mcg of molybdenum is probably the minimum necessary for most people, and up to 2,000 mcg a day may be called for if you wish to address some of the condi-tions just listed. If you eat a lot of protein or sulfur-containing foods, such as eggs, you'll need more than the minimum amount. So will people with a sweet tooth, because the body requires a molybdenum-dependent enzyme to metabolize fructose and sucrose. Consuming sugar, therefore, can lead to a depletion of the trace mineral. Alcohol consumption and excess copper intake also draw upon molybdenum stores.

Larger doses are very safe for most people, because the mineral is washed away easily in the urine. My only precaution is for people with gout. Molybdenum's ability to help create uric acid, which when elevated leads to gout, could prove prob-lematic. Supplementation could elevate uric acid to an aggra-vating level, although adverse reactions are rare, even with large dosages.[6] On the other hand, if you do not have gout and your blood uric acid level is low (below 3.6 mg per cent), there is a very good chance you are deficient in molybdenum.

I routinely prescribe 500 mcg of molybdenum whenever I see a patient whose uric acid is low. It plays so many useful roles in our bodies that I am inclined to correct the possibility of a deficiency just on face value.

BORON: *Sex hormone and bone provider*

Although it is almost as fundamental as calcium to the strength of a woman's bones, boron has yet to receive an RDA. This is despite the fact that the US government's own nutrient researchers have found that a deficiency of the mineral dulls thinking and interferes with hand-eye coordination, while other research shows a decided impact on arthritis.[1]

Because relatively little research has been done on boron, our conclusions are based upon just a few studies. So far, however, I'm impressed with what I've seen. According to one ground-breaking study, boron apparently can raise a woman's natural oestrogen level just as much as does hormone replacement therapy and is an equally effective safeguard against osteoporosis. Thus it's a terrific option for women who want to prevent osteoporosis but can't afford hormone replacement therapy's increase in cancer risk or its unsettling influence on blood sugar.

In the above-mentioned study, twelve postmenopausal women followed a low-boron diet for four months, then began to take 3 mg of the mineral every day. The results were impressive. Boron cut the women's urinary loss of calcium, the main component of bones, in half. It also raised blood concentrations of oestrogen and testosterone, which all women secrete in tiny amounts. The oestrogen levels climbed into the range normally reached by following oestrogen replacement therapy.[2] In addition, other studies have shown that boron enables the body to make better use of vitamin D, the nutrient responsible for calcium's accumulation in our bones. It has been shown to decrease the urinary output of oxalate, which, with calcium, causes kidney stones. This may make boron an essential element in the prevention of this extremely prevalent condition.[3]

Because it stimulates natural oestrogen production, boron can also be employed against other hormone-related health problems. It has enhanced the benefits of the therapies I use to alleviate hot flushes, vaginal dryness and other menopausal symptoms.

Male Hormone Deficiencies Since boron appears to raise DHEA (a male hormone precursor) and testosterone levels in women, it is logical to assume that it should also increase testosterone in men. If so, it could have the ability to shore up a waning libido or lagging sexual function. I have yet to locate a study proving that, however. Some bodybuilders, who believe that such a testosterone boost would help increase their muscle mass, have been taking boron supplements. But so far that belief seems to be unfounded, since the few studies conducted in this area have been unimpressive.[4] In fact, a 10 mg daily dose for one month raised men's oestradiol levels 40 per cent, but the testosterone levels rose only slightly.[5] However, because my patients' therapeutic goals are different, I still frequently offer boron supplements to older men, especially those whose dietary intake is very low. The majority notice a detectable increase in sexual desire.

Arthritis In countries where there is a greater dietary consumption of boron, it has been noted that the incidence of arthritis is lower. Taking 6 mg of the mineral daily for eight weeks, one study concluded, significantly improved arthritic symptoms and had a marked benefit against severe osteoarthritis.[6] With more research of this kind, we might find that boron affects other degenerative joint diseases as well.

Mental Performance Scientists at the US Department of Agriculture have established that a boron deficiency decreases our ability to concentrate. We become drowsy, less alert and slower to respond. The deficit impairs performance of a variety of tasks, from finger snapping to following a target on a computer screen, the government researchers found, and changes in brain wave patterns reflect the handicap.[7] The next research project should be to prove whether or not giving boron supplements would improve performance.

SUPPLEMENT SUGGESTIONS

We ingest anywhere between 1.7 and 7 mg of boron daily. Drinking water can sometimes provide a significant amount of the mineral. Fruits, vegetables, nuts and seeds are the primary food sources, while wine and beer have high amounts, too. Because Americans and Britons aren't noted for their consumption of vegetables, nuts and seeds, and the mineral content of water varies greatly, I suspect a considerable number of people fall into the lower ranges.

Dietary intake of up to 40 mg per day has not caused any toxic reactions in humans. This is because the mineral is poorly assimilated; 3 mg supplements increased the plasma boron levels by only 50 per cent. I believe most of us should get 3 mg of boron per day in addition to our dietary intake. For the 'target' groups – arthritics, those who want to prevent osteoporosis, or those who are dealing with sexual decline, menopausal symptoms or oestrogen replacement withdrawal – I prescribe 6–18 mg per day. This dosage was determined through my clinical use; it is the amount that allows my patients to reduce their hormone replacement therapy without experiencing any adverse symptoms.

SILICON: *Skin, hair and nails provider*

You probably won't find silicon in your typical multivitamin or multimineral supplement. Most nutritionists believe that diet satisfies our need for this essential trace mineral. There are, however, some prominent dissenters whose opinions I share, such as Forrest H. Nielsen, director of the US Human Nutrition Research Center.

In certain mammals, silicon affects a variety of substances necessary for healthy development of bones, blood vessels and the brain, including collagen, elastin and glycosaminoglycans.[1] It specifically helps animals develop better cartilage.[2] It helps bones to absorb calcium, evidenced by its presence around the calcification sites of growing bones. Lab animals deficient in silicon develop joint abnormalities,[3] and people, some research suggests, may lose bone density if they don't get enough.[4]

Epidemiologists have noted that fewer cases of arteriosclerosis exist in areas with a higher concentration of silicon in the water supply, just one piece of evidence that the mineral may help keep arteries strong and supple.[5] A deficiency also may contribute to high blood pressure and ischemic heart disease.

A Barrier Against Alzheimer's?

Newer research implicates silicon in the brain's absorption of aluminium, which might influence the risk of Alzheimer's disease. When the silicon concentration in soil is low, the aluminium concentration is frequently high, and some studies suggest that the same association may exist in the brain.[6]

Supplement Suggestions

The typical diet provides about 30 mg of silicon per day, which conventional thinking considers an adequate amount. Because most processed foods are virtually devoid of the mineral, as insurance against the loss of bone density, I recommend a 2 mg daily supplement. I would consider adding between 3 and 6 mg to a woman's nutrient programme. Instead of having to swallow an even greater number of pills, you may want to take an extract of horsetail, an herb rich in silicon that can be found in most health food stores. Other dietary sources include apples, unrefined grains, legumes and root vegetables.

GERMANIUM: *Oxygen deliverer*

Found naturally in such foods as garlic, ginseng, chlorella and various mushrooms, germanium stirred up considerable excitement in the medical community back in the 1950s, when its discoverer, Kazuhiko Asai, PhD, demonstrated that it delivers more oxygen to body tissues. Though the mineral is officially nonessential, he and other investigators have since learned that the element might help treat cancer, arthritis, osteoporosis, *Candida albicans* (yeast), AIDS and other viral infections.[1] It may also accelerate wound healing and decrease pain.

I have been using germanium for a substantial number of cancer patients, who consistently report an improvement in overall well-being. Scientific research indicates why. It shows that germanium, especially the sesquioxide, boosts the immune system, wards off free radical damage, helps the body rid itself of immune-weakening toxins and generates oxygen production inside tissue cells.[2] Each of these mechanisms represents a well-accepted approach for patients gaining the upper hand over the malignant process. Combine these effects with other natural, safe substances providing similar benefits, and you may begin to see how complementary cancer therapy achieves its many successes.

When we analyze the meaning of the word 'sesquioxide', we see that such a compound carries six oxygen molecules to whatever tissue it reaches. Now consider that oxygen is anathema to cancer cells; they demand an anaerobic (oxygen-free) environment to multiply. Germanium is uniquely suited to favour the growth of normal tissue over the invasive malignancy.

SUPPLEMENT SUGGESTIONS

Eating more garlic, chlorella and medicinal mushrooms are some ways to get germanium, but they're not the best. Supplements are the most reliable source, but not any bottle labelled 'germanium' will do. Consume only pure, organic germanium,[3] at a dosage of 25–300 mg or more per day. The safest, most effective form of the nutrient is germanium bis-carboxyethyl sesquioxide-132, or Ge-132, for short. Germanium dioxide, germanium lactate citrate and other inferior versions are inexpensive and widely available – but potentially dangerous. They've been blamed for two deaths[4] and have been linked to cases of kidney damage.[5] Pure Ge-132 is expensive, but it has never been shown to cause adverse effects.

CHAPTER 5

◆

AMINO ACIDS

INTRODUCTION

Drugs influence almost every bodily function. Some accelerate wound healing, others provide the raw materials for brain chemicals that may treat depression or a mental illness. The innumerable others juggle our internal chemistry in ways that prevent epileptic seizures, lower blood pressure, numb irritated nerves and wake up a sluggish immune system, to mention just a few examples.

Amino acids do precisely the same things. The only difference is that they work naturally by providing the body with what it needs to do its job, but without the ever-present risk of side effects from medications (which work by *preventing* the body from doing one of its jobs). To maintain health, improve health and correct illnesses, we need them, and in quantities and combinations that food can't provide. When a so-called nutrition expert contends that we get plenty of amino acids from the protein in our food, you can bet that the assertion is backed up by the latest cutting-edge knowledge of the 1950s. If the expert warns that amino acid supplements arc hazardous, you can interpret the statement as a roundabout admission of their therapeutic ability.

WHEN 'NONESSENTIAL' IS INDISPENSABLE

Without different combinations of amino acids, hair would be indistinguishable from the heart, among other unseemly possibilities. Just as letters of the alphabet form every word in the dictionary, these chemicals congregate in an endless array of ways to form protein molecules that influence and define the body's every cell.

You've all heard, I'm sure, of the eight 'essential' amino acids. I won't bother to list them. Their designation, in number and name, is misleading. Yes, those nutrients are essential, but medicine doesn't work from the same dictionary that you and I use. In the narrow official definition, the same one applied to vitamins, 'essential' means that the body can't manufacture the amino acids on its own from other raw materials. It must get them ready-made from food or supplements.

This characterization, besides making no allowance for quantity, implies that the other 'nonessential' amino acids are insignificant or of little importance. Few things could be further from the truth. Taurine, glutamine, arginine and the rest of this supposedly dispensable bunch are among our most valuable medicinal nutrients. Sure, the body manufactures them from other biochemicals, although only in amounts determined by the availability of the other ingredients. Often the raw resources are either in short supply or missing altogether.

We're going to take a close look at the remedial potential of many key amino acids, including more than the eight that we get only through diet. In addition to quantity, the key to these, well, essential substances is balance. Just as a football team can't show up for a game with extra strikers but no goalkeeper, so must the amino acids appear in proper proportions. In the wrong ratio, the body can't synthesize as much protein for our muscles, organs, skin and other lean tissue. If even one is undersupplied, the other seven will be metabolized inadequately.

Blood analyses are a valuable, albeit expensive and often impractical method for disclosing amino acid imbalances. A good rule of thumb is that animal protein, such as from beef, fish, fowl and eggs, provides a better balance than do vegetables, because meat contains each of the essential eight in the correct amounts. One or more of the octet will be missing from plant foods or won't appear in the necessary quantity. That's why vegetables are said to have a lower 'protein efficiency ratio'. For example, a diet centred around soya very well could be low in the essential amino acid methionine, giving you less of a complete protein bang for your mealtime buck. Many strict vegetarians, notably those who shun eggs and dairy products, frequently need amino acid supplements because their food choices don't supply enough lysine, thyronine and methionine to deal adequately with stress.

Some vegetarians advocate designing meals so that some foods compensate for proteins absent in others. A bean-grain casserole, for instance, supposedly gives the body a complete set of essential amino acids. This practice can provide a little extra complete protein, but animal food remains the wisest choice. And this brings me to my favourite protein choice: the egg. Maligned – wrongly – as it may be, the egg contains all essential amino acids in near perfect balance. Its amino acid ratio, in fact, is the officially accepted standard upon which all other protein sources are judged. For someone who lacks any given amino acid, eating eggs tops my list of dietary recommendations.

But we're getting ahead of ourselves. Allow me to backtrack and examine some of medicine's most vital prescriptions.

ARGININE: *Immune booster*

If this book had been written a decade ago, this section would only be a paragraph or two long. That was before researchers discovered that arginine regulates an amazing blood compound called nitric oxide, the compound responsible for regulating blood flow, immune function, communication among nerve cells, liver function, blood clotting and even sexual arousal. That's why, in 1992, boron won *Science* magazine's prestigious designation 'Molecule of the Year'.

Don't confuse nitric oxide with nitrous oxide, otherwise known as laughing gas, the anesthetic that a dentist might pump into you before extracting a tooth. Nitric oxide, chemically written NO and also referred to as 'endothelium-derived relaxation factor', is a key player in allowing blood vessels to relax and thereby controlling high blood pressure. Until the discovery of the arginine connection, science was unable to harness this substance. Now a mere nutrient, a simple supplement that's found on the shelf at any health food store, gives us the means through which we can better manage myriad cellular processes.

As with iron, however, arginine supplementation isn't as uncomplicated and innocuous as swallowing a handful of pills. Like so much in nutritional medicine, prescribing it, whether to manufacture nitric oxide or to take advantage of its other rewards, involves finding the right balance in the blood. While a nitric oxide deficiency carries definite risks, so, too, does a surfeit. Despite all its benefits, the compound is a free radical, which is capable of inflicting oxidative damage.[1] Ideally, doctors of the future will analyze nitric oxide levels in blood serum to determine whether you need more of this body chemical. If so, your arginine supplements should be accompanied by a broad spectrum of antioxidant protection, including coenzyme Q_{10} and lipoic acid, which will neutralize the potential harm.

CARDIOLOGY'S MIGHTIEST AMINO

Of the many ways in which arginine can improve heart health, almost all have been revealed only in the last few years. Even nutritionally oriented doctors may not yet be accustomed to prescribing the amino acid for heart problems and other conditions, but they should. Here's why:

Arginine itself (not the nitric oxide it produces) decreases cholesterol more effectively than any other amino acid. Daily doses of 6–17 grams a day have lowered LDL cholesterol without reducing the beneficial HDL cholesterol, and it did so without producing side effects. It also promotes healthy coronary microcirculation in people with high cholesterol,[2] and it deters the formation of blood clots, which can lead to heart attacks or strokes.[3]

The NO that is created by arginine is capable of much more. By relaxing arteries, thus permitting better blood flow, it can improve such circulation-related conditions as coronary heart disease with angina, intermittent claudication (poor leg circulation),[4] and high blood pressure. Disorders of brain circulation also may be helped. Arginine-induced vasodilation is detectable even in younger men, who typically don't suffer from impaired circulation,[5] and injections of the amino acid can strengthen the cardiac muscle in people with congestive heart failure.[6] In Japan and in Greece, cardiology teams are infusing the nutrient directly into the coronary blood vessels of angina patients and dramatically reopening their circulation.[7] Israeli heart doctors are improving the performance of the hearts of patients with congestive heart failure by administering 20 grams of arginine by vein over one hour's time.

A Multipurpose Benefactor

Arginine, of course, acts as more than the precursor of NO. In certain instances – examples include a growth spurt, recovery from trauma, wound healing and any need for a strong immune presence – the body can't satisfy its need for arginine, and arginine becomes 'essential'.

Like the other building blocks of protein, arginine participates in the maintenance of muscle and lean tissue throughout the body. It can be converted into ornithine, another amino acid. And its presence can stimulate the release of certain natural anabolic hormones, such as growth hormone and insulinlike growth factor.[8]

Muscle Preservation According to a small study of forty-five older people, a daily tonic containing 17 grams of arginine was shown to preserve lean muscle tissue. It also raised blood readings of insulinlike growth factor (a measure of human growth hormone) and lowered LDL cholesterol. The study volunteers who did not receive arginine actually lost lean muscle tissue.[9]

Immune Function Natural killer (NK) cells, a main component of our body's defence system, step up their activity dramatically with arginine's assistance. Taking a total of 30 grams over the course of the day, one study showed, expanded these NK cells' activity by a whopping 91 per cent. T cell function also improves.[10]

The rejuvenation could prove to be of great value to people afflicted with AIDS or any other virus or malignant disease.

Supplementation also can increase the weight of the thymus gland, where most immune function originates,[11] and strengthen the bacteria-killing power of neutrophils. At the same time, more nitric oxide becomes available to patrol the gastrointestinal tract, combating infections and quelling any overgrowth of *Candida albicans*.[12] Taking arginine with lysine, another amino acid, further augments the immune system's strength, especially in its battle against recurrent infections. In turn, this more potent immune system may account for the association between arginine supplements and a reduction in both tumour growth and the incidence of cancer, as has been documented in several studies.[13]

Male Sexual Disorders Nitric oxide is the decisive factor in a man's ability to achieve and maintain an erection.[14] Taking 2.8 grams of arginine per day, several studies show, generates enough of the vasodilating compound to help in the treatment of erectile failure. Enhanced genital blood flow probably facilitates sexual arousal in women, too.

Regular doses of the amino acid also invigorates sperm production. A daily supplement of 3–4 grams, according to other research, increased both sperm counts and overall sperm activity.[15] For a more thorough nutritional approach to infertility, nutritional doctors would add supplements of zinc, carnitine and coenzyme Q_{10}.

Bone and Tissue Injuries Burn researchers found arginine to be indispensable in restoring protein balance in severe burn victims. It also has been shown to speed the healing of wounds, fractures and diabetes-related foot ulcers.[16] It may heal and regenerate nerves.[17] Additionally, the success of an osteoporosis prevention programme also may hinge on arginine. Nitric oxide inhibits the loss of bone, while the release of growth hormone also may augment bone density.[18]

Reye's Syndrome In ways not understood, a deficiency of the amino acid may perhaps encourage the syndrome. Supplements may have preventive potential against this serious childhood illness.[19]

SUPPLEMENT SUGGESTIONS

I'm sure you'll see that the dosages of arginine required for many of its most valuable usages are unwieldy (it is difficult to swallow a 'vitamin pill' containing more than 1 gram of ingredients). Using this amino acid requires a goal-oriented mindset. I've prescribed arginine in dosages as low as 1 gram and as high as 30 grams. For wound healing, helping to restore sexual response and supporting the immune system, between 1,500 mg and 4 grams per day usually prove useful. As part of cardiovascular therapy, 15 grams or more a day might be necessary. You won't obtain that much from food or even from most amino acid supplements. For convenience and economy, get a pure, powdered form of the nutrient.

As with so much in nutritional medicine, the best therapeutic use of arginine involves finding the right balance. To help find your own ideal balance and to assure your safest use, follow a few guidelines:

- To avoid arginine's risk of promoting free radical oxidation, supplements should be accompanied by a broad spectrum of antioxidant protection, especially from coenzyme Q_{10} and lipoic acid.
- Don't give multigram doses to children under eighteen for any extended period of time. The release of growth hormone prompted by large doses is, in all likelihood, not appropriate for their young bodies.
- Take the amino acid cautiously if you have arthritis or an active infection, because an excess of nitric oxide can trigger inflammation.
- For immune strengthening, take additional lysine with arginine. While the amino acid offers some encouragement for AIDS or other causes of a frail immune system, some infections, including herpes, may become worse because their viruses like to feed on arginine. Adding lysine to the balance may neutralize any virus-sustaining effect.

GLUTAMINE: *Master protein builder, gut restorer*

Glutamine, the most abundant protein constituent in the body, may also be the most important. The secret to its significance is that it provides nitrogen more readily than any other amino acid. From treating intestinal maladies to calming addictive urges, few other substances offer as much to nutritional medicine.

To recover successfully from any of a variety of illnesses and injuries, the body needs certain proteins. No matter which are needed, all can be made with the help of L-glutamine. It possesses an extra nitrogen atom, which it readily offers for the synthesis of other amino acids. In this way it works as a kind of molecular Robin Hood that directs the distribution of our amino acid riches. In this 'nitrogen shuttle', as it's called, glutamine takes proteins from where it can be spared and delivers them to where they are most needed. In addition, it helps the body create other important nutrients, such as glutathione, glucosamine and vitamin B_3.

INTESTINAL FORTITUDE

Glutamine maintains the structural integrity of the intestines to such an extent that it has been dubbed 'intestinal permeability factor'. No other nutrient is as important for gastrointestinal health.

Every Atkins Center patient with a severe intestinal or inflammatory bowel condition gets a healthy daily dose of glutamine. Even though its primary benefit is directed to the small intestine, it rapidly facilitates healing and restores the health of mucous membranes inside the colon (large intestine). I first learned about its gastrointestinal impact from Judy Shabert, MD, RD,[1] and her husband, Douglas Wilmore, MD, a Harvard researcher investigating the value of the amino acid before and after surgery.

The nutrient's usefulness was recognized some forty years ago, when it was used in a dosage of just 1.6 grams per day, to treat peptic ulcers.[2] Much more recently, research proved that supplementation lessens stomach inflammation caused by chemotherapy[3] and can be useful in treating diarrhoea.

Surgical Recovery Following an operation or any other physically stressful event, the body can't synthesize enough glutamine to heal wounds, preserve lean tissue and nourish the immune system, among other needs. After draining its reserves, the body must then draw from muscles and the branched-chain amino acids. Providing supplemental glutamine avoids all of these complications, normalizes the amino acid levels, speeds the healing of wounds and burns and improves overall surgical recovery.[4] People whose intravenous feedings included glutamine also developed fewer complications and were discharged sooner.[5]

Immune System Assaults The immune system's primary source of energy is glutamine. While always high, the need for fuel skyrockets whenever we're subjected to stress, trauma or injury. Many forms of cancer, for instance, deplete the body of glutamine, one reason that people with the disease lose lean tissue and muscle mass. Polyps in the colon, a major precancerous lesion, have a significantly lower glutamine content than the healthy tissue around them.[6] Supplementation shields the liver from chemotherapy's toxic side effects, animal studies show, and might strengthen the cancer-killing ability of certain chemotherapeutic drugs.[7]

Viral infections also deprive the immune system of glutamine. When our reserve is low, a standard measurement of immune activity, the number of T cells declines,[8] while our toxic particle-attacking white blood cells, called macrophages, lose strength.[9] But when L-glutamine is given in dosages of 20–40 grams daily, the immune system responds, as demonstrated by the extra infection safeguard it provided in studies of patients with bone marrow transplants.[10] For all these reasons, glutamine is an essential treatment for AIDS or viral chronic fatigue syndrome.

Liver Diseases Glutamine can inhibit fatty buildups inside the liver and aid treatment of cirrhosis.[11] However, in the very late stages of liver failure, the advantage is lost, because the organ no longer can handle glutamine effectively.

Addictions Long before we knew about its involvement in tissue repair, I was using glutamine to help control cravings. I got the idea from Roger Williams, PhD, the nutritionist who inspired so many of us to pursue nutritional medicine. He used glutamine to curb the desire to drink alcohol, which it does quite well. A daily dose of 12 grams (about 3 teaspoons) did the job for 75 per cent of the people studied in one experiment.[12] Adapting the treatment to my practice, I decided to try the amino acid with my many patients who crave sweets. It worked, and it will probably work for you, too.

When a sugar urge emerges, take 1–2 grams of L-glutamine, preferably with some double cream and just a touch of nonsugar sweetener. The immediate desire to eat something sweet will pass. For a reference attesting to its efficiency, ask any of the eight thousand Atkins Center patients for whom I have prescribed it. It was quite gratifying to read not long ago that a research director at the US National Institute of Mental Health also acknowledged glutamine's influence on sugar cravings.[13]

Obesity It is possible that glutamine may help weight loss through other mechanisms. In addition to preserving lean tissue, which contributes to burning off fat, the amino acid helps cleanse the body and liver of waste products that are created by fat metabolism. It's also a readily available, carbohydrate-free energy source if you drastically cut your calorie consumption.[14]

Mental Instability Glutamine is the great natural balancer of excitement and lethargy. It's a major source of energy for the brain and an important building block for several neurotransmitters. Though some critics correctly note that the body may convert glutamine into glutamic acid, a so-called excitotoxin that overly stimulates and agitates brain cells, they fail to recognize that glutamine can also be converted to GABA, a natural brain tranquillizer that calms hyperactive cells. Nature wisely allows the body to manufacture either GABA or glutamic acid on an as-needed basis.[15]

Exercise Recovery The repair and preservation of muscle tissue makes glutamine a popular supplement among weight lifters and other dedicated athletes. Prolonged exercise causes microscopic injuries to the muscles and, for as long as two weeks after a workout, lowers the body's glutamine stores.[16] Taking supplements feeds the need for and replenishes the supply of glutamine, but that's not all. The extra nitrogen allows the body to build more lean tissue and helps fill stockpiles of glycogen, the form of carbohydrate stored in muscles and the liver for use during physical activity.[17] With enough glycogen on hand, less muscle tissue is broken down for energy. The amino acid also promotes the release of growth hormone, which can spur muscle growth.

Don't expect to look like Mr Universe, if that's your goal, simply by using supplements. And if you're taking glutamine for some other medical reason, don't worry about sprouting bulky bulges of muscle. The average person just maintains a healthy pace against the constant turnover of muscle tissue that occurs through normal metabolism. Gains are modest and hard earned, noticeable only with strenuous resistance training.

SUPPLEMENT SUGGESTIONS

Powdered L-glutamine is the easiest and most economical way to take the amino acid. A daily teaspoon, about the equivalent of 5 grams, is useful for maximizing gains from a weight-lifting programme. Treating disease demands far greater amounts, and the more severe the illness, the higher the dosage you should take.

To stimulate the immune system you'll need between 5 and 20 grams per day. Between 2 and 3 grams will suffice for counteracting a desire for alcohol or sugar. Take it as soon as the urge comes to mind. As a treatment for inflammatory bowel disease or leaky gut syndrome, I've prescribed as much as 40 grams a day. A similar amount could be required for wound healing or recovery from a prolonged hospital stay. These dosages are very safe; none of my patients have ever developed side effects.

LYSINE: *Herpes fighter*

Although best known among health food fans as a very effective herpes treatment, lysine is no single-purpose supplement. It also deserves recognition for its help in preventing osteoporosis and cataracts, preserving muscle tissue and helping us to recuperate from stress. In addition, it maintains energy levels and keeps the heart strong by providing the ingredients for the body to make the amino acid carnitine. And it may be a piece of the elusive puzzle called 'How to Control Lipoprotein(a)'.

Lysine is one of the eight essential amino acids that the body cannot manufacture on its own, but most people consume all the lysine they need. Red meats, chicken, turkey and other animal proteins provide ample amounts. Vegetarians and low-fat dieters, however, may not get enough. Milling strips grains of their lysine, leaving little in flour and other refined products. Cooking a protein food along with sugar also destroys lysine. That's one reason desserts and junk food raise the risk of a protein deficiency.[1] In the absence of even one of the essential eight amino acids, the body can't make protein efficiently enough to preserve our lean tissue.

THE BONES AND BEYOND

Until relatively recently, we weren't fully aware of lysine's contribution to bone health. Now, however, it's an established part of my osteoporosis programme. All postmenopausal women should take at least 500 mg per day, perhaps more if the diet is low in animal protein. The body needs lysine to absorb calcium and transport the mineral to the bones. A deficiency can increase the loss of calcium through urine.[2]

Cold Sores Lysine actually does not kill the herpes simplex virus, but a dosage of between 1 and 3 grams a day does hold back active symptoms, notably the blisters that emerge around the mouth or the genitals. Lysine works because it interferes with the absorption of the virus's favourite food, the amino acid arginine.[3]

Immune Strength Although the two amino acids vie for absorption, lysine and arginine become allies in the immune system. Consuming the two together, lab tests show, increases certain indications of better immune system vitality, such as the number and effectiveness of neutrophils, the most numerous of our white blood cells.[4] This provides a rationale for using lysine as part of the nutritional treatment for chronic fatigue viruses, hepatitis or HIV.

Cataracts In the eye, lysine slows the lens damage that high blood sugar inflicts. Anyone with Type I or Type II diabetes should take the amino acid for additional protection against cataracts.

Heart Disease At least one doctor-author, Mathias Rath, MD, feels that lysine may play a big role in reversing heart disease. Along with another amino acid, proline, and vitamin C, he feels it helps reverse the artery-blocking effects of lipoprotein(a).[5] Considerable reports of patient successes support his claims.

SUPPLEMENT SUGGESTIONS

A few researchers have linked a high-lysine diet to increased cholesterol, but I've never seen this occur in any of my patients.[6] In fact, dosages as high as 8 grams per day have been administered in some studies without ill effects. Nevertheless most of us do not need lysine supplements. We get quite enough from food. Supplements need to be considered only by vegetarians or anyone eating a low-protein diet, as well as by anyone attempting to combat a herpes outbreak or another lysine-responsive condition.[7]

For suppressing herpes, lysine, in a daily dose of 1–2 grams, works better if combined with a sugar-free diet and supplements of vitamin A, vitamin C, the bioflavonoids and bromelain. Taking lysine and arginine together in a daily dosage range of 1–3 grams each should provide immune support against viruses unrelated to herpes.

PHENYLALANINE: *Be happy, feel no pain*

Almost all of the amino acids convert into some important biochemical compounds that play specific roles in maintaining health. If you know what the body chemicals are and what they do, you can get a pretty good idea of what might happen upon consuming a large amount of the amino acid. Phenylalanine (PA) is the primary building block for neurotransmitters that promote alertness, a positive disposition, and, perhaps, pain relief. Therefore it is only logical that this amino acid produces these same qualities in the human body.

Depression Imipramine, one of the major antidepressant drugs, isn't as effective as PA, according to several comparative studies. In a dose of 500–3,000 mg, the amino acid, along with vitamin B_6, produced an almost immediate improvement in thirty-one out of forty depressed patients[1] The D- and DL- forms of phenylalanine were used in the studies, even though the L- form is the natural one, a fact that holds for all amino acids. The depressive states most influenced by PA are those in which there is an associated apathy and lethargy.

Several mechanisms help explain PA's effect. In addition to phenylalanine's role in making adrenaline mimickers, it provides spirit-boosting endorphins. Phenylalanine is the only substance that the body can use to make phenylethylamine (PEA), the slightly stimulating but mind-mellowing chemical in chocolate that's said to re-create the feeling of being in love. The low PEA levels in depressed subjects show that phenylalanine is not being metabolized. Both pharmaceutical antidepressants and PA will raise PEA levels, demonstrating that they accomplish the same thing.[2]

Caffeine Withdrawal You probably won't sink into the depths of depression if you try to kick the coffee habit, but you will initially feel fatigued, particularly upon awaking in the morning. Phenylalanine is a very good substitute eye-opener. Anyone who wants to enhance alertness can try it. Studies repeatedly show that it works under a variety of conditions.[3] Take 500–1,000 mg on an empty stomach, or you may divide the total dose with a matching amount of L-tyrosine, an amino acid with very similar biochemistry. In all cases, note that PA is capable of raising the blood pressure or pulse rate, so it requires a doctor's supervision.

Pain Relief A considerable amount of research backs the use of phenylalanine to alleviate arthritis aches, back pain and menstrual cramps, especially in the DL- form.[4] It slows the body's breakdown of endorphins and other natural painkillers, so their effects will last longer.[5] It also controls inflammation and may even enhance the work of analgesic medications. Daily doses of 1–3 grams work better, I have found, when combined with a diet free of foods that foster inflammatory reactions, including sugar, safflower oil, sunflower oil, corn oil and overfried foods. (This contrasts with omega-3 oils, which are anti-inflammatory.) A number of patients tell me they feel DL-phenylalanine's effect the first day they try it. The relief from dietary restrictions takes somewhat more time to notice.

Vitiligo A number of studies have concluded that L-phenylalanine can promote skin repigmentation, helping to diminish the faded blotches caused by vitiligo.[6] Phenylalanine has about the same impact against vitiligo as does L-tyrosine. Creams that contain the amino acid work rather well. To enhance the results, use the nutrient with some copper, which the body needs to produce melanin, a natural pigment.[7]

Neurological Diseases With some verification of the encouraging results exhibited in a few isolated studies, we might be able to use phenylalanine against multiple sclerosis[8] or Parkinson's disease. More than two decades ago researchers found that the amino acid significantly reduced the severity of Parkinson's symptoms like depression, speech impediments, limb rigidity and walking difficulty. The hand tremors characteristic of the disease, however, continued unabated. The participants in this experiment took 1,250 mg of the amino acid twice a day for just four weeks.[9] Problem is, I haven't seen the study replicated.

Appetite Suppression While phenylalanine is used to control the urge to eat, the results aren't consistent or predictable, ranging from significant appetite suppression to no effect. When it does work, however, it shares with diet pills their intolerable disadvantage: when you stop them, your appetite returns greater than ever.

SUPPLEMENT SUGGESTIONS

You might have received a bad impression about phenylalanine from a widely seen but little understood package label warning: 'Phenylketonurics: This product contains phenylalanine.' (So do many foods, including pork, poultry, wheat germ and cheese.) PKU, as it is abbreviated, is a problem only for those people who have the genetic defect that causes severe retardation because they cannot metabolize PA. Therefore people with this disorder should avoid the supplement and all phenylalanine-containing foods at all costs. In an interesting side note, however, some research suggests the similar amino acid tyrosine might provide some relief, implying that the retardation in PKU is actually a consequence of a tyrosine deficiency.

The vast majority of people, though, don't have PKU, and except for the aforementioned caveat about blood pressure or heart rate, and in cases of tardive dyskinesia or of skin cancer (melanoma) or a brain cancer called gliobastoma multiforme, people can take full advantage of the supplement. To overcome lethargy, depression, fatigue or pain, try taking 250–1,000 mg before mealtime. A similar dose may also help suppress appetite. If you don't notice an effect, match the nutrient with an equal amount of tyrosine before concluding that it doesn't work for you.

TYROSINE: *Antidepressant*

Mainstream medicine teaches us that the best treatment for depression comes from psychopharmacology. But for my patients it comes from a bottle of tyrosine. The amino acid works better than the majority of antidepressant drugs, costs less and helps all of us think better when we're under stress.

Our reserves of the neurotransmitters that allow us to fend off stress, such as adrenaline and noradrenaline, depend to a great degree on tyrosine. The amino acid also supplies us with a message-relaying brain chemical, L-dopa, whose deficiency is associated with Parkinson's disease.

Tyrosine and Acetyl-Tyrosine: The Happy Makers

The more tyrosine we have on hand, the better we handle stress and the better able we are to resist dips in mood. Despite what some old-time nutritionists might say, the amino acid does reach the brain once it gets into the bloodstream, although a form of it called acetyl L-tyrosine (ALT) travels there with more certainty and is the form I generally use.

I often suggest up to a gram of ALT whenever someone needs a short-term day brightener. Its impact on clinical depression, though, is a more significant contribution to nutritional medicine. The most pronounced effect is on depressive states characterized by apathy, lethargy and listlessness. For the agitated, overwrought type of depression, different amino acids, tryptophan and 5-hydroxy-tryptophan, work better. Both sets of symptoms often coexist in people who are depressed, which makes both nutrients, when taken together, valuable tools of healing.

Studies that verified tyrosine's psychological lift, even against serious cases of depression, used doses of 600–2,000 mg per day. Some people showed signs of feeling better within a week.[1] Dosages can be scaled down, to perhaps 300 mg once or twice a day, by using acetyl L-tyrosine.

In conjunction with tryptophan, tyrosine affects several other illnesses that stem from a brain chemistry imbalance, including attention deficit/hyperactivity disorder,[2] Parkinson's disease,[3] hypothyroidism and withdrawal from cocaine addiction.[4] Though doctors usually prescribe the drug L-dopa, an amino acid that the body makes from tyrosine, to help control the trembling, rigidity and other symptoms of Parkinson's disease, some research suggests that tyrosine supplementation, along with other medications, could improve the therapy.[5] A doctor must supervise the treatment, however. Very large doses of tyrosine are necessary, and they should not be administered at the same time L-dopa is taken.

Tyrosine also lends itself to the production of thyroid hormone, leading some to reason that supplements might increase the gland's low output in cases of hypothyroidism. Though this is good reasoning, it would work only for the few cases in which hypothyroidism occurs because of an actual tyrosine deficiency.

SUPPLEMENT SUGGESTIONS

One of the most prevalent concomitants of depression is fatigue. But there are millions of people who are not clinical cases of depressive illness yet experience fatigue and melancholy as everyday symptoms. For such people, 1,000–2,000 mg of ALT is a most reliable treatment. Higher doses should be given under a doctor's observation because it shares phenylalanine's warnings about increasing high blood pressure or rapid pulse, or the caveats about MAO inhibitor drugs, migraines, melanoma or gliobastoma multiforme. The amino acid does not cause these forms of cancer, but their tumours feed on it.

This caveat does not apply to everyone else, but then most of us won't need to take tyrosine unless seeking a mental boost or a lift out of depression. When you do call upon its help, remember that proper absorption depends on knowing how to take supplements. The presence of other amino acids interferes with its transport into the brain, so it's best to take tyrosine on an empty stomach, along with some vitamin B_6 and vitamin C.

GABA (GAMMA-AMINO BUTYRIC ACID):
The perfect tranquillizer

Imitation may be the sincerest form of flattery, but for pharmaceutical companies it's also an easy way to profit at the expense of a nutrient. GABA is an effective, thoroughly safe nutritional tranquillizer that some people need to control seizures or rise above depressive feelings.[1] However, the drug industry chose to invent Valium, an addictive medication that merely mimics how GABA works in the brain.

Gamma-amino butyric acid is both an amino acid and a neurotransmitter, one of the chemicals that enables the transmission of nerve impulses between cells in the brain. Few people, in theory, need to worry about taking supplements, but the reality may be different. Exposure to oestrogens, free radicals, salicylates or food additives can affect our internal supply. A low-protein diet can also hinder production, as can an insufficient amount of zinc or vitamin B_6, both of which help the body to make the nutrient.

THE GIFT OF GABA

When the brain is confronted with a lack of its most widely distributed neurotransmitter, several GABA-related disorders may develop.

Anxiety In their heyday, Valium and the other drugs in the benzodiazepene family were used by some 15 per cent of all Americans and was widely taken in the UK too. They induce the same changes in brain chemistry that nature intended GABA to perform. The only difference is that GABA isn't addictive or otherwise harmful. A natural relaxant and tranquillizer that won't knock you out, GABA is entirely safe to use during waking hours. How unlike the prescription pretenders! I prescribe GABA quite often for patients who seem nerve-racked. At the next visit almost all of them comment on their improvement.

Depression Whether as an independent emotional disorder or a comparatively minor side effect of premenstrual tension, depression seems to be associated with a low GABA level.[2] Women whose hormonal changes caused depressive feelings, one study found, had significantly lower GABA measurements compared with women whose moods were unaffected by menstrual changes.[3] Restoring the supply has helped to lift spirits.

Convulsions Especially in children, seizure disorders frequently coincide with a low GABA level. Taurine's seizure-controlling ability probably stems from its ability to raise GABA levels in the brain.[4] The anticonvulsant drug valproic acid works through the same mechanism. But GABA itself has been shown to be useful in seizure control.[5]

In other therapeutic areas, 2 grams of GABA per day have helped to improve speech and restore memory loss in people who have had a stroke. The same amount has been found to decrease high blood sugar, while a daily 3 gram dosage appeared to reduce blood pressure[6] and bolster overall heart function.[7] Further research on GABA, if there would be someone willing to fund it, promises to prove it to be one of our most useful amino acids.

SUPPLEMENT SUGGESTIONS

Independent of diet but with the assistance of a few other nutrients, the body usually manufactures all the GABA it requires. A lack of either zinc or vitamin B_6 could reduce the brain's GABA concentration enough to prompt convulsions or another neural disorder. The vast majority of us, however, will be taking zinc and B_6 supplements for other health reasons (part of the beauty of Targeted Nutrition is its ability to fill several nutrient needs simultaneously).

To take the edge off of anxiousness and irritability, a dosage anywhere between 500 mg and 4 grams a day usually works well. Beyond that amount, especially for seizure disorders or depression, see a doctor. Large doses can cause nausea and other side effects.

METHIONINE: *Antidepressant, liver helper*

When my mainstream colleagues read about a new drug that is a supposedly effective treatment for a given condition, they often await the okay to use it with the excitement of a child looking forward to birthday presents. I experience a similar enthusiasm with any word of a new, possibly groundbreaking natural substance. As this book goes to press, I'm anxiously awaiting the arrival of SAM.

SAM is s-adenosyl methionine, a metabolite of the standard amino acid L-methionine. In Italy, doctors have been administering it with good results to alleviate depression, inflammation, liver disease and, sometimes, certain muscle pains. The US Food and Drug Administration, however, has not yet authorized the import of SAM, so I cannot personally confirm its value or recommend its use. I can only report, with ever-growing anticipation, the success of its use abroad.

Like taurine, N-acetyl cysteine and glutathione, methionine contains sulfur, which is as vital to our lives as any vitamin. Without enough sulfur, our bodies would be less able to make and utilize a number of the antioxidant nutrients. Methionine is also one of the body's most important methyl donors. This means it is capable of giving off a single carbon atom with three tightly connected hydrogen atoms, a molecule we need for a diverse array of biochemical conversions throughout the body. Methionine reaches its full clinical potential, however, once the body transforms it into SAM, a much more effective methyl donor that seems to yield better clinical results.

Methionine itself remains valuable because our liver uses it to make SAM, as much as 8 grams of it every day, when conditions are ideal. We know, though, that conditions are rarely ideal. Liver disease, osteoarthritis and the overuse of prescription drugs or over-the-counter medications can diminish the body's SAM production. When that happens, supplements could prove to be of enormous value.[1]

Depression SAM's major application is probably in alleviating depression. A dose of 800–1,600 mg per day helped to elevate mood and disposition among people who were moderately clinically depressed.[2] Even major depression, once thought to be the exclusive domain of drug therapy, has responded remarkably well.[3] Methionine itself has been widely used by nutritionally oriented psychiatrists for treating depression for several decades now.

Liver Disease Supplements of both methionine and SAM can

measurably improve how well the liver functions. For women who are on oral contraceptives or oestrogen replacement therapy, the nutrients help the liver to convert the stronger, more carcinogenic oestradiol into oestriol, a safer form of the female hormone that is associated with a lesser cancer risk.[4]

A daily 1,600 mg dose of SAM has been remarkably effective against hepatitis or cirrhosis, according to the research.[5] Because of its benefit to the liver and to emotional health, the amino acid would make a good addition to a nutrient-oriented rehabilitation programme for alcoholism. It helps even in advanced cases of liver disease (in a German case report, it reversed liver failure, a dreaded complication that threatens any hospitalized patient on total intravenous feedings).[6]

Osteoarthritis While they temporarily relieve aches and pains, aspirin and other analgesics often inflict gastric side effects and contribute to the deterioration of joints. Not SAM. Its anti-inflammatory effects are well proven. In studies of more than twenty-two thousand people with osteoarthritis, it both decreased pain and encouraged joint healing. But no SAM takers complained of gastric side effects at therapeutic dosages.[7]

Brain Disorders Both methionine and SAM have demonstrated their worth in treating various neurological abnormalities. Methionine apparently enters the brain more easily, but SAM gets higher therapeutic marks. For a small group of people with Parkinson's disease, a daily 5 gram methionine dosage reduced limb rigidity and, to a lesser degree, tremors, two common symptoms of the affliction.[8] Adding some SAM to the prescription might have improved the results, because it is better at helping to make dopamine, the brain chemical that people with Parkinson's lack.[9]

Though far more investigative work is required, SAM also might offer hope to people with multiple sclerosis. One researcher noticed a low level of the nutrient in the spinal fluid of three children with MS and speculated that SAM is somehow linked to the erosion of the protective myelin sheaths around the nerves of people with the disease.[10]

Fibromyalgia SAM's anti-inflammatory influence would be appreciated by anyone who experiences these muscular pains of unclear origin. A daily 1 gram dosage worked for a sizable number of fibromyalgia sufferers in one study.[11]

Chronic Fatigue Fibromyalgia is a common complaint of people with chronic viral fatigue syndrome. A fascinating British study pointed to methionine and SAM as part of the right treatment. More than half of the twenty-one chronic fatigue sufferers were deficient in methionine, while no more than three of them lacked any other amino acid.[12] Though I've been replenishing the methionine stores of my chronic fatigue patients, I wonder whether SAM might work better. At the very least, it promises to raise the depressed spirits of many people who suffer from this often neglected and dismissed condition.

SUPPLEMENT SUGGESTIONS

Most of us don't need methionine supplements. Possible exceptions include strict vegetarians and anyone who follows a low-protein diet. People who use soya foods exclusively to meet their protein needs may also develop a methionine deficiency, because soya is low in the amino acid. For them and for anyone with a methionine-related illness, supplements could restore an important part of the body's nutritional armour. It wouldn't hurt to add taurine, cysteine and the other sulfur-containing amino acids, as well as vitamin B_6 and folic acid.

Should you want to take advantage of SAM's potential help against depression, Parkinson's disease, liver disease, arthritis and the like, use methionine until SAM becomes generally available. For these serious conditions, you may have to take 1,500–4,000 mg of L-methionine in divided doses over the course of the day. When SAM is available, the dosages will probably be half that.

GLUTATHIONE, N-ACETYL CYSTEINE (NAC):
Master antioxidants

Just about everyone knows about the antioxidants – at least the ones that mainstream medicine and food manufacturers promote. There's beta-carotene, of course, as well as vitamin C and vitamin E. You obtain them by eating fresh fruit, vegetables and all of those specially marked fortified foods. Although knowing about the trio is better than nothing, it is nevertheless important to be aware of the other nutrients that populate the antioxidant world. It certainly would be important for the medical mainstream to be aware of them.

One of the best antioxidants is an amino acid called glutathione. I'm not alone in considering it one of the most powerful cancer-curbing, age-slowing nutrients ever discovered. However, because of the way the body metabolizes and manufactures related nutrients, glutathione cannot be discussed apart from N-acetyl cysteine (NAC), a form of the amino acid cysteine. NAC raises glutathione levels in the body, something that even oral supplements of glutathione itself cannot do.

THE UPS AND DOWNS OF DISEASE RISK

The prevalence of a wide spectrum of illnesses rises and falls directly with the amount of glutathione the body holds. Name a major disease, and chances are that research has determined that a lack of glutathione is one of the causes. People with cancer, for example, usually fare far worse when their glutathione readings are low.[1] Among older people, lower levels are closely associated with greater risks of heart diseases, diabetes and arthritis. Conversely, taking NAC supplements corresponds to improvements in blood pressure, body fat and the cholesterol ratio.[2] Additionally, no other antioxidant works so dramatically to reverse blood clotting inside blood vessels.

AIDS Glutathione's apparent ability to resuscitate a frail immune system and, at least in the test tube, suppress the HIV virus has attracted the attention of researchers at Harvard, Stanford and across Europe. Since people with AIDS have extremely reduced amounts of the nutrient in their bodies, and since glutathione suppresses the HIV virus in test tube studies, a clinical trial was suggested.[3] The first such study reported that the group with extremely low T helper cell counts who were given 3–8 grams of NAC daily had double the number of two-year survivors as the untreated group. Sadly, the article reported, no companies were willing to fund further trials.[4]

Detoxification Mainstream medicine acknowledges NAC for one indication: it is the generally accepted treatment for a type of liver failure that sometimes results from acetaminophen (paracetamol) poisoning.[5] This ability to detoxify some chemicals makes it a lifesaver against certain drug overdoses and toxic metal poisoning.[6]

Heart Disease NAC is becoming an indispensable heart supplement for reasons entirely separate from glutathione. Perhaps better than any other therapy, nutritional or pharmaceutical, it eliminates the cardiovascular threat posed by lipoprotein(a), a product of cholesterol metabolism recognized only within the last few years as an independent risk factor in heart diseases. In doses of 2–4 grams a day, NAC brings lipoprotein(a) down to a less threatening level. Traditional medicine has yet to introduce a treatment for dealing with this hazard.[7]

NAC reduces hypertension by relaxing blood vessels and improving blood flow. It might also be useful in treating congestive heart failure. It works well in conjunction with the heart drug nitroglycerin; the combination opens up the blood vessels three times greater.[8] During the initial treatment of an evolving heart attack, Australian cardiologists have discovered quite recently that a dose as high as 15 grams allows more of the heart muscle to remain intact than was the case in those who were not treated.[9]

Breathing Problems NAC helps you cope with respiratory impairments in several ways. Conventional medicine uses it widely in inhalants to ward off asthma attacks.[10] It's effective against simple colds and bronchial infections, too, complementing vitamin C by working to break up mucus. In a dosage of 1.8 grams a day, NAC was shown to help people with pulmonary fibrosis.[11] And it may prove to be the treatment of choice in the often fatal adult respiratory distress syndrome (ARDS).[12]

Colitis The colon tissues of Crohn's and ulcerative colitis patients are depleted in glutathione, proportionately to the severity of the condition.[13] Glutathione restoration is an important part of Atkins Center protocols for these inflammatory bowel diseases.

Women's Hair Loss One of the consequences of our low-fat obsession is a lack of sulfur, and one of the consequences of a sulfur insufficiency, particularly for women, is hair loss. NAC is one of the best of a short list of sulfur-containing supplements, and dosages as high as 5 grams per day can stop hair from falling out. Sometimes the hair may even grow back. Eating more eggs and meat, our best food sources of sulfur, is also effective. Remember, however, that the nutrient may help only when the hair loss originates with a sulfur deficiency. Supplements won't affect male pattern baldness.

SUPPLEMENT SUGGESTIONS

Researchers aren't asking whether we should try to raise our glutathione levels. We certainly should, because most of us, especially as we age, don't have as much as we need for optimum health. The more difficult question is how best to raise the concentration of glutathione in our tissues. The nutrient is abundantly available from fresh fruit, vegetables and meats. In general, however, we don't eat enough of the right foods to make an appreciable difference. The body also manufactures it from a handful of nutritional building blocks, namely the amino acids cysteine, glycine and glutamic acid, plus selenium and vitamins B_2 and B_6.

The trick is to use all these building blocks, because consuming more glutathione may not be the answer. Scientists disagree whether or not glutathione-rich foods and glutathione supplements actually elevate the level found in blood. Some test results failed to show any impact from doses as high as 3 grams, while other research concludes that the body does absorb the antioxidant. What accounts for the difference? Success, I'm all but convinced, hinges on the method of supplementation.

It's quite possible glutathione capsules alone may be futile. The nutrient has a short shelf life and begins to lose its antioxidant ability when exposed to air. That which remains active at the time we swallow it would be broken down by the digestive system into its individual proteins before it could be absorbed intact.

In light of these facts, I favour intravenous infusions of 'reduced glutathione', the nutrient's active form. For the do-it-yourself nutritionist, however, the most practical and reliable way to obtain the antioxidant is through supplements of its building blocks. This is the formula I currently favour. Let me give an example of how I would treat an adult who is at high risk for recurrent cancer, because I consider it an absolute mandate to provide the full spectrum of antioxidant nutrition for such people.

In addition to the 'traditional' antioxidants, natural carotenoids, selenium, tocopherols and tocotrienols, vitamin C and assorted flavonoids (pycnogenol, grape seeds, bilberry and turmeric are all glutathione boosters), I try to create an optimal blood level of glutathione. Even though I do prescribe 150 mg of reduced glutathione daily, I rely on the following supportive nutrients: NAC 3,000 mg, lipoic acid 300 mg, selenium 300 mcg (worth a second mention), riboflavin 100 mg, pyridoxine 200 mg and L-glutamine 3,000 mg.

The dosage is usually divided into three equal portions and taken near meals. For those with less urgent conditions, the dosage is scaled down to one-third or one-half; in treating advancing cancer, I would be inclined to double these doses.

TAURINE: *Oedema, high blood pressure, seizure fighter*

When I first realized that many vita-nutrients, because of their extremely high benefit-to-risk ratio, really deserved to be considered by all doctors as the 'treatment of choice' for certain medical conditions, the one that immediately came to mind was L-taurine. For conditions as varied as congestive heart failure, fluid retention, high blood pressure, asthma, seizure disorders and macular degeneration, complementary doctors time and again turn to this amino acid. If the rest of the medical profession acknowledged or understood its value, taurine would consistently place as one of the top three best-selling 'drugs'.

Unlike other amino acids, taurine does not become part of our protein supply. Instead it polices our cell membranes, keeping potassium and magnesium inside the cells and keeping excess sodium out. In this way the nutrient works like a diuretic. But unlike prescription diuretics, taurine is not a cellular poison. It does not act against the kidneys. In fact, because it improves kidney diseases in experimental animals, it was proposed as a treatment for several kinds of human renal disorders.[1]

For any condition in which tissue swelling or fluid accumulation must be diminished – heart failure, liver disease and ovarian cancer, among them – taurine is the best resort. Even for those harmless instances when you get a little puffy, such as after a long plane flight or as menstruation nears, a few doses of taurine will do the job without any fear of side effects. That's more than can be said for pharmaceutical diuretics, which have been accused, in recent years, of *causing* the very tissue swelling and water retention that they purport to relieve.

The 'side effects' of taurine, in contrast, amount to even more additional benefits. Regular supplements contribute to our antioxidant defenses, reinforce the immune system, strengthen the heart muscle, stabilize heart rhythm, prevent blood clots, guard against diabetes and aid digestion.

Heart Disease Thousands of my patients with high blood pressure have taken taurine supplements over the years, and almost all of them benefit. In addition to encouraging the excretion of excess fluid, which takes pressure off our blood vessels, the amino acid dampens the sympathetic nervous system (which can constrict blood vessels), thereby relieving arterial spasms that cause blood pressure to rise.

The nutrient's impact on congestive heart failure is extraordinarily well documented. In one placebo-controlled study, 79 per cent of a group of heart patients derived some benefit from taking taurine.[2] Why does it work? Aside from the diuretic action, taurine strengthens the heart muscle and maintains the calcium balance. It plays a major role in regulating the heart's contractility,[3] and it guards against the toxic threat of drugs like doxorubicin, a medication used in chemotherapy that frequently causes heart attacks, cardiac arrest and arrhythmia.

Arrhythmia, a disturbance in the heart's regular rhythm, often coincides with a loss of both taurine and magnesium. Supplements of magnesium taurate or taurine plus magnesium play a key role in stabilizing heart rhythm. They also help prevent cholesterol from sticking to artery walls, promote the excretion of harmful blood fats and discourage blood platelets from clumping together, thereby reducing the risks of blood clots.[4]

Seizure Disorders For me, seeing is believing. What I know without doubt is that my patients with epilepsy or similar brain irritability remain free of seizures when they take taurine regularly. When they neglect to do so, the seizures return. Seizures caused by the swelling of brain tissue such as occurs with brain tumours are relieved by taurine. Certain excitotoxic chemicals, such as monosodium glutamate and aspartame, lower the body's concentration of taurine, which may be one reason why these food additives are associated with seizure activity.

Occasionally an editorial is published that disputes taurine's value as a seizure treatment. My response is the Atkins Center's consistent clinical success with taurine therapy. Patient observation is a scientific study. My patients' successful discontinuation of seizure medication is a scientific fact.

Vision Impairment The rods and cones in our retinas contain the highest concentration of polyunsaturated fats of any other cells in the body. These fats need constant antioxidant protection provided by nutrients, including taurine. A deficiency damages the retinas of both animals and people.[5]

By administering taurine intravenously, Robert Bradford, PhD, has been achieving dramatic improvements in vision for people with macular degeneration. It's proved to be one of the few substances, natural or synthetic, that can influence this virtually untreatable retinal disease.[6] Sometimes the amino acid can also be useful against another cause of blindness, retinitis pigmentosa.

Immune Weakness Intravenous infusions of taurine can also masterfully help to rebuild a suppressed immune system. The most abundant amino acid in our white blood cells, it protects these infection fighters from self-destruction as they battle invading microbes. When taurine is in short supply, white blood cells often won't fire at all, greatly weakening the immune system.

High Blood Sugar Although Type I and Type II diabetes are two distinct diseases, taurine helps stabilize blood sugar in both. For people with Type II, it improves cellular sensitivity to insulin; for people with Type I, a daily 1.5 gram dose keeps blood sugar lower over the long term and reduces abnormal platelet activity.[7] People with diabetes frequently have below normal blood levels of taurine, which might compound their susceptibility to retinopathy and heart damage.

Fat Metabolism To break down cholesterol, the body needs bile, an enzyme manufactured in the liver with taurine's help. In taurine's presence, bile remains in a liquid state and is less likely to form gallstones. The process is of notable concern to anyone whose gallbladder has been surgically removed or whose liver may not function optimally. Additionally, people with cystic fibrosis can digest fats more successfully when they take taurine supplements.[8]

Breathing Constrictions Our lungs are exposed to more free radicals than any other part of the body. Taurine plays a major role protecting these tissues. According to animal studies, taurine offers nearly complete protection from respiratory hazards such as ozone.[9] Anyone with asthma should keep taurine as a constant companion. Asthma attacks are diminished significantly when a daily 500 mg dosage is taken as a lung aerosol.[10]

SUPPLEMENT SUGGESTIONS

Because it's produced in the body (albeit in small amounts), taurine is another of the many nutrients branded by mainstream medicine as 'nonessential'. But the possibility of a deficiency exists, especially if you don't eat shellfish, the nutrient's most abundant source. The two sulfur-containing amino acids that can be turned into taurine are cysteine and methionine, found most often in egg yolks and animal meats. However, these are rare ingredients for anyone who follows the conventional low-fat diet.

Oestrogen replacement therapy blocks the manufacture of taurine, as will chemotherapy or a lack of good bacteria in the gastrointestinal tract. (Supplements of beneficial bacteria and vitamin B_6 can restore the proper balance.) In infants, taurine may be an essential nutrient; mother's milk is rich in it, but cow's milk is not. Fortunately most infant formulas now contain taurine.

Few adverse reactions are associated with taurine supplementation. However, the amino acid should not be used indiscriminately by people with ulcers because it can increase the secretion of stomach acids. Everyone else should easily tolerate between 1 and 3 grams every day. In some people, doses of 5 grams or higher may occasionally loosen stools. For treating seizure disorder, oedema, high blood pressure or the like, the therapeutic range is 1.5–4 grams daily, in divided doses.

VALINE, LEUCINE, ISOLEUCINE (BRANCHED-CHAIN AMINO ACIDS): *Muscle fuel*

Meat, eggs, fish and the other protein foods offer us about twenty different amino acids, yet just three of them constitute almost half of our entire daily protein consumption. In this case the ratio isn't nutritionally unbalanced. The trio's preponderance points to the importance of all three.

Valine, leucine and isoleucine are the muscle-sparing amino acids. Also known as the branched-chain amino acids (BCAA), they preserve our muscles and all other tissue except bones and fat from the constant breakdown that occurs as a natural part of metabolism. Normally the body regenerates these tissues, using amino acids as the building blocks of new protein. But the breakdown often outpaces the repair, such as when we don't eat enough protein, when we exercise excessively, when we're under stress, or when we're sick. The process is especially accelerated when the individual is afflicted with cancer, end-stage kidney failure, AIDS or another so-called wasting disease. BCAA, along with glutamine and medium-chain triglycerides, is considered by progressive surgeons to be important intravenous support for critically ill patients.[1]

All of us stand to benefit from taking branched-chain supplements. For instance, after a group of average, healthy people received a single intravenous infusion of the amino acids, the amount of tissue breakdown that normally occurs overnight decreased by 50 per cent.[2] A daily dosage of 7.5–12 grams per day spared muscles completely for a group of marathoners and cross-country runners.

SUPPLEMENT SUGGESTIONS

Don't worry about any side effects from keeping more lean tissue than you metabolize. You won't suddenly possess greater muscle mass, although bodybuilders and weight lifters use branched-chain supplements for this very reason. For the best therapeutic effect, the three nutrients should be taken together, along with L-glutamine, another essential amino acid. Good therapeutic dosages are 4–5 grams of valine, 3–4 grams of leucine, 2–3 grams of isoleucine and 4–6 grams of L-glutamine.

HISTIDINE: *Arthritis aid*

The next time you pop a cold capsule or spritz an allergy medication up a nostril, think of histidine. In essence you'll be counteracting the histamines that this amino acid allows the body to make.

Although the nutrient is considered essential for infants, the rest of us generally need not worry about how much we consume. The body gets all that it requires to synthesize histamines. Only on a few occasions do we need to raise blood pressure, constrict the lungs' bronchial muscles or induce any other effect commonly associated with these allergy-exacerbating substances.

Nothing to Sneeze At?

On the other hand, histidine appears to be linked in some way to rheumatoid arthritis. In a 1969 experiment, daily supplements of 1–5 grams quite demonstrably improved joint flexibility and grip strength for people with inflammatory joint disease.[1] At the time, the study piqued my curiosity, and some years later I asked a writing colleague of mine to contact the author for an update on his work. What my colleague learned spoke volumes about the relationship between the pharmaceutical industry and the direction of medical research. Essentially the doctor was told that his sponsoring medical institution preferred that his research go in another direction.

In the years since, only a few studies have investigated histidine's effect on arthritis. The amino acid may work by regulating the immune system in a way that reduces inflammation; it also might interfere with oxidation[2] and lower any accumulation of toxic heavy metals. More lab and clinical work needs to be done before we can know histidine's full therapeutic reach. Some practitioners have suggested that by releasing histamines, supplements of the amino acid might encourage enough extra blood flow to improve libido and facilitate orgasm.[3] Again, though, clinical experiences and research offer nothing conclusive.

Supplement Suggestions

Food generally satisfies the body's minimal requirement for histidine. In the absence of allergies, though, people with rheumatoid arthritis might want to see if the amino acid has any effect on joint pain. I would not, however, experiment without some guidance from a nutritionally oriented doctor. Besides aggravating allergies, supplements might increase blood pressure.

TRYPTOPHAN: *The best sleeping pill not on the market*

Tryptophan was nutrition's superstar, the dietary David that single-handedly took on the lucrative Goliath-like market of sedatives, tranquillizers and antidepressants. More and more doctors felt it was a hands-down winner. It relieved depression, induced sleep and soothed anxieties with the best of them.

But to the pharmaceutical industry, this marvellously effective, remarkably safe and freely available nutrient threatened to be a billion-dollar pain in the balance sheet. Industry moguls must have privately wished for tryptophan to be discredited. So, after an improbable event, it was: scandalized, tried, convicted and banished by the very people entrusted to police – not to enrich – the pharmaceutical business.

DANGERS: REAL AND CONTRIVED

Investigators first traced the illnesses to the use of tryptophan supplements, then to a single contaminated batch of the supplement made by one Japanese company that had inexplicably changed their manufacturing procedure. In November of that year the American FDA recalled tryptophan from all over-the-counter shelves. Since then the agency has refused to lift the ban, even though several additional probes of EMS outbreaks in both the United States and Germany later reaffirmed that all of the illnesses and deaths stemmed from that one contaminated batch. Tryptophan itself poses no inherent danger, the research concluded,[1] and its prior and subsequent use by tens of millions of people for decades has harmed no one.[2]

Prohibiting the use of trytophan, in fact, presents a more dangerous scenario for people who take pure crystalline amino acid formulas. These forms upset the body's amino acid balance by forcing a drop in blood levels of tryptophan, which can exacerbate symptoms of premenstrual tension in women.[3] In men, according to another study, the imbalance created by taking tryptophan-free supplements increased anger, annoyance and other indicators of aggression and hostility by as much as 30 per cent.[4]

THE SEROTONIN BUILDING BLOCK

The key to tryptophan's success is its ability to influence brain chemistry. In our bodies' own chemical factory, it is the biochemical that is converted directly into serotonin, a neurotransmitter that relaxes the mind and instills a sense of emotional well-being. The same qualities account for its therapeutic effect on depression. People who are depressed have low blood levels of both serotonin and tryptophan. Prozac, Zoloft, and other members of this family of mood-elevating drugs work by extending the life of serotonin (whatever little of it there may be) in the brain. Tryptophan attacks depression more safely, allowing the body to increase its production of serotonin in the brain.

Tryptophan is also useful against other emotional disorders, such as premenstrual anxiety and depression[5] and seasonal affective disorder.[6] It also could play a role in treating eating disorders,[7] alcohol addiction,[8] Down's syndrome, aggressive behaviour,[9] attention deficit/hyperactivity syndrome, schizophrenia,[10] sleep paralysis and pain syndrome. I find it useful in obsessive-compulsive disorder, and it is perhaps the treatment of choice in Tourette's syndrome.

Tryptophan may have other uses. It and its 5-hydroxy variant have been helpful in fibromyalgia and chronic fatigue syndrome.[11]

SUPPLEMENT SUGGESTIONS

There are abundant sources of tryptophan in all meats, especially pork, duck and wild game. However, supplements are far more effective than food. A 2 gram dose taken right before bed will safely and effectively overcome insomnia.[12]

I remain ever optimistic that the over-the-counter prohibition will be lifted. Until it does, find an alternatively oriented doctor who prescribes it, or present your own doctor with the exonerating evidence (compounding pharmacies will fill a doctor's prescription). People with asthma should probably avoid it, because any serotonin precursor could make their breathing worse, and high doses may lead to a noticeable sense of fatigue following exercise.[13] Otherwise it's entirely safe.

Two prescription types are available – L-tryptophan, the natural amino acid, and 5-hydroxy-tryptophan, which is the immediate biochemical precursor of serotonin. I generally prescribe 2–4 grams of L-tryptophan daily, more in severe cases. For the 5-hydroxy version, only a 300–400 mg dose is needed. For either kind, take most of the daily dosage before going to bed, but if daytime anxiety or depression is the problem, it should be taken throughout the day. Always take it before meals, because to be effective the trytophan or 5-hydroxy must be connected with an amino acid transport system that delivers it to the brain, and the protein in your food will compete with it. Accompany the amino acid with some niacinamide to extend its action. We need tryptophan to manufacture our own niacinamide, and supplements of the B-complex nutrient spare tryptophan for other important tasks, like keeping you happy and relaxed.

CARNITINE: *The fat burner*

Do you want to know which vita-nutrient I personally take in greatest quantity every day? It's carnitine. For a substance that is supposedly nonessential, carnitine is as necessary a nutrient as you'll ever find. While it's quite true that our bodies make this amino acid, rarely do we have enough to keep us at our healthiest.

The heart is completely dependent upon carnitine; two-thirds of its energy supply comes from the fats that carnitine allows the body to burn. The release of fat for use as fuel also makes this nutrient an important adjunct to any weight-loss or exercise efforts. That's why I never forget my carnitine.

Heart Disease After a heart attack, several complications are likely, including chest pains (angina), heart rhythm disturbances and heart failure. Taking 2 grams of carnitine per day for four weeks, hospital-based studies show, can cut the number of those complications in half.[1] That's a better performance than standard drug therapy.

Cardiomyopathy, a disease of the heart muscle, becomes a distinct possibility without carnitine. The amino acid protects the heart muscle from damage when a heart attack or a spasm cuts off the oxygen supply.[2] It also helps correct that most devastating of blood lipid profiles, the combination of high triglycerides and low HDL cholesterol. An irregular heart rhythm will also quickly deplete carnitine stores in the body, creating a deficiency precisely when an optimal amount is most needed. Congestive heart failure flaws our ability to make carnitine, too.[3] However, taking 900 mg per day improved the health of one group of congestive heart failure patients, significantly increasing both their energy and their ability to exercise.[4]

Energy and Endurance Anyone who uses carnitine will get an energy boost from the amino acid, which also helps convert body fat into readily available fuel and elevates levels of certain enzymes needed to metabolize sugars, starches and other carbohydrates. Whether you're a casual exerciser or a more dedicated athlete, compensating for the greater amount of carnitine lost through physical activity extends your stamina and reduces the accumulation of lactic acid, the by-product of heavy-duty exertion that's responsible for the 'burn' felt inside the muscles.[5] This may enable exercisers to get the 'gain' without the 'pain', as one study confirmed.[6] Carnitine also clears the bloodstream of ammonia and aids in creating glycogen, the form in which the body stores glucose. Even marathon athletes can improve their stamina. A daily intake of 2 grams of taurine increased their treadmill performance by nearly 6 per cent,[7] enough to turn an 'also ran' into a gold medalist.

Muscle Loss Anyone with a severe degenerative disease, such as cancer or AIDS, stands to gain from carnitine supplementation. It's a key nutrient for helping to prevent muscle atrophy.[8] The AIDS drug AZT depletes carnitine, as does Valproate, an antiepileptic drug. Such drug-induced carnitine deficiency can be life-threatening.

Infant Health Although considered 'nonessential' for adults, carnitine is officially classified as indispensable for infants. So critical is this early need that researchers once proposed naming the amino acid 'vitamin Bb'.[9] Babies usually get carnitine through breast milk or fortified formulas – but not always. Most infant formulas contain carnitine, but it's best to check the label. Breast-feeding mothers who follow a vegetarian diet almost certainly need to take supplements. Carnitine may also be a very important nutrient for protecting children against Reyes syndrome.[10]

Other Conditions People with low thyroid function need carnitine to help them overcome diminished energy levels and the tendency to gain weight.[11] Kidney dialysis rinses away stockpiles of the amino acid, another reason people who undergo the procedure are often weak, tired and threatened by high triglycerides. Other published studies suggest that carnitine may be of some value in treating diabetes, hypertension, liver disease and immune problems.[12] It may also protect the liver from alcohol and other challenges.

One reason Atkins Center doctors prescribe carnitine so frequently is that it seems, in our experience, to be the nutrient most likely to overcome that bane of many dieters' existence – metabolic resistance to weight loss. For fat to be used up as fuel, carnitine is essential.

SUPPLEMENT SUGGESTIONS

Most of us consume about 30–50 mg of carnitine a day, hardly an optimum amount. While beef is the largest, best source (with chicken, fish, eggs and milk containing smaller amounts), we can't rely simply on eating more red meat. High-protein, high-fat meals stimulate carnitine excretion. High-carbohydrate eating is even more futile, because grains and vegetables contain negligible amounts.

To make up for the carnitine gap, a supplement of between 500 mg and 1 gram is the minimum amount we need to take for preventive purposes. For a heart problem, I normally recommend 1–2 grams daily. If you are on heart drugs, you may need less medication, which calls for the supervision of a nutritionally aware cardiologist. People who get stuck on truly effective diets, such as the Atkins diet, may need 1,500–2,500 mg to break the log jam. To support the body's own synthesis, make sure you take additional amounts of vitamin C, lysine, methionine, iron, vitamin B_3 and vitamin B_6.

ACETYL L-CARNITINE: *Brain energizer*

Suppose we had a simple treatment for slowing the downhill progression of Alzheimer's disease or for speeding up the often lengthy recovery process after a stroke. Happily, we don't need to suppose; we have it available in health food stores.

Acetyl L-carnitine (ALC) is a sort of 'supercarnitine', in many ways still similar to the original amino acid, but in other ways far different. Better absorbed and probably more active than plain carnitine, it can refresh mental energy, improve mood, slow the aging of brain cells and impede the advance of Alzheimer's. By energizing and balancing the central nervous system as a whole, it also strengthens our defences against infections and immune problems.

NEURAL NECESSITY

Supplementation will compensate for the natural decline of ALC production that starts around the age of forty and continues as we grow older. It's a significant loss, because ALC contributes to our stores of some of our most valuable nutrients, including glutathione, coenzyme Q_{10} and acetylcholine. Melatonin also depends on it. Restoring the optimal amount improves health against a variety of neurological and immune-related afflictions.

Stroke Supplements of ALC can accelerate recovery from stroke, according to researchers who gave daily dosages of 1,500 mg over a nine-month period to a group of people who, because of a stroke, had lost the use of one side of their bodies.[1]

Alzheimer's Disease The modern-day equivalent of the Holy Grail could easily be an effective treatment for this terrible memory-robbing condition. ALC is the first compound, drug or nutrient, that has both improved the symptoms of Alzheimer's and reversed the imbalances in brain chemistry that coexist with it.[2] People who took 3 grams of ALC per day for a year, to cite one study, displayed far less mental deterioration than did a similar number of people who did not take the supplement.[3] ALC has performed well in controlled studies involving more than six hundred people afflicted with the disease, and at least one large study showed it to be effective in non-Alzheimer's mental decline in elderly people.[4]

For many of my patients with senile dementia, ALC seems to slow the disease process significantly. Colleagues have also reported that some of their patients have regained some memory ability and kept themselves better grounded in reality. Though ALC is not a 'cure', it often does temporarily reverse the downhill course of the disease, especially when combined with high doses of vitamin C and vitamin E.

If ALC helps to fight Alzheimer's, what about Parkinson's disease? Primate studies from this field of research are showing promising results thus far.[5]

Immune Disturbances Results are preliminary, but ALC could contribute to strengthening the immune system or shielding it from viral attacks. People with chronic fatigue syndrome, whose immune systems have clearly broken down, have lower than expected levels of ALC. Replenishing the supply alleviates symptoms, such as fatigue and brain fog.[6]

Establishing an optimal physiological amount of ALC stimulates the overall activity of immune cells in both younger and older adults. A dosage of 2 grams a day for thirty days, according to one study, improved immune function in people with active pulmonary tuberculosis.[7]

SUPPLEMENT SUGGESTIONS

Vigorous exercise will aid the body's natural conversion of carnitine into ALC, but taking carnitine supplements is not an effective substitute. Only ALC increases the brain's energy and protects nerve cells from the harm inflicted by stress and free radicals. For anyone older than forty, in fact, ALC is clearly the preferred form of carnitine. A generally healthy person who wants to improve mental and physical performance should take about 500–1,000 mg of both carnitine and ALC. To reinforce the immune system, an amount in the 1,500–3,000 mg range is necessary. Because ALC invigorates the brain, don't take it in the evening; it may interfere with sleep. People with epilepsy should use it with extreme caution, because their brains already are overly sensitive to neural stimulation.

I take both ALC and carnitine every day, as do hundreds of my patients. In the optimal dosages, I noticed a subtle metabolic effect: my energy level is steadier, and I have more stamina. I also get greater weight-loss rewards from my dietary efforts, and I make fewer trips to the fridge. On my one hundredth birthday, I'll be happy to let you know whether it retards aging.

CHAPTER 6

◦

FATTY ACIDS

ESSENTIAL FATS: *Our greatest deficiency*

Sit down in your most comfortable reading chair and get ready for what may be this book's most significant message: *Many diseases are caused by deficiencies of certain fats, and many of the same diseases can be overcome by supplying the essential fats missing from most people's diets.*

Our fear of fat is reinforced with an unchallenged fanaticism by our mass media, our advertising, our medical authorities and undercritical medical reporters. Worst of all, there is no differentiation between the truly dangerous fats – the trans-fats in margarine and overfried foods, for example – and the wonderful, healing fats found in flaxseed oil and salmon and sardines. These fats have about as much in common as Charles Manson and Mother Teresa, respectively, yet our fat-phobic media tells you both are equally dangerous. In so doing, it prevents us from understanding how to obtain optimal health.

Such ignorance has propelled us from the frying pan right into the fire. Our low-fat nations have never been more overweight, and we're falling prey to the very diseases that the low-fat, high-carbohydrate liturgy preaches we can deter. In the search for answers, we've looked everywhere except the most logical place – our scientific community. These researchers have amassed a rock solid body of evidence that shows we are not just eating too much fat; we're eating the wrong kind and missing the right kind. And we're not getting enough of the vitamins and minerals needed to enhance their beneficial effects.

Relearning the ABCs: Fats as Vita-Nutrients

Apparently, everyone seems to know that there are just three kinds of fat – saturated, derived from dairy products and red meat, and is supposedly bad; unsaturated, derived from vegetables and vegetable oils, and is good; and monounsaturated, derived from fish or olives, and is best. Except that is not the way it really is, and in fact, there is a much more useful way to classify fats.

First of all, most fats are not essential. We can dispense with many of them, because they are either harmful or, to give a nod to our fat-obsessed culture, a source of unneeded excess calories. Two fatty acids, though, have been deemed essential. They're like vitamins in that they cannot be made by the body, and a lack of either one of them will cause disease. But in the insanity of our pathological fat phobia, we're throwing the baby out with the bathwater, creating fatty acid deficiencies that are in part responsible for epidemic levels of cancer, heart disease, inflammatory ailments and a host of other degenerative illnesses. What is becoming inescapably clear is that the essential fatty acids are collectively the number one missing nutrient in many Western diets. By the end of this chapter, you will understand why I prescribe or recommend supplements of these essential substances to every patient.

Meet the Omegas

Although we need fat for a number of reasons (it is our primary source of reserve energy fuel, it's part of every cell membrane in the body and it also cushions our organs), the essential fatty acids are indispensable because they provide the building blocks for the body's numerous eicosanoids. These hormonelike chemicals, many of which are also called prostaglandins, have an enormous influence on health. Eicosanoids are the power brokers of the body. They can lower blood pressure, raise body temperature, open or constrict bronchial passages, stimulate hormone production and sensitize nerve fibres. And that's just for starters. They are so dependent on dietary fat that we can directly attribute the specific activity of a particular eicosanoid to the class of fats from which it is derived.

Therefore it follows that we have the power to greatly enhance our health by picking fats that in turn create beneficial eicosanoids. Dividing them in this manner gives us the three fat families: the omega-3s, the omega-6s and the omega-9s. Fats in the first two classes contain the strongest power to generate eicosanoids; omega-9s are weaker and not labelled as essential but are helpful nevertheless. The real secret to good health is keeping a dietary balance between the two major classes, the omega-3s and the omega-6s, so that the body's eicosanoids are balanced. Think of the brake and accelerator pedals in a car: we need both to drive. Having just one or the other would create serious problems.

So it is with fats. What kind, therefore, is more important than how much we eat. Our biggest problem is that during the course of the twentieth century, we have eaten too many omega-6 fats – safflower, sunflower and corn oil – and have virtually eliminated foods high in the omega-3s, such as flaxseed oil and cold-water fish. Reclaiming our health means striving to tip the balance towards these omega-3s. Before examining the essential fats in all their medicinal detail, let's look at the general health purposes of the three classes and their best food sources.

THE WONDERFUL OMEGA-3S

Cancer, rheumatoid arthritis and other inflammatory conditions, arterial plaque, blood clots, immune system weakness – it's no coincidence that some of our most prevalent diseases also are some of the most serious health problems associated with a lack of omega-3 fats. Omega-3s are both America's and Great Britain's principal essential fatty acid deficiency, and it's not too difficult to understand why. Most of the best dietary sources – fish and fish oils, flaxseed oil, rapeseed oil, chia seeds, soyabean oil, walnut oil, eggs from flaxmeal-fed hens and wild game –

are either rarely consumed, improperly prepared, or ridiculously branded as unhealthy.

Three specific essential fatty acids are found in omega-3 fats and oils. They are alpha-linolenic acid, eicosapentaenoic acid (EPA), and docosahexaenoic acid (DHA). Flaxseed oil is a very good supplement source of alpha-linolenic acid. To a lesser extent, so are rapeseed oil and walnut oil. For EPA and DHA, nothing beats cold-water fish and fish oil supplements.

Omega-6s: Don't Get Too Much of a Good Thing

The other essential fatty acids come from this class – linoleic acid and superhealing version gamma-linolenic acid. Linoleic is found in safflower, sunflower and corn oils. GLA is found in supplements of evening primrose oil and borage oil and is a tremendous asset when faced with arthritis, diabetes, skin disorders and multiple sclerosis. However, don't go overboard on the ordinary omega-6s. This is especially important, since corn oil and its cohorts are already widely consumed. This can give rise to an excess of certain inflammatory eicosanoids that can, among other undesirable things, constrict blood vessels, narrow bronchial passages and raise blood pressure. Overconsumption of these oils correlates strongly with depressed immune function, cancer and inflammatory diseases such as asthma and arthritis.

Don't rush to a hasty judgment about these fats and oils. It's important to understand that they are not inherently hazardous. You should not conclude that 'omega-3s are good' and 'omega-6s are bad'. This is the kind of oversimplification that helped to get us in the trouble we're now in with cholesterol. (Remember: dietary cholesterol is harmless.) Both omega-3 and omega-6 fats are in our bodies for a reason: to create a balance, a sort of yin and yang. Sometimes bronchial constriction or tissue inflammation is necessary; more often we're better served by a reduction in inflammation or a relaxation of our hearts' arteries. My nutritional health strategy tips the balance towards omega-3s mainly because we eat so little. (To be sure, in practice, a fatty acid profile that overdoes omega-3s is difficult to achieve, and the people who come closest, the Eskimos, display surprisingly good cardiovascular health.)

Omega-9 Fatty Acids The omega-9s may be the most recognizable subgroup, because they are, in fact, the monounsaturated fats and are found in olives, almonds, macadamias, hazelnuts, peanuts, sesame seeds and avocados. The pressed oils from these foods are especially rich in omega-9 fat, which is excellent for cooking. The omega-9s, with olive oil a featured performer, explain the famed Mediterranean diet's all-around superiority. It is a very stable fat that helps keep cholesterol from sticking to artery walls. Diets high in these fats have been repeatedly shown to be far more protective than the high-carbohydrate, ultra-low-fat diet currently being touted as best for everyone.

For all of their healthful attributes, though, omega-9-rich foods are actually quite low in essential fatty acids. Omega-9s are not essential, for the body can make them. Indeed, their health benefits pale in comparison with the therapeutic power of omega-3s and omega-6s. In a diet well fortified in these incredible essential fats, the omega-9s are just part of the support staff. If monounsaturate-based eating can outdo the low-fat diet in health benefits, it should come as no breach of logic that a diet rich in essential fatty acids would provide even greater health returns.

THE BAD AND THE UGLY

An omega imbalance isn't the only way in which dietary fat can endanger us. Often the problem is in the way fats and oils are made or used. Without margarine and the hydrogenated oils in vegetable shortening, to give one stark example, Americans and Britons could cut their heart attack risk in half. Margarine is but one example of nutritional errors that contribute to the harmful consequences of our intake of fat.

Processing and Packaging In refined vegetable oils, which generally are any of the brands at a supermarket, the essential fatty acids have often been destroyed or damaged by harsh chemical processes. In addition, the vitamin E and carotenoid content is almost always removed. Further, the oils' glass or plastic containers are usually clear, which exposes the product to light damage that further deteriorates the oil. Even worse, they are rarely organic. You'll do better by buying oils at health food stores, where the products are much more likely to have been prepared more responsibly and naturally.

Heat Fats Minimally

High heat initiates a variety of distinct molecular changes in food and creates disease-promoting elements like free radicals and lipid peroxides. Deep-frying, no matter what oil is used, turns a fat into a health threat. Stir-fried foods are better, as long as you avoid soya and other delicate oils that burn easily. Oils from peanuts and coconut are more stable and can better handle the higher heat used in stir-frying.

Not Margarine – Please!

I haven't knowingly eaten anything that contains margarine since the 1970s, when Dr Carlton Fredericks first warned me of the threat it presents. Margarine is a primary cause of atherosclerosis and heart disease – not butter, as the American Heart Association would have you believe. Dr Fredericks, Adelle Davis, and other progressive nutritionists tried to alert the public back in the 1940s, but their words were ignored. After animal experiments in the 1970s demonstrated that margarine can cause hardening of the arteries, the scientific community picked up the scent. The truth eventually came with all the authority of the most comprehensive health survey in medicine, the Harvard Nurses Study of 85,095 women.[1] Margarine, because of its trans-fatty acids, correlated with the risk of heart disease more strongly than any other food – including butter, beef, pork and lamb. Eating other foods high in partially hydrogenated vegetable oil such as vegetable shortening, biscuits, cakes and chips also was significantly linked to a higher risk of heart disease.

Keeping Their Heads in the Sand

Since then the evidence has mounted into a near overkill, with countless studies showing that the trans-fatty acids in margarine and vegetable shortening increase LDL cholesterol, lower the beneficial HDL cholesterol[2] and raise the overall risk of coronary artery disease[3]. Medical journals now almost routinely warn doctors of the danger in margarine consumption[4], but nutritional policy makers are still reluctant to warn the general public. It is still the only fat recommended in diets created by the US National Cholesterol Education Program (NCEP). Most people still innocently believe they are being virtuous by using margarine. And many of them still innocently fall victim to hardening of the arteries, heart attack and premature death. Why do consensus panels engage in such a denial of the evidence? Compare the US response to that in Europe, where most countries have enacted stiff laws to limit the amount of trans-fatty acids in food. Many of the margarines sold in the United States are illegal in Europe.

Another way that fats can be processed to sabotage your health is through hydrogenation. This is another process that makes margarine worse than butter, but margarine is not the only example of a hydrogenated fat. Far from it: partially hydrogenated fats (because of their physical properties of providing long shelf life, which cannot be duplicated with natural substances) are ubiquitous in our diet. Cereals, breads, prepackaged mixes, heat-and-serve meals, crackers, biscuits, shortening and almost all vegetable oils are partially hydrogenated to some degree. Many products sold in health food stores contain hydrogenated fats.

If you cannot avoid them, make sure they are not near the top of the list of ingredients (the ingredients list is arranged in order of decreasing quantity within the 'recipe'). These hydrogenated fats worsen the lipid profile (HDL and LDL) and interfere with omega-3 and omega-6 metabolism[5], and they do so in proportion to the amount consumed.

HOW SUGAR BECOMES A BAD FAT

This is as good a place as any to plug my favourite dictum: avoid sugar. It, like any other carbohydrate or starch, will create bad fats when consumed beyond what the body needs. Sugar is broken down into small molecules and is reassembled as fats.

These fats are called triglycerides. These are the fats that fill our fat cells, impair blood flow inside blood vessels and raise the risk of coronary artery narrowing. Sugar also raises insulin. When too much insulin is circulating in the bloodstream, our triglycerides jump astronomically and our cholesterol ratios also worsen, with HDL falling and LDL rising.

As will be evident, the triglyceride-LDL cycle is of profound importance. You cannot escape this bad fat trap merely by not eating bad fats. You have to avoid sugar and limit carbohydrates as well. Remember, the prime steak that frightens fat-phobic folk was created by feeding a steer all the grains it wanted.

THE OMEGA-3S: *The very good fats*

If doctors truly believe in 'evidence-based medicine', they obligate themselves to put into practice what scientific evidence has determined to be beneficial. As a descriptive word, 'beneficial' doesn't do justice to the incredible therapeutic action of omega-3 oils. Our two supplemental sources are fish oils and flaxseed oil. Although both are high in omega-3 fatty acids, they often can't be used interchangeably, so it's best for us to consider them separately. Let's start with fish oils, which I consider the most important nutritional prescription we have for preventing heart disease.

Nothing Fishy About It

Because of a diet that consists almost exclusively of seal meat and blubber, the Eskimo people of Greenland are 'probably the most exquisitely carnivorous people on Earth', according to no less an authority than physiologist August Krogh, MD, who won a Nobel Prize for his work on preventing heart disease. At the same time, Eskimos have one of the lowest rates of heart disease in the world. Their LDL cholesterol is low, and their HDL readings are high.[1] One very likely reason is that they eat no refined sugars or carbohydrates. The other reason, also supported by scientific evidence: their diet is high in fish fat and fish oil, both rich sources of two essential fatty acids – EPA (eicosapentaenoic acid) and DHA (docosahexaenoic acid).[2]

Since the early surveys of the Greenlanders, countless scientific efforts, including a Dutch study conducted for twenty years, have shown that by increasing our consumption of cold-water fish and fish oils, we can dramatically reduce the risk of heart disease.[3] Another major study calculated a 50 per cent reduction in fatal heart attacks for people who consume more salmon and other cold-water fish.[4] Supplements are similarly effective, according to a group of scientists who compared fish and fish oil supplements. The overall reduction in mortality for the fish oil group was extraordinary. The number of total deaths dropped by 29 per cent. The results were so amazing that the study was stopped so that the good news could be spread.[5]

If you are a heart patient, I must ask you this: Why hasn't your doctor prescribed fish oil to you? Perhaps you should demand that your cardiologist read two recent review articles, one coauthored by Jorn Dyerberg, MD, the Danish researcher who broke the Greenland Eskimo story a generation ago. The articles' bibliographies provide all the medical justification any doctor could ever need.[6]

HOW FISH OILS WORK

How do these fish oils do it? In a variety of ways. EPA and DHA help keep blood platelets from clumping, thereby preventing the formation of clots that could cause a heart attack.[7] Their effect on platelets makes them the number one alternative therapy to warfarin (Coumadin) anticoagulation and provides a far safer (although less well documented) option than the extremely toxic drugs in general use. Even in high concentration there is no increase in abnormal bleeding.[8] EPA and GLA also lower blood pressure and appear to protect arteries from a buildup of plaque.[9] In short, they do many of the things that prescription heart drugs do, and without any of the side effects so commonly caused by pharmaceuticals, particularly the lipid-lowering medications.[10] For these reasons, fish oil, with its two omega-3 fats, stands as the single most important nutrient for the prevention of heart disease.

Keeping the Blood Fats Low

Much of the latest research is finally corroborating what the more perceptive heart scientists have known for years: elevated triglycerides are more strongly associated with heart disease than is elevated cholesterol. Even a triglyceride reading of 100 mg/ml, once thought to be 'normal', now is associated with twice the heart risk of a lower reading. Fish oils very reliably lower the triglyceride threat. Success has been achieved with daily doses of as little as 1 gram each of EPA and DHA.[11] At last count, more than seventy studies documented that omega-3 oils can be counted on to lower triglycerides by an average of 25–35 per cent.[12] Combine EPA and DHA with a sharp curtailment of carbohydrates and you can expect your triglycerides to plunge 75 per cent.

Arrhythmia Heart doctors should also use fish oils for what may be their most lifesaving mechanism – the prevention of an irregular heartbeat.[13] A number of my cardiac patients have come to me after their own doctors have unsuccessfully attempted to control their arrhythmias. A regular rhythm is reestablished in a majority of them with fish oil supplements[14], and they work especially well combined with magnesium, potassium, taurine and a sugar-free diet.

Coronary Large doses – up to 10 grams per day – have lowered the number of angina attacks by 41 per cent. Exercise tolerance also increases. And this dose cuts the risk of sudden cardiac death in half.[15]

Blood Pressure Fish oil's ability to lower blood pressure is well documented, even at a dose of just 2 grams per day.[16] Early studies yielded inconsistent results, but more recent experiments, using 4 grams of EPA and DHA daily, have been quite successful.[17] Although EPA and DHA alone may not reduce hypertension sufficiently, they nevertheless support our better nutritional treatments. Magnesium, potassium, CoQ_{10} and taurine, taken within the overall context of a sugarless diet, will regulate blood pressure and avoid the need for drugs more than 80 per cent of the time.

Diabetes Triglycerides pose a greater than normal cardiovascular danger to people with diabetes, making fish oil a particularly valuable treatment. Still, there are those who question its role in diabetic therapy since some studies show that EPA may raise blood glucose.[18] Others have found no impact at all[19], while yet others indicate that the disease may interfere with how EPA is metabolized.[20]

It is my considered judgment that fish oil's overall benefit far outweighs any modestly elevating effect it may have on blood sugar. The more recent research tends to agree that fish oils consistently diminish the triglyceride threat faced by most diabetics.[21] In addition, fish oil maintains arterial flexibility, important for preventing the plaque buildup that leads to hardening of the arteries. Finally, in an area outside of heart disease, fish oil supplements can cut in half the pathological finding of protein in the urine of people with diabetic kidney disease.[22]

Best of all, EPA's edge need not come at the risk of higher glucose. A mere 500 IU supplement of vitamin E, research demonstrates, can prevent most EPA-produced elevations of blood sugar.[23] Vitamin E and fish oils should, in any event, be used together. They have the synergistic effect of helping to magnify insulin's effectiveness and increase the fluidity of the body's cell membranes – both vital for the health of diabetics.

Cancer Cultures known to have consumed significant amounts of EPA and DHA have had low levels of cancer – at least they did until 'civilized' man arrived with sugar, white flour and refined omega-6 oils. Until the introduction of these refined foods, cancer was rare among the Greenland Eskimos. Diabetes, tooth decay and a whole range of other ailments were also not known before they were given junk food.[24]

Omega-3 oils have a particularly inhibitory effect on cancers of the breast[25] and colon[26]. Women who eat fish high in EPA, for example, have a significantly lower rate of breast cancer. Additionally, women who have been diagnosed with a tumour typically display a smaller concentration of omega-3 fats in their breast tissue than do their healthy peers.[27]

While many people speculate that a high-fat diet may increase the risk of colon cancer, such an association simply does not exist when the fats are EPA and DHA. For example, among people who took omega-3 supplements, one study found a decline in premalignant changes in the mucus lining of the colon, a sign of decreased cancer risk and, in all likelihood, an indication that fish oil might prevent the appearance of precancerous polyps.[28] When an adenoma (a precancerous lesion) was present, supplements normalized cell proliferation in the rectal lining in twelve weeks.[29] Fish oils block tumour-stimulating hormones that come from omega-6 fats.

Treating Cancer Fish oils are valuable in treating established cancer; they can cut down the number of T suppressor cells (the cells that turn off the immune response) when 18 grams daily are given.[30]

Besides preventing and reversing different varieties of cancer, EPA and DHA may serve as a breakthrough treatment combination to stave off something that all people with cancer face – cachexia, the tissue-wasting, life-threatening loss of body mass. Halting that loss and keeping body weight up is critical to any cancer patient's survival. A group of patients with pancreatic cancer were experiencing this loss of body mass at a rate of about 2.7 kilograms a month when researchers began to give them 2 grams of EPA per day. Study participants didn't merely stop losing weight; they actually gained a few kilograms. More significantly, blood tumour markers that reveal the disease's progress were improving, a suggestion that the EPA was having broad anticancer effects in addition to the weight gain. This effect may represent an entirely new application for EPA and its wider use in cancer treatment.[31]

Joint Diseases As you will see, the most oft recurring theme of all is fish oil's consistent ability to suppress inflammation and benefit everyone with illnesses in which inflammation plays a major role. For example, in arthritis, fish oils effectively replace nonsteroidal anti-inflammatory drugs (NSAIDs), the painkilling medications that lead to thousands of deaths every year and cause gastrointestinal bleeding for millions.[32] EPA supplements both decrease pain and increase ease of movement.[33] Eicosanoids created by our overconsumption of omega-6 fats encourage the inflammation responsible for rheumatoid arthritis, so it makes thorough sense to offset them with omega-3 eicosanoids from fish oils.[34] They're safe and nontoxic, free of the gastric blood loss and other NSAID side effects. Fish oil's success in inflammatory arthritis is a splendid example of a well-documented[35] nutritional treatment deserving, but still awaiting, mainstream acceptance.

Fish oil won't work as fast as an NSAID. You can't pop a capsule or two and watch the clock, waiting for a little temporary relief. A daily dosage of 3–4 grams is necessary, and improvements may take months to appear. Full modification of immune function towards less inflammatory reactions may continue slowly for up to nine months or more. The reward for patience, though, is more effective pain relief without any NSAID-like risk.[36]

Autoimmune Diseases Rheumatoid arthritis is just one of several autoimmune disorders benefitted by fish oils. In such diseases, the immune system attacks components of our own bodies as if they were invaders, but EPA and DHA, in doses of 3 grams per day for just three weeks, can suppress this self-destructive process. This is one reason I find them invaluable for any patient with lupus, scleroderma, multiple sclerosis, thrombocytopenia and other autoimmune diseases. Clinical studies showing the ability of EPA/DHA to produce remissions in lupus are beginning to appear.[37]

Inflammatory Bowel Disease Every colitis and Crohn's disease patient we see gets all of the omega-3 fatty acids for reasons that are well supported by research.[38] Fish oils markedly decrease the damage these disorders can cause the colon wall. They do this by reducing the overproduction of inflammatory compounds that are associated with colitis.[39] In a year-long double-blind study of seventy-eight people with Crohn's disease, the proportion of those who remained free of a relapse jumped from

26 to 59 per cent once they began to take a daily dosage of nine fish oil capsules.[40] I've seen scores of people with these two inflammatory bowel diseases, and I always ask how their gastroenterologists had treated their disorders. I'm still waiting to hear someone mention fish oil. I am at a loss to understand why EPA and DHA are not yet mainstream medications for these bowel disorders.

Skin Disorders An imbalance in the production of inflammatory hormones in the skin may cause any number of reactions, including atopic eczema and acne. All of these can be helped by fish oil supplements. EPA and DHA are especially effective in psoriasis. When omega-3s were emulsified and given by infusion in a German experiment, twenty people with acute cases of psoriasis improved dramatically in just one week.[41] Daily dosages of 10 grams or more are required, however, for lower amounts do not always help.

Pulmonary Disorders There is plenty of evidence that EPA and DHA relax the lungs and help them work better. Since there is a strong inflammatory component to asthma, I've given fish oils to hundreds of my patients with this disorder, and they experience far fewer attacks. Surprisingly, little published research has covered this treatment area until recently.[42] Much of the work that has been done comes from Australia, where the incidence of asthma, especially among children, has been increasing rapidly. This is probably a result of the dramatic rise in the consumption of the omega-6 fatty acids down under, one researcher speculates.[43] American and British kids share this trait. Breathing difficulties appear less frequently among children who more often eat fresh oily fish. And taking fish oil supplements for nine months improves results of pulmonary function tests for asthma patients.

It has been proved that heavy smokers can protect themselves from emphysema with a high dietary intake of omega-3s. The oils, according to University of Minnesota researchers, interfere with inflammatory products produced by their omega-6 fats in meats and vegetable oils.[44]

Kidney Problems I always include fish oils in my treatment of inflammatory and autoimmune kidney disease, and a few studies support this practice. Six grams per day of EPA can improve recovery and restore renal function in recipients of a kidney transplant,[45] as well as in people with nephritis[46] and lupus nephritis.[47] The most common form of glomerulonephritis, IgA nephropathy, is usually accompanied by an omega-3 deficiency. Giving EPA and DHA caused a major improvement in kidney function in fifteen patients with this condition.[48] Further, EPA can protect the kidneys from the toxic effects of such medications as cyclosporine. Healthy people can also support proper kidney function by taking fish oils.

Chronic Fatigue Syndrome Even in small doses, EPA can correct the fatty acid deficiencies present in chronic fatigue syndrome, which is more accurately termed 'postviral fatigue syndrome'. Adding GLA and other essential fats will probably enhance the improvement, as shown by a three-month study in which the fatty acid combination of fish oils and GLA helped 85 per cent of the participants feel better and more energetic.[49] I hope such investigations continue, and with larger doses of these crucial fats.

Mood Disorders Since the advent of the ultra-low-fat diet, which fails to provide enough omega-3 oils for healthy brain function and good mood levels, EPA and DHA have become critically important to the treatment of depression. I prescribe them routinely for all mood disorders. Depression is more strongly correlated with coronary artery disease than any other personality variable, probably because both conditions are caused by lack of omega-3s.

DHA: *Brain fat*

I've been considering EPA and DHA as one because they exist together as constituents of fish oil. For the most part, they also have been studied together. But researchers are discovering that the two fatty acids have their own 'personalities'. DHA may have some real value when taken alone.

What we're seeing is that EPA demonstrates stronger anti-inflammatory actions, while DHA seems to be more important for brain health, particularly brain and eye development in infants. In fact, the supplements with EPA probably should be restricted during infancy, since it may suppress the action of other essential fats such as arachidonic acid, which the baby needs for growth. DHA not only preserves these essential fats, but it also improves upon the benefits that arachidonic acid alone provides to infants. Mother's milk is rich in omega-3 fatty acids, notably DHA. Among infant experts, a consensus is growing that all babies should be getting optimal amounts of DHA either through breast milk or fortified formulas.[1]

THE BRAIN AND RETINA'S BEST FRIEND

The foetus's nervous system depends critically on the omega-3s for correct development, and DHA is the omega-3 required by the brain and retina. Research has linked a better DHA intake with, among other benefits, a smaller chance of neurological disorders. Eyesight also relies on a healthy supply. Premature infants who don't get enough omega-3 fats, for example, could suffer from poor retinal development, while infants who receive an adequate amount of DHA have better visual responses. (This also suggests they have better neuronal development.) Premies given DHA-supplemented formulas had better visual acuity than those getting standard supplements.[2] The most exciting avenue of research into fatty acids and infancy is that breast-fed babies are smarter. They have a better vocabulary and display better behavioural development, according to a study of 13,135 tykes.[3]

For adults, DHA alone may improve schizophrenia treatment. People with this emotional disorder have particularly low levels of the essential fat, and in one study supplements reduced symptoms impressively.[4] And, DHA may be given alone (1,250 mg daily) to lower triglyceride and raise HDL.[5]

FLAXSEED OIL: *The king of the vegetable oils*

Fish oil may be the Hercules of omega-3 health supplements, but flaxseed oil also serves us very well. An extract of the reddish brown flaxseed that grows in the northern part of the United States and throughout Canada, flaxseed oil is an extremely important source of an omega-3 fat called alpha-linolenic acid (ALA). This eicosanoid precursor possesses many of fish oil's immune-enhancing and anti-inflammatory effects. It is also a good protector of the cardiovascular system, deterring the clotting tendency of platelets, lowering cholesterol and reducing blood pressure. Many benefits of the Mediterranean diet may stem from its rich content of the omega-3s like those found in flaxseed oil. While fish oil may be more potent, flaxseed may be a little more affordable for people to use on a daily basis.

While the oil is remarkable, don't discount the value of the entire flaxseed. An excellent source of fibre, flaxmeal contains cancer-opposing compounds called lignans, which work to de-activate the more cell-stimulating forms of oestrogen. At the very least, this helps to mitigate the hormone's monthly influence on premenstrual tension, but a more dramatic result could be the power of the antiestrogenic lignans, along with additional support from the omega-3s, to help prevent breast tumours and other hormonally based cancers. I also give fresh flaxmeal to many of my colon cancer patients, encouraging them to consume at least 85 grams of the freshly ground meal per day.

SUPPLEMENT SUGGESTIONS FOR ALL THE OMEGA-3S

Fish or flax? When should you take supplements of flaxseed oil, and what occasions call for fish oils? The body will convert flax oil's fatty acids into EPA and DHA, but this may take weeks. Even when it does occur, the blood's DHA concentration won't equal that achieved by fish oils. Therefore fish oil is the better choice for a more immediate response or for easing inflammation or lowering triglycerides.

To safeguard all of the essential fish oils, you need to take vitamin E. DHA and EPA are extremely unstable and prone to degradation, both in the supplement bottle and in your body. If this occurs, they can actually be harmful. To minimize this peroxidation threat, take at least 400 IU of vitamin E along with your fish oils.

Given DHA's importance to babies, mothers-to-be should take supplements for the duration of their pregnancy. However, the baby's need is most critical from the beginning of the last trimester through at least the first three months of life. If the omega-3s are in short supply, the baby could be born with a low birth weight. DHA supplements further enrich breast milk with omega-3 fats, and they manage to reserve some of their therapeutic assistance for Mum. Without them, postpartum depression is more likely. Mothers-to-be should take at least 1,000 mg of DHA per day along with at least 1 teaspoon of flaxseed oil. In one study, 1,000 mg of DHA and 1,600 mg of EPA were provided by supplements and sardines; in two months they raised the plasma DHA by 45 per cent.[6]

For those who want to maintain a vegetable-based omega-3 presence in the body, take between 1 teaspoon and 1 tablespoon of flaxseed oil daily. When a therapeutic effect is needed, you may need to take up to 3 tablespoons per day. Make sure to purchase an organic oil that comes in a black opaque container. As I've mentioned, light and heat oxidizes and destroys it, so never use it in cooking. It's fine for a salad, though.

With virtually no exceptions, save the few just mentioned, nearly anyone can safely take either of the two omega-3s in the quantities suggested. But if you were to take prodigious quantities (over 5,000 mg) for six months, you would then oxidize the fats in your red blood cells. The 'if some is good, then more is better' school of thought rarely applies in nutrition. Because fish oil so powerfully inhibits platelet clumping, some have cautioned that it may lengthen the time it takes for a cut to stop bleeding. Research shows, however, that no danger exists for greater blood loss. In fact, fish oil can be taken in low doses even before surgery. Even those on warfarin-type blood thinners need not avoid fish oils or vitamin E, because the platelet-separation system and the vitamin K antagonist system (conventional anticoagulants) use completely different mechanisms and their effects are not additive.

The most ideal treatment for my patients is to take both fish oil and flaxseed oil (and – as you will soon learn – GLA). On page 000, you will learn about the essential oils formula I prescribe to almost all my patients. If we learn anything about essential fatty acids, it is that health depends on balance. Now that the omega-3 fats are becoming more widely accepted and considered by scholars to be a part of every good medical practice, the research papers will convince our primary care doctors to prescribe them.

GAMMA-LINOLENIC ACID: *The good omega-6 fat*

Without any doubt, the typical Western diet's lopsided over-consumption of omega-6 fats is a significant cause of premature aging and our almost epidemic rates of arthritis, cancer, heart disease and other illnesses. Yet the members of this fatty acid class remain essential to our good health and even to life itself. Only the omega-6s can convert themselves into gamma-linolenic acid (GLA), which while not technically an essential fatty acid is an essential nutrient for all practical purposes. Without it we could not manufacture the eicosanoid superstar, prostaglandin E_1. PGE_1, as it's known for short, is one of the body's greatest natural therapies for fending off premature aging, heart disease, cancer, arthritis, allergies, asthma and autoimmune diseases, among other disorders.

Obviously there must be a hitch somewhere. How can an excess of omega-6 oils correspond with a higher risk of certain diseases, while a fatty acid derived from the omega-6s provides therapeutic assistance against the very same health problems? There is a rub, and it goes by the name of delta-6-desaturase (D6D). Without this enzyme, omega-6s won't transform themselves into GLA. Many of us do, in fact, lack a sufficient amount of D6D. We lose it as we grow older and suppress it if we consume a lot of sugar, alcohol, margarine or other partially hydrogenated oils. Certain saturated fats also may lower its activity. Additionally, the loss of this enzyme may be caused or exaccrbated by diabetes, hypothyroidism, a viral infection or cancer. The enzyme is made with the help of vitamin C, vitamin

B_6, vitamin B_3, zinc and magnesium; a low amount of any of these nutrients will decrease the amount of D6D the body makes. The great majority of us fall into one of these D6D-robbing categories, and 100 per cent of us could probably use more of its valuable end product: GLA.

A DEPENDABLE SUCCESS

One of my life's most rewarding insights into nutritional medicine came some fifteen years ago at a weekend seminar conducted by the world's foremost authority on GLA, Dr David Horrobin. Under his aegis, many well-performed double-blind studies have been done to demonstrate GLA's clinical uses. To my chagrin and surprise, though, mainstream medicine has been uninterested in replicating or even challenging Horrobin's work. This is especially bewildering because fish oils, which play a parallel role, have been thoroughly studied and widely accepted. What I can relate, then, comes primarily from a body of published research that is not as well replicated as it deserves to be, and from my own experience. The inescapable conclusion is that GLA is ready for use as a mainstream therapy.

THE POWER OF GLA

Immune Weakness Viral infections have a penchant for blocking the body's ability to make GLA. The resulting GLA shortage greatly impairs our immune defences. For people with chronic fatigue (or postviral) syndrome, GLA along with EPA brings about clinically measurable improvements.[1]

High Cholesterol For nearly two decades, patients at the Atkins Center have been reducing their cholesterol levels by taking GLA, among other supplements. Lipid profiles improve or worsen directly with a corresponding increase or decrease of the GLA dosage. (The benefit is even more pronounced when EPA is added.) This success is predictable, and I see the results every day. The fatty acid's conversion into PGE_1 is the reason for this benefit. In cells that lose the ability to synthesize the prostaglandin, cholesterol production becomes uncontrollable.[2]

Taking 400 mg of GLA daily for twelve weeks sufficiently restores the body's PGE_1 stores and significantly lowers cholesterol.[3]

Cancer Extremely large amounts of GLA have tripled life expectancy for people with terminal pancreatic cancer, according to research cited by Horrobin.

Arthritis The fatty acid's best-documented role is the amelioration of inflammatory conditions, principally arthritis. After taking a daily 10 gram dose of borage oil (providing 800 mg of GLA) for twelve weeks, members of an arthritis study group enjoyed an increase in joint mobility and a reduction in morning stiffness. Their sleep patterns improved, too, while side effects were minimal.[4] Other studies corroborate these results, although at a far higher dosage – typically about 1.4 grams of GLA. Taking that amount enabled rheumatoid arthritis patients in a pair of University of Massachusetts studies to reduce assessments of joint swelling and tenderness by more than 40 per cent over their placebo-using counterparts.[5]

Multiple Sclerosis Not everyone afflicted with MS responds to GLA. However, for the 40 per cent or so who do, it is frequently one of their most valuable treatments. GLA doses from 500 to 1,000 mg slow or even halt the progress of the disease in those who respond. The other essential oils, such as EPA and flaxseed oil, are also necessary to get maximum benefit, I've discovered, as is the strict avoidance of fried foods and anything made with or cooked in trans-fatty acids.

PMS Virtually every practitioner of complementary medicine offers GLA to women bothered by premenstrual tension. The treatment is nothing short of remarkable. Some published work does substantiate the treatment, usually at a daily dosage of 300 mg.[6] Levels of the fatty acid are greatly reduced in women with PMS, probably because of an impaired ability to manufacture GLA (which in turn is due to intense monthly hormonal fluctuations). Irritability, cramps and breast tenderness[7] often are eliminated on GLA therapy after three months.

Diabetic Complications Science has established rather conclusively that GLA halts the otherwise inevitable advance of nerve damage caused by diabetes. GLA helps the nerves to heal. As one study of 111 patients showed, people with either form of diabetes, Type I or Type II, can benefit, using a dose as small as 480 mg of GLA (from evening primrose oil) per day.[8] Other research suggests that the fatty acid may even prevent the nerve deterioration from starting up.[9]

Some kind of abnormality in fatty acid metabolism is very likely involved in the development of diabetic complications and maybe even the development of diabetes itself. People who have the disease seem unable to make GLA from dietary fats and therefore may suffer from an insufficiency of PGE_1. Coincidentally enough, this substance can potentiate the work of insulin and exerts insulinlike actions of its own. Therefore diabetics need all the PGE_1 that GLA can help them make.

Healthy Skin GLA is legendary for creating smooth, supple skin, and supplements will easily correct brittle or split nails. I have often said many cosmetic companies would go out of business if the general public knew of its remarkable effects. Ironically, essential fatty acids were once a mainstay of dermatological treatments for a number of skin disorders until the advent of the more toxic, more costly and, I might mention, less effective topical steroids.

Nine studies show that GLA is useful for treating eczema. With dosages between 300 and 500 mg, results may take three to six months to appear, but they are worth the wait. Other research shows that the fatty acid reduces the need for medications to manage atopic dermatitis. The skin condition improved for 111 of the study's 179 participants, who took four evening primrose capsules with meals twice a day for a total GLA dosage of 360 mg.[10]

Overcoming Dryness As we age, our bodies tend to lose the ability to secrete natural fluids and lubricants. Even among younger people on a disciplined low-fat diet, dry eyes and dry mouth are common problems. Antihistamines or other drugs also can dry out tear ducts and salivary glands. GLA is an almost certain remedy.[11]

In the study demonstrating the fatty acid's effect on brittle nails, daily 270 mg supplements (from evening primrose oil) allowed participants to shed tears for the first time in years. The month-long nutrient protocol also included vitamin B_6 and vitamin C.

Obesity The influence of essential fatty acids on metabolism is a relatively new area of investigation. Although the early research was promising, I have not seen any benefit in the usual dose, but several callers on my daily radio show describe 13.5 kilogram weight losses without changing their diets. In the one successful study, half of the overweight people lost weight without any conscious effort to diet, just by taking 400 mg per day of GLA.[12]

Other Illnesses The research, both published and unpublished, is far from conclusive, but GLA might offer some help against neuropathy-related kidney abnormalities, *E. coli* bacterial infections and schizophrenia. Preliminary work with lab animals suggests it cuts down on calcium excretion, suggesting it may figure into treatments for kidney stones and osteoporosis.[13] A recent paper describing an 86 per cent improvement rate in migraine headache involves giving GLA, 1,800 mg, combined with alpha-linolenic acid.[14] But it also required an extremely high carbohydrate diet. More work is needed to learn how best to do the programme.

SUPPLEMENT SUGGESTIONS

For a good number of years, evening primrose oil was thought to be our sole source of GLA (this is why most of the medical research I've cited used the oils extracted from seeds of this wildflower). We now know that GLA also exists in two other plants, namely black currant seeds and borage seeds. I'd go so far as to say that no one's usual diet includes healthy servings of any of these three plants, which makes supplements mandatory.

Borage oil appears to be the most economical and practical choice. A single capsule usually contains at least four times the GLA of an evening primrose capsule, which generally contains only 45 mg of the omega-6 fatty acid. Borage capsules usually contain 240 mg of GLA. For a therapeutic effect, about 240 mg of GLA daily is the minimum requirement; as we've seen, though, some conditions, such as rheumatoid arthritis, need at least 1,400 mg per day in order to improve.

Though some have argued that GLA competes with omega-3 oils and renders them less effective, in reality their effects are synergistic. I, as well as most other practitioners who endorse the essential fats, use both omega-3s and GLA, giving the body all the raw materials to make whatever eicosanoids it needs most. In most instances I prescribe six capsules a day of an essential oils formula that contains 400 mg each of borage oil, flax oil and a fish oil supplement rich in EPA. This translates into 576 mg of GLA, 720 mg of EPA and 480 mg of DHA, in addition to 1,080 of linoleic acid, 984 mg of alpha-linolenic acid and 912 mg of monounsaturated oil – which, not surprisingly, covers all the bases.

The differential effect on serum lipids (GLA has a cholesterol-lowering effect and EPA has a triglyceride-lowering effect) serves me as a guide for individualizing dosage. For those whose cholesterol is high and more than double the triglycerides (the usual ratio), I tend to give extra GLA; for those whose triglycerides are high and more than half the cholesterol number, I may prescribe extra EPA.

CHAPTER 7

◦—◦—◦

FAT-BASED NUTRITION

MEDIUM-CHAIN TRIGLYCERIDES:
Fats for energy and weight loss

When we talk about the cardiac dangers of high triglycerides, we are referring to long-chain fats: fatty acids that, biochemically speaking, have a long chain of carbon atoms attached to them. Because of this chain, they aren't metabolized very well and are thus able to accumulate in the bloodstream. Worst of all, they are stored in fat cells.

However, when the carbon chain is a little shorter, the triglycerides behave in an entirely different manner. They're absorbed rapidly and transported directly to the liver for use as energy. These medium-chain triglycerides (MCTs), as they're called, don't get rancid, won't linger in the blood, and won't build up in fat tissue. Such properties don't qualify MCTs as essential fats, but they do present enough therapeutic might to be regarded as a valuable supplement.

MCT oil, the most common and versatile supplemental form, provides a rapid source of sustained energy. That's why it's popular among athletes. Rats that were fed MCTs, for example, significantly increased their swimming endurance compared with rats that were fed long-chain triglycerides. As a supplement, MCTs will also figure into your weight-loss programme. They share with dietary fats the virtue of providing satiety and not affecting blood sugar. But because they are burned almost immediately, they won't deposit themselves on your abdomen or hips. Additionally, some research suggests that they might increase the body's resting metabolic rate, which burns off additional fat.[1]

Medicinally, MCTs can contribute to cancer therapy, particularly brain malignancies. Cancer cells feed on sugar, and MCTs help the body to mimic a ketogeniclike metabolic state that deprives cancer cells of nourishment. Other research has suggested an MCT role in managing cystic fibrosis, epilepsy, cholesterol gallstones[2] and cirrhosis. Because they're absorbed so quickly from the intestines, these nonstorable fats have also become an established part of nutritional therapies for digestive disorders.

Supplement Suggestions

Though MCT oil is available in 1,000 mg capsules, the liquid form offers more palatable consumption possibilities. Substitute the oil any time you otherwise would use butter (or margarine), vegetable oil or salad dressing. With a high smoke point and thin consistency, it's perfect for a quick sauté and can be mixed with virtually any spice. Butter-flavoured MCT oil is delicious when spritzed on a bowl of popcorn. For more mundane supplemental purposes, such as a general increase in energy, a standard daily dosage is 1 teaspoon or five 100 mg capsules, taken with meals. To enhance endurance for sports, try taking 1–3 teaspoons of the oil a day. The upper dosage range has a self-limiting drawback; if you take more than your intestinal tract can handle, you will experience diarrhoea and loose stools or perhaps a little nausea. So build up your quantities slowly.

SQUALENE: *Oxygenator, cancer fighter*

Oxygen is the great forgotten nutrient – and the great forgotten nutrient deficiency. A lack of it has been pinpointed as a cause of or contributing factor to nearly all our degenerative diseases.

Squalene is the closest thing we have to an oxygen supplement.

This remarkable compound imbues the tissues and organs of our bodies with the life-sustaining element through a simple chemical interaction with water. The process has nothing to do with lung respiration, so don't mistake squalene for a better-breathing nutrient. It won't alleviate asthma, reduce shortness of breath or allow you to go scuba diving without a snorkel, although by releasing oxygen inside body tissues, it does contribute to one of the lungs' functions.

A thin, oil-like extract, squalene was first isolated from the liver of a rare species of deep-sea shark, although it's found naturally in the human body, too, principally the skin. We now know that olive oil is a rich source as well. In fact, the substance may account for a good deal of olive oil's heart-protecting qualities.

Sharks use squalene to manage the limited amount of oxygen in their deepwater environment. Above sea level, our atmosphere has lost some of the oxygen content it had a century ago, which could in part explain our almost epidemic rates of cancer, heart disease and immune system malfunctions, to name just a few illnesses. In Germany, Japan, Korea and other nations, squalene supplements fortify treatment programmes for hardening of the arteries, ischemic heart disease, high cholesterol, liver disorders and skin problems.[1]

Cardiovascular Disease Heart cells may suffer most from the lack of oxygen. For this reason I'll sometimes give squalene to patients with congestive heart failure, who need all the help they can get in delivering oxygen to starved cardiac muscle. Life's dependency on oxygen does, however, come at the cost of oxidation. Squalene helps to offset any possible additional risk because it's an antioxidant, working with vitamin E and similar nutrients in guarding cells from the damage that allows cholesterol to build up inside arteries.

Supplement cynics might point out that squalene is one of the very ingredients that the body uses to manufacture cholesterol in the first place. This is true. But supplements do not elevate blood levels of cholesterol. To the contrary, research suggests that the compound *lowers* high blood concentrations of cholesterol and triglycerides. A daily 860 mg dosage, one study found, augmented the ability of cholesterol medications to decrease LDL and increase HDL cholesterol.[2]

Cancer Both a deficit of oxygen and the cell damage of oxidation are major reasons for the development and spread of tumours, so squalene's anticancer properties should come as no surprise. Progressive doctors, myself included, and many of their cancer patients the world over are convinced that squalene further controls the spread of malignancies. Animal research backs up the belief. In one such laboratory study, squalene, along with vitamin E and aloe vera, shrank tumours by more than 33 per cent.[3]

Immune Weakness Our general ability to fight off illnesses ultimately depends on a vibrant immune system, which in turn relies on a steady supply of oxygen. Squalene improves several measurements of immune system strength, especially against cancerous tumours and overall activity. As the dosage increases, so do the results of the immune tests.[4] Squalene wards off cancer-causing substances, bacteria, fungi, the herpes virus, the Epstein-Barr virus and such autoimmune diseases as leukaemia. Squalene detoxifies several chemicals capable of hurting us. Its presence also has prevented the deaths of experimental animals given lethal doses of theophylline, phenobarbital and strychnine; they survived when protected with the oil. Lab mice exposed to a lethal level of radiation survived longer when squalene was given.[5]

Skin Problems Squalene's abundance in the skin is proof enough of its need there. It holds moisture, which helps to keep skin smooth and supple. Studies have found good indications that it may guard against ultraviolet radiation and, along with its anticancer and proimmunity influence, forms of skin cancer.

Supplement Suggestions

Neither I nor any published studies have found any detrimental effects from long-term squalene supplementation, so safety problems are not a consideration. To oxygenate the body and as a general health enhancement, I normally recommend a daily dosage of 1–3 grams. I prescribe 2–4 grams for people with cancer. Judging from the number of European oncologists who also use it, I expect to see a major paper soon chronicling squalene's clinical success.

GLYCEROL MONOLAURATE: *Antiviral therapy*

One of my prescriptions for certain viral infections is a special kind of fatty acid whose deficiency may partly account for the rampant growth of infectious diseases around the world.

THERAPEUTIC TARGET: THE ENVELOPE PLEASE

Glycerol monolaurate, a chemical compound of glycerin and a medium-chain fat called lauric acid, first proved its might more than a decade ago. Besides knocking out the influenza virus, it attacks herpes 1 and 2 viruses and the three major microbes seen in chronic fatigue syndrome: the cytomegalovirus, the Epstein-Barr virus and the herpes 6 virus. In lab experiments done at the US Centers for Disease Control, it killed respectable numbers of fourteen different so-called envelope viruses.[1] These various bugs are distinguishable by their surrounding coats of fatty acids, which allow them to latch on to and infect cells in our bodies. Glycerol monolaurate dissolves the fatty acid 'envelope', rendering the virus incapable of grabbing on to cells and spreading.

LAURIC ACID IS EFFECTIVE

We've known about the completely safe, infection-fighting power of certain fatty acids for a long time. Lauric acid fell victim to a bad rap, though, because its chief sources include palm oil, coconut oil and butterfat – all saturated fats that traditional medical wisdom claims will raise cholesterol. Though this is still the official line, more sophisticated research now tells us that these fatty acids in fact raise the level of desirable HDL cholesterol.[2] Among Polynesians, whose typical diet includes a plentiful amount of lauric acid from tropical oils, rates of heart disease are very low.

The presence of infectious diseases around the world seems to correspond to the declining consumption of medium-chain fats, leading some researchers to speculate that fats such as lauric acid may afford some protection against viruses. Others point out that HIV and HTLV, the pathogens associated with AIDS, are envelope viruses and more likely to spread in a medium-chain fat-deficient world.

SUPPLEMENT SUGGESTIONS

I am not enthusiastic about routinely administering flu shots every winter. As often as I can, I tell patients to avoid them. The best protection from colds and more severe viruses is a well-nourished immune system, combined with the strategy that a team of targeted vita-nutrients will be used at the first symptoms of a flulike illness. Glycerol monolaurate, which you might see in health food stores under the trade name of Monolaurin or Lauricidin, is a vital member of that team, along with vitamin C, vitamin A, zinc, oregano oil and olive leaf extract. Glycerol monolaurate should be given at the first sign of a viral infection. On day one I prescribe four to six capsules of 300 mg each. When the illness begins to subside, I cut down to two to four capsules per day.

ALKYLGLYCEROLS: *Inflammation, cancer fighter*

You probably have never heard of these fat-soluble compounds, but if you know anyone who is enduring a round of radiation treatments or chemotherapy, you might want to read up on them. Alkylglycerols both improve orthodox cancer therapies and spare the body from some of their inherent damage. These remarkable compounds can also deliver a little more immune system protection from colds or the flu. And because they aid in reducing inflammation, they might be useful for arthritis and psoriasis. They also boost the ability of other cells to protect themselves from free radical damage.[1]

I've limited my use of alkylglycerols mainly to cancer patients, based on Swedish research that dates back to the 1970s. One study found that chemotherapy, especially as a treatment for uterine cancer, shrinks tumours more significantly when the patient is taking alkylglycerol supplements.[2] At the same time, alkylglycerols protect healthy cells from some of the damage inflicted by radiation therapy.

For older people or anyone else with a weak immune system, supplements offer a little resistance to a cold, the flu or a bronchial infection. Their contribution to immune strength comes from their creation and support of the white blood cells, which fight off bacteria, viruses and other invaders. Unlike drugs, they are completely nontoxic and can be used for as long as you'd like. The body never develops an immunity to them.[3]

Alkylglycerols, found naturally in the spleen, the liver, bone marrow and breast milk, help the body to produce white blood cells, red blood cells, and blood platelets. Whenever any of these blood components is low, supplements can come in handy.

Supplement Suggestions

For daily health maintenance, I usually recommend 500 mg of shark liver oil extract, which yields 100 mg of alkylglycerols. If a serious infection, cancer or HIV demands a stronger immune response, I'll prescribe 1,000–1,500 mg.

Few companies can correctly perform the delicate, difficult extraction of alkylglycerols from shark liver, so the quality of many supplement brands cannot be assured. Rather than take your chances with an off-the-shelf product, you probably should consult a complementary doctor.

CETYL MYRISTOLEATE: *The real arthritis cure*

In addition to medical journals, the ideas for the vita-nutrient therapies I use in my practice and report on in this book often come from the medical meetings I attend. Two organizations – FAIM (Foundation for the Advancement of Innovative Medicine), of which I was the founding president, and ACAM

(American College of Advancement in Medicine) – provide excellent forums where breakthroughs in complementary medicine are first presented.

Doctors at both recent meetings were abuzz with reports that a new natural, nontoxic treatment was now available that will replace the standard pharmacological treatments for all forms of arthritis.[1] The nutritional substance is called cetyl myristoleate, or CMO, for short.

I asked its proponents to show me the literature published about CMO, and they said that although none had yet been published, an interesting study was awaiting publication. I reviewed that paper and found it to be so promising that, having ascertained that CMO was perfectly safe, I began using it on those patients of mine who were still handicapped by rheumatoid or osteoarthritis.

THE EUROPEAN STUDY

Over four hundred patients entered the study, and two hundred of them were treated with CMO. About one hundred of the latter also were given companion treatments (glucosamine sulfate, cartilage extract and sea cucumber). Patients with osteoarthritis and rheumatoid arthritis were in both groups. Compared with untreated arthritis patients, only 14 per cent of whom showed any improvements, the CMO users benefitted 63 per cent of the time.

When the three helpers were added to the treatment, the improvement rate soared to 87 per cent. Side effects were minor at worst. If the results hold up, this programme alone could qualify as the treatment of choice for all forms of arthritis.

CMO comes from such animal sources as sperm whales, mice and beavers. The compound, a union of the fatty acid myristoleic acid and cetyl alcohol, lubricates joints, suppresses inflammation and curbs the autoimmune reaction that targets the body's own joints.

CMO may prove useful in a variety of inflammatory conditions. Since none of the patients I have prescribed it for experienced any adverse reactions and many have reported rather gratifying symptom relief, I feel it is quite appropriate to explore these possibilities with patients experiencing major discomfort.

SUPPLEMENT SUGGESTIONS

I have been using the same protocol as in the European study, which involves a total of 180 capsules, each containing 100 mg of cetyl myristoleate per capsule. The capsules may be administered in a course of thirty to forty-five days (six to four daily would be used) along with the companion nutrients. After two weeks some relief of symptoms is usually noted. The initial teaching was that CMO treatment need not be resumed unless or until symptoms return, but I am more inclined to prescribe a maintenance dose of two to four capsules daily.

CHAPTER 8

<figure>◇</figure>

DIGESTIVE AIDS

There is a wide range of digestive aids, from the much discussed value of fibre to little-known sugars that offer special benefits. Let's begin with fibre.

FIBRE: *Roughage to live well*

Dennis Burkitt, a brilliant British doctor who worked in Africa for twenty years, noticed something extraordinary in the rural areas where he worked – a nearly complete lack of diabetes, varicose veins, appendicitis, heart disease, colon cancer, irritable bowel, gallbladder disease, constipation and hiatal hernia. After carefully examining the African diet, he noticed that they ate one thing in far greater quantities than the 'civilized' world did: fibre.[1] Though it is tempting to conclude from his findings that fibre corrects the entire spectrum of modern disease, Burkitt's discoveries were simply epidemiological observations. This type of research can find correlations between possible causes and results, but correlation is not causation. These findings could be explained in another way: perhaps the refining of foods in Westernized countries is removing key nutrients needed for health. (Surgeon-Captain D. L. Cleave confirmed the identical African disease pattern but saw refined carbohydrates as the villain.)

Although this is an equally compelling explanation, other research has demonstrated that fibre is an integral part of a healthy diet. It plays an important role in maintaining the health of the digestive system and seems to have tangible value for the prevention of cardiovascular disease, cancer, diabetes and other ailments.[2] Dietary fibre, in a recent very large Finnish epidemiological study, was found to be asociated with a 30 per cent reduction in heart-related deaths.[3]

WHAT IS FIBRE?

Fiber is the portion of plant food that is not digested by the body and is often referred to as roughage. Because the body does not absorb the substance, it took much effort on the part of Dr Burkitt and others to convince Western medicine that this unused portion of food serves an important purpose. Fibre cleanses our intestinal tract and enhances its function, thereby benefitting nearly every digestive ailment. Metabolized by intestinal bacteria into substances that prevent colon cancer, fibre also dilutes and speeds the removal of carcinogens and other toxins in food so that they spare the delicate lining of the GI tract. It also helps achieve optimal blood sugar control and cholesterol levels by slowing digestion and maximizing cholesterol excretion. Fibre is found in whole grains, beans and legumes, fruits, vegetables, nuts and seeds, but not in meat, fish, eggs, cheese or dairy products.

WHERE DID THE FIBRE GO?

The twentieth century has witnessed both a great reduction in fibre intake and a dramatic increase in our intake of refined carbohydrates. There can be no question that the general frightening escalation of degenerative disease is a result of both of these related phenomena. In America, the large-scale refining of grains began in the 1890s, and grains like whole wheat were turned into white flour on a massive scale. In the same decade sugar consumption increased dramatically – as the rage for drinking Coca-Cola swept the nation – to the point where Americans now consume more fibre-free sugar in a week than their nineteenth-century counterparts did in a year. And alarmingly, the 50-gram-per-day increase in carbohydrate intake over the past decade is due entirely to an increase in these fibre-free carbohydrates.

THE DARK SIDE OF REFINEMENT

The devastating effects of these refined carbohydrates first began to materialize in 1920, when a new word entered medical lexicons – 'myocardial infarction', the scientific term for heart attacks. Hard as it may be to believe, heart attacks were unknown before the twentieth century (the first description of a heart attack in a medical journal appeared in 1912), and we have the food refiners to thank for its appearance. The clutching chest pain of angina, also a rarity, became much more common by the 1920s. And as refined carbohydrate foods like white bread and spaghetti made greater inroads on to dinner tables, our risk for a variety of digestive problems, including appendicitis, hiatal hernia, haemorrhoids, constipation and diverticulosis increased. Low-fibre, high-sugar diets also increase the risk for colorectal cancer, breast cancer and, especially, diabetes and hypertension and their many consequences.

Because low-fibre foods provide less long-term satiety, we began to overeat. The not very surprising result is that the twentieth century has become the era of obesity. Americans literally take the cake as the most overweight people in the world owing in large part to their overconsumption of refined, low-fibre foods. The obesity, in turn, has contributed to the epidemic status of all the problems I just listed.

RETURNING TO WHOLE FOODS

For decades I have been urging my patients both to restrict carbohydrates (if they are overweight) and to consume more fibre. For many of them, this poses a dilemma and requires a personalized strategy. They need fibre sources that contain small to moderate amounts of carbohydrates, so I often recommend leafy green vegetables, freshly ground flaxmeal, nuts and seeds. For people who need not restrict carbohydrates, whole grains, fruits and legumes are excellent sources. Just don't think the benefits of fibre mean that you can eat all the whole-grain, high-carbohydrate foods you want. Even though they are far better for you than refined grains like white flours and pastas, many people are stuck with the fact that too many carbohydrates will make them fat. For those of you facing this dilemma, my strategy for solving it is this: the best way to increase your fibre intake is to use fibre supplements.

Getting fibre in supplement form means that you can avoid the increased intake of carbohydrates and still get all of the nutrient's benefits. Wheat bran, oat bran, guar gum, apple pectin and all of the pure fibre supplements contain very little digestible carbohydrates and therefore do not count as calories or towards your total carbohydrate intake. Now you know why I prescribe fibre supplements!

FIBRE: SOLUBLE AND INSOLUBLE

Fibre comes in two basic forms: soluble (meaning it dissolves in water) and insoluble (it doesn't). Foods high in soluble fibre include oats and oat bran, barley, psyllium husks, flaxmeal, beans, peas, carrots, citrus fruits and apples. This form has been shown to lower cholesterol and triglyceride levels, and stabilize blood sugar by slowing the absorption of sugar from the digestive tract. This makes soluble fibre useful for diabetics, especially since it has been shown to help lower insulin and triglyceride levels. Soluble fibre also has the advantage of being free of the phytates, found in insoluble fibres, which tend to block mineral absorption.

Insoluble fibre is found in such foods as wheat bran, corn bran, celery and the skins of fruits and root vegetables. Its impressive list of benefits include reducing the risk of intestinal cancers, helping prevent constipation and diverticulitis, absorbing toxins from food and reducing the production of bacterial toxins in the GI tract. Ideally one should balance both soluble and insoluble fibre to get the different benefits they confer.

Psyllium Husks One of my favourite fibre supplements, psyllium husks, help to alleviate both constipation and diarrhoea, especially when combined with rice or wheat bran. Psyllium husks are an excellent source of soluble fibre, and many studies have shown that they lower cholesterol and triglycerides.[4] Don't confuse psyllium husk powder with psyllium seeds. I find the husks more effective (and unlike the seeds, they don't contribute to carbohydrate intake).

Pectin Amply supplied in apples, strawberries and citrus fruits, pectin has been shown to be one of the most reliable forms of fibre for lowering cholesterol and triglyceride levels.[5] By slowing the absorption of sugars from the digestive tract, pectin also helps balance blood sugar levels in diabetics and in those with low blood sugar. Animal studies suggest that pectin can also reduce the accumulation of plaque on the walls of the heart's arteries.[6]

According to animal studies, pectin seems to improve the intestinal tract's ability to function and even its size[7], a benefit that may be important for those with impaired digestive ability. Pectin may also be an important fibre supplement for those who experience a thinning of the gut wall, due to the effects of such medications as antibiotics and anti-inflammatory painkillers. Pectin supplements also proved valuable to survivors of the Chernobyl radiation disaster by keeping their antioxidant levels normal and thus protecting them from the radiation they had absorbed.[8] This is probably the result of its ability to prevent absorption of toxins.

Pectin does not have the bulking effect that other fibre sources do because it is completely metabolized by bacteria in the intestine.[9] Therefore you shouldn't take pectin to relieve constipation. Do take it if you want to balance blood sugar, lower cholesterol, help your body remove toxins and promote the health of your GI tract.

Flaxmeal Though used frequently as a supplement, flaxmeal is technically a food because it consists of nothing more than ground flaxseed. Although it contains carbohydrates, the percentage is quite low when compared with other high-fibre foods. At the same time, its health-enhancing benefits are impressive.

The various fibres and fatty acids in freshly ground flaxmeal are extremely effective in relieving constipation and inflammatory bowel problems. Even better, these pulverized seeds contain lignans, compounds that help promote female hormone balance and reduce the risk of female hormone-related cancers.[10] This dual action makes flaxmeal my fibre of choice for the management of such cancers, as well as PMS, fibroids, endometriosis, menopausal symptoms and a range of other problems related to female hormonal imbalance.[11]

To make your own flaxmeal, buy organic flaxseeds and grind them in a small coffee grinder or food processor. This is important for optimal freshness and benefit. A few companies have come out with ground flaxmeal that is reasonably stable when kept refrigerated. Those with weak digestive tracts may want to soak their flaxseeds in water overnight before grinding them. (This will help you digest them more easily.) I usually recommend 1–3 tablespoons per day dissolved in water or mixed with semisolid food such as soured cream. It's better to take them early in the day, for these energizing flaxseeds make it difficult to fall asleep if ingested towards evening.

Low-carbohydrate dieters should note that 25 grams of flaxmeal contains 11 grams of carbohydrates, 6 of which are fibre, leaving only 5 grams of digestible carbohydrates.

Guar Gum A gel-forming fibre extracted from the Indian cluster bean, guar gum, like other soluble fibres, has been shown to lower cholesterol, and does so by up to 28 per cent.[12] Because it helps slow the release of sugar from GI tract, it therefore may be useful for Type I[13] or Type II diabetics[14] who want to keep their blood sugar and insulin levels under better control. High blood pressure levels also decrease on guar gum supplements.[15]

I would prescribe guar gum routinely in diabetic patients were it not for one side effect: gas. In addition, the trade-off for guar gum's slower release of sugar is a longer digestion process. Users of guar gum can counter this delay by taking some insoluble fibre.

Oat Bran According to numerous studies done over many decades, both whole oats and the bran extracted from it lower cholesterol. Though the effect is a mild one, it is nevertheless well established.[16] The active agent in oat bran that lowers cholesterol appears to be beta-glucan, which is also found in barley. This substance increases the body's excretion of cholesterol.[17] Perhaps beta-glucan supplements will display even more cholesterol-lowering power than oat bran.[18] However, whole oat bran may be more helpful than the extract and has the added benefit of being an easy-to-use ingredient in many recipes.

Wheat and Rice Bran The soluble fibre in wheat bran is excellent for eliminating constipation and softening the stool. It may also help to raise levels of the beneficial HDL cholesterol. Most people tolerate wheat bran well, including those with wheat allergies. Why? Because the protein that triggers these allergies is not present in the bran portion of the plant. (However, if you are severely wheat sensitive, use wheat bran only under the supervision of your doctor.) Wheat bran also helps regulate oestrogen levels and, like flaxmeal, may be useful in the prevention and treatment of such hormonal-related disorders as uterine fibroids, endometriosis and breast cancer.[19]

Another excellent source of insoluble fibre is rice bran, which also contains valuable compounds such as gamma-oryzanol and tocotrienols.

Modified Citrus Pectin A special form of soluble fibre, modified citrus pectin (MCP), has been shown in animal studies to help prevent the spread of cancer in the body, particularly prostate cancer.[20] MCP is made by breaking down pectin's long-chain molecules into smaller ones that the body can absorb. Once absorbed, these short-chain molecules appear to stop the growth and progression of cancer in the body. Regular pectin cannot do this because it is not small enough to be absorbed.

In lab animals given MCP, cancer metastasizes or spreads to new places at only half its usual rate.[21] In humans, MCP enhances the action of natural killer cells, important members of our immune system. (Though additional human research still needs to be done, some research shows that MCP stimulates the immune system. This suggests that MCP may prove valuable in the fight against other cancers besides prostate cancer.)

Treatment doses are high – about 15 grams per day, usually in powder form to help keep down the cost of this expensive supplement. At the Atkins Center, MCP is used routinely for patients in all stages of prostate cancer, and a very small percentage of them develop disseminated disease. Our experience, however, was meant to be simply good patient care, not a scientific study.

FIBRE DECEPTIONS

Please do not be victimized by ad campaigns for cereals, breads or other foods fortified with psyllium, oat bran or some other fibre. Despite their healthful aura, these foods are typically high in sugars. Adding fibre to a snack cake doesn't make it healthy, and many of these foods are not too far afield from that. Look at all the ingredients on the label, not just the fibre content. Appropriate high-fibre breakfast foods are pure, unadulterated whole grains – for example, porridge oats and brown rice cooked as a hot cereal, preferably with freshly ground flaxmeal on top. Beans are another good source, especially black-eyed peas. For those who are on a low-carbohydrate eating plan, nuts and leafy greens are good sources.

SUPPLEMENT SUGGESTIONS

How much fibre should you eat? The average American or Briton consumes about 10–12 grams a day, although I am not sure that even 30 grams a day is enough. (Some communities in rural China eat as much as 75 grams a day.) At the very least, try to take 1–3 tablespoons of a blend of psyllium, wheat bran, rice bran and flaxmeal per day, beginning with perhaps just 1 teaspoon and working up from there over a course of a few weeks. It's best to introduce fibre slowly. A sudden increase in fibre can stress the digestive tract, causing an uncomfortable bloating, especially in those who have not consumed much fibre for years.

I strongly prefer the powdered forms over capsules and tablets. They're easier to ingest and are essential to obeying the cardinal rule of fibre supplementation: take fibre along with plenty of water. In the intestine, fibre sucks up water like a sponge. If you already have capsules or tablets, stir them into a glass of water and let it stand for a minute before drinking.

For a better balance of health attributes, take both soluble and insoluble fibre, emphasizing whichever suits your own objectives. Finally, don't take fibre at the same time as the other supplements in your nutrient programme. It may interfere with their absorption.

BENEFICIAL BACTERIA: *Our gut's true protectors*

FRIENDS ON THE INSIDE

Louis Pasteur long ago theorized that having the right bacteria in the digestive tract was essential for good health, and modern science proved him right. But even Pasteur did not comprehend the full involvement of these 'friendly flora' in disease and illness. Beneficial bacteria represent a minority among the trillions of organisms in the human intestines. The entire bacterial colony, which weighs up to 1.35 kilograms, is so fundamental to overall health that it has been referred to as the 'forgotten organ'.

For most of history the significance of the bacterial community within our gut might have remained unknown, for nature intended the balance within it to be self-correcting. However, during the past fifty years the Western world has brought upon itself a new form of pathology whose consequences have forced the good bacteria on to centre stage. The main villains in this drama are antibiotics, which indiscriminately destroy both bad and good bacteria. Their casual overuse upsets the digestive tract's delicate bacterial balance, giving an edge to certain of the more harmful microorganisms such as yeast, as well as enabling mutant microbes to emerge. Other disturbers of the bacterial balance are bad diet, stress and environmental chemicals: for example, the chlorine and fluoride added to tap water that have the nasty habit of killing off our most beneficial bacteria.

The Good Guys

To compensate for the negative effects of antibiotic therapy, wiser practitioners now advocate treating patients with 'probiotics', the name given to beneficial bacteria. Besides promoting digestion and overall intestinal health, these organisms support our immune defences and actually manufacture certain nutrients, including folic acid, biotin and vitamin K. A deficiency of good bacteria may cause or exacerbate a number of ailments, such as food allergies, as well as the many ensuing health problems. Repopulating the gut with good bacteria is vital for overcoming diarrhoea and other bowel disorders and often will alleviate lactose intolerance as well.

The Three Musketeers

There are many kinds of friendly flora, but I have three favourites: *Lactobacillus acidophilus,* bifidobacterium and *Lactobacillus bulgaricus.* Studied more extensively than the others, these three appear to be associated with the most health benefits and are the ones I use most often in my practice. Let's take a quick look at each:

• *Acidophilus* This probiotic inhibits the growth of the *Candida albicans* yeast, *E. coli* and other harmful bacteria.[1] By helping the body to make interferon, it also augments immune function. Though primarily a resident of the small intestine, acidophilus also is part of the protective flora in the vagina, where it's central to warding off yeast infections. Research demonstrates that eating yogurt containing active acidophilus cultures can decrease the incidence of vaginal yeast infections.[2] In my mind, given the high sugar and carbohydrate content of most commercially available yogurts, acidophilus supplements are clearly a better choice.

• *Bifidobacterium* The most important and most populous of the friendly flora, bifidobacterium contributes to lowering cholesterol levels, preventing food poisoning, digesting lactose and making many B vitamins.[3] From its main residence in the large intestine, this probiotic also lowers blood levels of ammonia (which is toxic to the body) and wards off many other harmful compounds. It may be extremely helpful in combating lactose intolerance.[4] Before taking a trip to a foreign country, load up on bifidobacterium supplements. They offer your body maximum protection against the many strange or new bacteria that can cause traveller's diarrhoea.

• *Bulgaricus* This probiotic may stimulate the immune system more than acidophilus. In an encouraging study of one hundred cancer patients, the bulgaricus strain known as LB-51 showed very impressive results as an adjunct treatment for a range of cancers. It enabled the patients to live longer, stopped or slowed tumour growth, and halted the cancer's spread through the body.[5]

RESCUING THE DIGESTIVE TRACT

Beneficial bacteria are a cornerstone of my treatments for nearly all bowel disorders, including Crohn's disease, colitis, irritable bowel syndrome and *Candida albicans* overgrowth. Almost every one of these ailments is caused, in part, by a deficiency of good bacteria.[6] Whenever a food allergy is felt to be behind a medical problem, probiotics will prove beneficial. A recent study on infants with atopic eczema made that point very well.[7]

Constipation is perhaps the most common intestinal problem that stems from a bacterial imbalance. While fibre, magnesium, vitamin C, water intake and proper thyroid function are important for reestablishing regularity, the most valuable tool for getting things moving again is probiotic supplements. I have seen people, constipated for decades, who have ingested heroic amounts of fibre to no avail. After taking the probiotic trio for a week, they return to my office with many 'moving' stories. Why? Much of the stool is made up of bacteria, and increasing the number of these good guys in the intestines will increase its bulk significantly, allowing the gastrointestinal tract to function normally once again.

WIDE SPHERE OF INFLUENCE

It stands to reason that intestinal problems would be linked to constituents of the intestinal tract. It may surprise you, however, that other illnesses throughout the body are also influenced by our friendly flora.

Arthritis For reasons that scientists do not fully understand, the wrong bacteria in the digestive system can cause or worsen arthritis.[8] This ailment is strongly associated with such gastrointestinal problems as Crohn's disease, colitis and celiac disease. Beneficial bacteria are a crucial part of the management – and perhaps even the prevention – of joint disorders. The overuse of antibiotics, which kill the friendly flora, is probably one of the causes of the arthritis epidemic in the United States and Great Britain. Older people are more likely to be low in beneficial bacteria, which might explain why they're more prone to arthritis as well.

Brain Dysfunction Research has suggested that an overload of toxins in the digestive tract and liver could be a cause of Alzheimer's disease and Parkinson's disease.[9] Harmful bacteria in the digestive tract create many toxins whose excess in the body may kill brain and nerve cells and in turn lead to these ailments. Hyperactivity in children may also be caused by such toxins from the gut. Probiotic supplements, happily, can reduce the buildup of these metabolic poisons.

Oxidation Damage We know that antioxidant nutrients like vitamin C and vitamin E fight off the unstable free radical compounds that both damage tissues and cause or worsen virtually all of our modern plagues – including cancer, heart disease, arthritis, scleroderma and sickle cell anaemia. A better idea than beating back the free radical attack might be to prevent free radicals from forming in the first place. The number one site of free radical production is the large intestine,[10] where they are created by harmful bacteria. By inhibiting the growth of these bad guys, the friendly flora add to our antioxidant defences.

SUPPLEMENT SUGGESTIONS

There are ways to support the growth of beneficial bacteria besides taking supplements. First, make sure that the yeast *Candida albicans* does not overgrow in the colon, crowding out the probiotics. You'll need a medical evaluation to know for sure. Second, remember that fibre, especially the insoluble forms from corn and wheat bran, can feed the beneficial bacteria in the large intestine, although you need not overdo it. Avoiding alcohol, antibiotics and foods high in sugar are other ways to prevent an overgrowth of harmful bacteria, as is minimizing stress. FOS (see page 266) is a specific promoter of bifidobacteria.

These support strategies, despite their importance, are no substitute for the use of high-quality probiotic supplements. Just about everyone – even those who do not have GI problems – should take supplements of acidophilus, bulgaricus and bifidobacterium. They not only represent one of the most important antiaging, disease-fighting strategies we can mount, but they probably ensure better absorption of all vita-nutrients, both dietary and as 'vitamin pills'. For maximum benefit consume them regularly, at least once a week. Their use is absolutely crucial if you have been on a course of broad-spectrum prescription antibiotics.

Potency and purity are important for all nutrients, but this is especially so for beneficial bacteria. They are, after all, alive. When shopping, look for a 'use by' date and for an assurance concerning the number of viable bacteria and the strain. As I have mentioned, the LB-51 bulgaricum strain seems to have the most benefit. Certain strains of acidophilus (DDS-1) and bifidobacteria (the North Carolina strain) also are better than others. The manufacturer should be able to attest that the strain is beneficial for humans.

Better bacterial supplements will be in the refrigerated section of the health food store, for a cool climate helps beneficial bacteria supplements retain their potency. Cultures can be grown on a variety of media, including milk, rice and soya. Avoid the milk-based variety. I usually use the powdered forms of beneficial bacteria because they are easier to take when treating digestive disorders. For most therapeutic applications I recommend taking between 1/2 and 1 teaspoon each of acidophilus and bifidobacterium. Mix each in a glass of unchilled water and take them daily, preferably in the morning and about twenty minutes or so before eating. Bifidobacteria usually are taken in a two-to-one ratio to the acidophilus. If you take 1/4 teaspoon of acidophilus, you should take 1/2 teaspoon of bifidobacterium. Bulgaricum should be taken before meals as well, and in a dose similar to acidophilus.

Do not conclude that the trinity of probiotics I have discussed in this section represent the entire list of beneficial bacteria. There are dozens of other possibilities. For example, many patients with candida overgrowth have done well with the administration of a laterospora species. The important lesson is that we all can benefit from a frequent dosing of a variety of probiotics.

DIGESTIVE AIDS: *Make our food available*

Most traditional nutritionists, in surveying a person's dietary adequacy, estimate the nutritional content of the foods taken in and start adding up the numbers. Their assumption, that people will absorb whatever they take in, is far from true. In fact, facilitating this absorption may be one of the best strategies in all of nutrition. Food and nutrient absorption is often obstructed, and correcting it can make a big difference.

You will need the help of a nutritionally oriented doctor to find if there are weak links in your digestive chain. If the doctor's lab tests reveal that your nutrient levels are below what should be expected, there are several digestive aids you might consider.

HYDROCHLORIC ACID

Symptoms such as fullness or flatulence or nausea after taking vitamins may provide you with the first clue that you have a deficiency of hydrochloric acid (HCl), our main stomach acid.

A lack of stomach acid is commonplace, the result of aging, genetics, use of certain medications and a variety of other factors.

Up to half of all people older than sixty do not secrete enough HCl, which provides the initial step in the digestion of protein. An insufficient amount of this acid can cause or aggravate all sorts of problems – including asthma[1], diabetes, food allergies, osteoporosis[2], iron-deficiency anaemia, pernicious anaemia and *Candida albicans* overgrowth.[3] Observations dating back seventy-five years link low HCl levels to rheumatoid arthritis, intestinal infections[4], and such skin conditions as psoriasis, vitiligo[5], hives, eczema, dermatitis, herpetiformis and acne[6]. It also may increase the risk of gastric cancer.

Low HCl also impairs the absorption of minerals and other nutrients, notably folic acid. If we do not thoroughly digest protein, to which folic acid is bound, we won't absorb it. The best way to determine your HCl need is through a Heidelberg test, or gastrogram, in which you will swallow an electrical transmitter (safe, small and disposable) that provides information about how well your stomach makes digestive acid.[7] A magnesium hydrogen breath test also can assess your need for the acid.[8]

Although replenishing HCl makes for a very valuable treatment, you should do this with a doctor's supervision. HCl, consumed in excess or when not needed, can irritate the gastrointestinal tract, cause ulcers or allow for a loss of minerals. The most commonly used agent for replacing stomach acid is a compound called betaine-HCl, which if taken just before eating will release enough HCl to replace a part of what is missing. It carries a risk of an overdose, which if not followed immediately by food can irritate the stomach lining. People with low HCl output can notice measurable benefits from taking two to four betaine-HCl tablets spaced throughout a meal.

PANCREATIC ENZYMES

Most nutrients enter the bloodstream from the small intestine, a coil some 6 metres long with a total absorption area roughly the size of a tennis court. After the stomach, the small intestine is the next stop along the digestive tract. Food (whether protein, fat or carbohydrate) is absorbed successfully here only if first broken down by pancreatic enzymes. Gas or bloating an hour or so after eating may signal a lack of these substances, but again, the best way to know is to take a laboratory test.

While enzymes that are derived from animals may be somewhat more effective, those derived from plants are better tolerated and remain active throughout the gastrointestinal tract. Animal-derived pancreatic enzymes work only in the alkaline environment of the small intestine; plant enzymes are also activated in acidic and neutral settings.

The failure to digest food will frequently lead to serious problems coming from an opposite direction. Many times we absorb large undigested particles, called macromolecules, which can do serious damage to our health. The condition, called 'leaky gut syndrome', leads to common problems such as food allergies, colitis and immune system weakness.

A fungal enzyme (the one best studied comes from *Aspergillus oryzae*) seems best equipped to correct the leaky gut phenomenon. It benefits the many gluten-intolerance, lactose-intolerance, food allergy and malabsorption-based symptoms that are so prevalent. In addition, it even helps dissolve clots in blood vessels, making it a candidate to replace standard anticoagulant therapy.[9]

SYSTEMIC ENZYME THERAPY

The three-thousand-plus enzymes in our bodies do more than digest food. They contribute to building DNA, reducing inflammation, strengthening immunity and fighting cancer, among other activities. Proteolytic enzymes, which digest protein, are of special therapeutic renown. The subject of some twenty-five years of research, much of it done in Germany, where they became known collectively as Wobenzyme therapy, the enzymes can foster healing in such problems as arthritis, immune insufficiency, pancreatitis and certain sports injuries.[10] Early laetrile investigators, followed by successful alternative cancer specialists such as William Donald Kelley, DDS, and Nicholas Gonzalez, MD[11], all incorporated these pancreas-derived enzymes into their anticancer protocols, and our doctors at the Atkins Center now administer them routinely to fight malignancies.

Achieving better digestion is not the objective here. If present in the bloodstream at a high round-the-clock level, according to the theory, pancreatic enzymes can erode the shield that tumour cells use to guard themselves from the immune system. A similar mechanism may work against autoimmune diseases. Taking my lead from German research demonstrating some help in controlling the acute setbacks suffered by many people with multiple sclerosis, I lob a preotolytic salvo whenever a flare-up strikes one of my MS patients. Many times the response is quick and dramatic.

Severe diseases such as cancer and MS require enzyme dosages that are extremely high. I may prescribe six to twenty tablets of crudely refined animal pancreas extracts so as to provide maximum potency in treating these patients. For digestive uses, one or two capsules of pancreatic enzymes with each meal is an appropriate dose. I must warn you that there is considerable variation from product to product. Therefore giving dosage advice might prove misleading.

FOS (FRUCTOOLIGOSACCHARIDES):
The beneficial sugars

For twenty-five years I've been warning people that long-term consumption of sugar is the surest way to create disease. Yet a special sugarlike digestive aid called FOS (fructooligosaccharides) may offer some benefits that table sugar could never provide: it might help lower high blood sugar and, equally improbable, aid in preventing cavities.

FOS turns these tricks because it's not absorbed by the body. Instead it's fodder for the friendly flora in our intestines. Consuming the compound allows our beneficial bacteria to grow and proliferate. The term applied to such benefactors of probiotics is 'prebiotics'. FOS is the most important of this group.[1] As they flourish, so can our health. Besides controlling cavities and bringing down diabetic blood sugars[2], FOS may favourably influence blood pressure, cholesterol and triglycerides, according to the small amount of research conducted so far. Again by

nourishing the friendly bacteria, it also can alleviate both constipation and diarrhoea.[3] I have found FOS a useful treatment for
relieving ulcer symptoms.

FOS is found naturally in many fruits and vegetables,
including bananas, onions, barley, tomatoes, asparagus and
garlic. You cannot obtain a therapeutic amount from food,
however, and the presence of other sugars diminishes or negates
its effect. For any possible health benefit, you need to ingest a
pure extract, either as a syrup or a powder.

SUPPLEMENT SUGGESTIONS

First-time FOS users should start off slowly. The body needs
some time to adjust to it. If the number of beneficial bacteria
in your intestines is low, big doses may cause diarrhoea. For a
better introduction, begin by taking 1/4 teaspoon daily with a
beneficial bacteria supplement. As the good bacteria population
increases, you'll more easily tolerate higher doses.

In the absence of major health problems, keep the daily dosage
at 1/4 teaspoon. If you have diabetes or high blood pressure,
build up to a dose of 1/2–1 teaspoon per day. Ulcer relief may
require 1–2 teaspoons daily. Be careful if you have a severe yeast
overgrowth; its most characteristic symptom is lower abdominal bloating and the gaseousness that accompanies it. A tiny
fraction of FOS's sugars (up to 3 per cent) will be digested;
some people may be extremely sensitive even to that small
amount.

To the taste buds, FOS is about half as sweet as other sugars,
so it can replace up to half of the sugar specified in many recipes.
You'll discover that the extract, especially the syrup, does a
terrific job of keeping foods moist.

CHARCOAL: *Poison absorber*

Every household should have some charcoal on hand. No, not
for an impromptu barbecue. For the medicine cabinet. Though
it should never be considered a daily supplement, charcoal is
the best poison remedy available, especially for drug overdoses.

Families that keep a ready supply of edible charcoal on hand, studies prove, are far better equipped to treat accidental poisoning in children.[1]

Charcoal will absorb just about anything – including, unfortunately, nutrients. That's why it can't be an everyday supplement, as well as why it can't be considered an antidote for dietary indiscretions (eating a lot of sugar or drinking too much alcohol, for example). It's an excellent emergency treatment for food poisoning, however, especially when combined with 2–4 drops of oil of oregano.

Many people take charcoal-based remedies to relieve flatulence, and it certainly is a blessing for occasional instances when intestinal gas is excessive or embarrassing. But charcoal is only a temporary palliative, addressing just the symptoms of a problem, not the cause. Flatulence is caused by poor digestion in the intestinal tract and the presence of bad bacteria. In the long run, supplements of digestive enzymes and beneficial bacteria are a more effective approach.

Supplement Suggestions

For a case of suspected poisoning, whether from food or a drug overdose, do not take some charcoal and assume everything will be okay. You still need to contact a doctor, a hospital accident and emergency department, or the local poison control centre. Taken repeatedly in *large doses,* charcoal may cause intestinal problems, which can be mitigated by consuming it along with some high-fibre food. As first aid for poisoning, a typical one-time dose would be 1 gram per kilogram, or 0.5 gram per 450 grams of body weight.

CHAPTER 9

◦◇◦

NUTRIENT-DENSE SUPERFOODS: ALL OF NATURE'S NUTRIENTS

While nature typically endows vegetables and other foods with generous amounts of individual nutrient complexes, some seem specially favoured and contain unusually broad arrays of nutrients in high concentrations. These nutrient-dense 'superfoods' provide for the growth of future generations of each species by gathering together every single nutrient expected to play a role in propagating the next generation. Seeking out such germinative foods would not only provide all synergistic nutrients without a single missing link, but would also supply any yet to be discovered nutrients. Especially if you don't eat a wide variety of protein foods and fresh vegetables, you should be sure to take advantage of at least one of these superfoods.

Supplements of these unique sources of nourishment are quite popular of late, although the concept is hardly new. The broad blend of nutrient complexes in brewer's yeast and liver extracts appealed to nutritionists two generations ago. Sadly, our antibiotic indulgences and other factors have given rise to millions of people with an overgrowth of the *Candida albicans* bacteria who cannot tolerate yeast in any form. Liver extracts, a concentrated source of most nutrients, have also fallen into disfavour, tainted by their association with the panoply of pesticides, hormones and toxic chemicals flooding our livestock and the earth's ecosystem.

Fortunately nature distributed the nutrient wealth to many other substances. Of them, I've selected a few favourites – barley and wheat grass, chlorella, spirulina, bee pollen, bee propolis and royal jelly.

BARLEY AND WHEAT GRASS JUICE:
The essence of sprouting grains

King Nebuchadnezzar of ancient Babylonia ate nothing but grasses for seven years to regain his health and mental clarity. I don't know if he started the first fad diet, but I do suspect that his meal plan represented the first medicinal use of cereal grasses.

Right out of the ground, wheat, barley, kamut and other grains are extraordinarily high in vitamins, minerals, chlorophyll, amino acids and other nutrients. As the grains grow, their carbohydrate counts increase and the nutrient concentration declines considerably. By the time they're harvested, milled, processed and packaged, they hold little or none of their initial nutritional value. However, ingesting concentrated forms of the young sprouts gives us a wonderful array of the whole food's therapeutic support.

Lab analyses show that extracts of wheat grass and barley contain compounds that may help protect cells from becoming cancerous.[1] Although we don't know if long-term use will actually prevent cancer in people, scientists have verified that the protective action is unique to the grasses and independent of any nutrient. The immune system also benefits.[2]

SUPPLEMENT SUGGESTIONS

Barley and wheat grass extracts are available in tablet and powdered form, but devotees insist that freshly juiced beverages, often called 'green drinks', are more therapeutic. The taste can be hard to take, yet many of my patients have reported overcoming serious illnesses by going on a fast that's punctuated with green juices. The powders and juices usually contain other health-promoting ingredients, such as herbal extracts and chlorella.

The concept of green drinks blends well with my overall dietary recommendations, although I suggest checking labels to see that the tonics or powders are low in carbohydrates and do not contain apple juice or other natural sweeteners. Even people who are sensitive to wheat can consume these products, because the proteins that might trigger allergic reactions have not yet formed in the young grasses.

CHLORELLA: *The chlorophyll connection*

A single-cell alga originally cultivated for third world countries as an inexpensive substitute for animal meats, chlorella turned out to offer us far more than protein. It could be the perfect antidote to some of the health problems caused by refined foods, nutrient-poor diets and our toxic environment.

Chlorella is loaded with nutrients and other unique compounds, including the B vitamins (it contains more pantothenic acid than any other natural source), magnesium and other trace minerals. Its high concentration of chlorophyll, a green pigment with remarkable cleansing qualities, is needed in any body detoxification or purification programme and as a source of organic iron. It also helps the body to eliminate cadmium and uranium, two toxic metals.[1] The alga's full spectrum of carotenoids is superior to beta-carotene alone for defending cells against oxidation. Another chemical constituent, chlorellan, fortifies our immune system by contributing to the production of interferon.

By stimulating the growth of beneficial bacteria in the intestines, chlorella promotes healing all along the gastrointestinal tract. Ulcers, colitis, Crohn's disease and diverticulosis all seem to improve when chlorella is added to the diet. Animal studies confirm that it helps to heal ulcers. For reducing high cholesterol, the alga (in a daily 5 gram dosage for three months) is as effective as many drugs – and free of side effects.[2] It's an excellent facial cleanser and can be applied directly to the skin to help wounds to heal. Some people claim that chlorella suppresses their appetites, although I haven't noticed the effect. Others find that it increases their energy and sense of well-being.

SUPPLEMENT SUGGESTIONS

For general health, most people can take just $1/2$ teaspoon of chlorella per day. If an ailment just mentioned is being dealt with, use 1–2 teaspoons. Bigger doses may be necessary for degenerative conditions, but take them only under the care of your physician. Don't start off by consuming larger amounts. The intestinal tract needs to get accustomed to chlorella.

Many strict vegetarians rely on chlorella and other such seaweed and algae for protein and vitamin B_{12}, based on the facts that the alga contains molecules similar to the B-complex nutrient and that it can elevate blood levels of the vitamin. But although half of chlorella's dry weight is easily assimilated protein, don't consider it a reliable source of B_{12}; strict vegetarians should still take supplemental B_{12}.

SPIRULINA: *The blue-green algae*

When sixteenth-century Spanish explorers saw the Aztecs harvesting this nutrient-dense alga, they dubbed it 'blue mud'. Spirulina, a name that encompasses a few thousand species of blue-green algae, has served people's health needs at least since the Aztecs' time. Cancer management might be the strongest therapeutic role of this wonderfully concentrated source of nutrients.[1] More research is clearly needed, but the initial studies have attracted some interest from scientists and nutritionists alike.

According to the results of animal experiments, spirulina enhances immune function, especially by stimulating the macrophages, special white blood cells that help eliminate waste from the body.[2] Some human research suggests that the alga may fight off oral malignancies. Scientists found that mouth lesions that are usually cancer precursors regressed completely for almost half of the tobacco chewers who took spirulina supplements for a year-long period.[3] The spirulina takers' blood levels of beta-carotene, one of the many nutrients in the algae, did not rise, which suggests that something else is deterring cancer.

SUPPLEMENT SUGGESTIONS

In addition to protein, B-complex vitamins, gamma-linolenic acid and a highly absorbable form of iron, spirulina contains what would seem to be vitamin B_{12}, a nutrient not otherwise found in plants. But as with chlorella, you cannot rely on the algae to satisfy the body's demand for this crucial nutrient. This form of B_{12} is not easily assimilated. The usual doses are 1–2 teaspoons or 6–9 tablets.

BEE PRODUCTS: *Pollen, propolis and royal jelly*

When you learned about the birds and the bees, were you told about the special link between nutrient supplementation and the reproductive system? This is essentially what bees do, helping to implement nature's master plan of concentrating nutrients in the reproductive systems of plants and animals. We're more familiar with germinative foods like nuts, seeds, roe and egg yolks, and they are indeed among the best food sources of nutrients. But by not taking advantage of the three bee products – pollen, propolis and royal jelly – we're depriving ourselves of the best of the best.

Bee Pollen Between the flower and the hive, pollen becomes a complete source of protein, vitamins, minerals and fatty acids, nourishing enough to sustain lab animals' lives over many generations.[1] It's an especially good source of rutin, a bioflavonoid that helps strengthen capillaries and treat glaucoma. Some research also suggests that bee pollen contains natural antibiotic compounds that may ward off salmonella and other harmful bacteria.[2]

The most exciting application, however, has been the treatment of benign enlargement of the prostate, prostatitis and other disorders of the gland. An extract from flower pollen has been used successfully in Europe for thirty years. And bee pollen could find itself alongside saw palmetto and pygeum for relieving the symptoms caused by prostate disease.[3] We're not sure yet what component of bee pollen possesses the therapeutic qualities. The nutrients, while plentiful, don't appear in sufficiently high amounts, so a unique compound as yet unidentified may in fact be responsible.

Bee Propolis Although considered a bee product, propolis is really a plant substance modified by bees. Flavonoids provide most of its healing activity, so think of it as a potent flavonoid extract prepared for us by our buzzing friends.

Bees use this sticky, resinous substance structurally, as an aid in constructing hives and plugging up holes. We can take advantage of its microbial protection, too. Research has documented its worth against parasites, fungal infections and viruses, especially herpes[4] and the flu.[5] Its antibacterial abilities are of significant value against upper-respiratory infections.[6] Probably because of the flavonoids, it's also an antioxidant.

Topically, propolis helps wounds heal; on the gums, it could be particularly useful for fighting periodontal disease. Applying it directly on cancerous cells, some animal studies have found, inhibited the malignancy and decreased the size of tumours by as much as 74 per cent.[7] When ingested, it can help heal ulcers. Although there's a paucity of clinical research on people, the initial work is encouraging.

Royal Jelly With her astounding size, longevity and reproductive assets, the queen bee doesn't rule by accident. She reigns over her parade of worker bees because they feed her nothing but royal jelly. Whether in the world of apians or *Homo sapiens,* this highly concentrated superfood is indeed fit for a queen.

Royal jelly has become a popular supplement for boosting energy, strengthening the adrenal glands and supporting the immune system. Of its many health-promoting advantages, the most important may be the ability to increase our nutrient absorption, allowing our bodies to get the most out of the food we eat. It's also a concentrated source of nutrients, including minerals, B vitamins and compounds unavailable anywhere else. For example, scientists have identified two unique antibacterial substances that reside within it: a protein called royalisin and a fatty acid dubbed 10-HDA. Other, perhaps stronger, bacterial killers may await our discovery, because the whole royal jelly displays ten times the disinfectant power of either isolated compound. I think it's another testament to the therapeutic whole being greater than the sum of its nutrient parts.

Included among the chemical components of royal jelly are precursors to human hormones, which validates the substance's traditional use as a fertility-enhancing food. It also works somewhat like insulin in the body.[8] Other research has affirmed its ability to lower total cholesterol and improve the LDL-HDL ratio.[9] In addition, when injected into the body, according to animal experiments, royal jelly opposes cancer. Lab mice with cancer remained alive and healthy for more than twelve months after receiving shots of either 10-HDA or whole, unprocessed royal jelly. Mice that didn't receive the supplement died within twelve days.[10]

SUPPLEMENT SUGGESTIONS

Given my oft repeated concern about natural sugars and their deleterious effects on our health, you may wonder how I can recommend other products from nature's honey makers. Some manufacturers may add honey or other sweeteners to their products, but in their natural forms, bee pollen, propolis and royal jelly don't contain appreciable amounts of honey or carbohydrates (although in a few unusually sensitive cases of diabetes or insulin resistance the food supplements may not be advisable). Most people can take full advantage of them, based on the following guidelines:

- *Royal jelly* Looking more like a yellowish paste than jelly and with a slightly bitter taste, it usually is stocked in the refrigerated sections of health food stores. Local beekeepers also supply it. Get minimally processed royal jelly that is not freeze-dried;

its proteins and delicate fatty acids are more likely to be intact. Avoid honey-laden mixtures that are more sweetener than substance. I'd recommend a dosage of 1/4 teaspoon per day, taken on an empty stomach. Weeks or months may pass before you notice an increase in energy or other benefits, but it is worth the wait.

• *Bee pollen* If you are at all sensitive to pollens, use care in taking these supplements. Bee pollen can provoke an allergic reaction like any other pollen. Most pollen devotees take 1 teaspoon of the granules every morning. Its high nutrient density makes a good addition to a health shake.

• *Bee propolis* Alcohol tinctures may be the most powerful way to get propolis's anti-immune and anti-infection protection. The usual preventive dose is 1/2 dropperful of the tincture stirred into tea or water. For a cold, the flu or another respiratory infection, I'd suggest 2 droppersful. You may also want to try an herbal propolis spray or cough syrup. Some people are sensitive to it, however, and may occasionally develop contact dermatitis. Apply a little of it to a small area of skin to make sure you are not overly sensitive.

Some pollen-producing companies use all three apiary products together. One such product administered together in large doses in a single morning played an important historical role in creating the US federal Office of Alternative Medicine (OAM). The beneficiary was Senator Tom Harkin of Iowa, and the quick eradication of his allergies led him to conclude that alternative therapies may be worth looking into. Harkin has since become the US Senate's foremost champion of alternative medicine and the driving force behind the OAM.

CHAPTER 10

VITA-NUTRIENTS WITH UNIQUE ROLES

COENZYME Q$_{10}$ (UBIQUINONE): *The vital nutrient*

When I coined the word 'vita-nutrient', I was thinking of co-enzyme Q$_{10}$, or CoQ$_{10}$. It is neither vitamin (the body can make it from other nutrients) nor mineral nor amino acid, yet it is absolutely vital to our health and vital that we get enough of it. CoQ$_{10}$ is essential to energy production in our every cell, allowing the cells to live longer. It is universally present in the body, so much so that science formally named it 'ubiquinone'.

Focused on their circumscribed methodology, early research-ers never asked why a supposedly 'nonessential' biochemical was ubiquitous. Fortunately some progressive investigators did ask, and they eventually learned the answer: in high enough amounts it performs an entire gamut of functions essential to optimum health. Nature, it seems, must want it to be made available to all part of our bodies.

Far beyond producing energy, CoQ$_{10}$ can protect the body from destructive free radicals and enhance our immune defences, making it extremely important in preventing and treating heart disease, diabetes, periodontal disease, high blood pressure, obesity, cancer and a growing list of neurological conditions.

On top of all this, it may help put the brakes on the aging process.

All the benefits on this laundry list are attainable – but only when we provide ourselves with an optimal amount of CoQ_{10}, which can be attained only with supplements. Food contains only trace amounts, and our bodies manufacture it in sometimes adequate, but never optimal, quantities. Deficiencies, unfortunately, are quite common.

Health Starts with the Heart

All organs with high energy demands need a lot of CoQ_{10}, and the most important is the heart. At the beginning of 1990, some fifty studies around the world attested to CoQ_{10}'s impact on cardiomyopathy, arrhythmia, coronary artery disease, congestive heart failure, mitral valve prolapse and hypertension.[1] When people who needed heart transplants took the nutrient, their conditions improved so remarkably that transplant surgery was no longer necessary.[2] When administered following a coronary bypass operation, CoQ_{10} reduces recovery time. And three separate studies showed that when 100 mg was given daily to several thousand people suffering from heart failure, more than 75 per cent displayed improvements in pulmonary function, oedema and heart palpitations – with no side effects.[3] Nothing in mainstream cardiology comes close to this kind of success. I am at a loss to explain why CoQ_{10} is not prescribed routinely to every heart patient.

I'm particularly impressed by CoQ_{10}'s therapeutic strength in treating cardiomyopathy, a mixed bag of conditions impairing the heart muscle that collectively are the third most common form of cardiovascular disease. Cardiomyopathy often is the most life-threatening of all heart conditions, and it's probably the number one reason that people undergo a heart transplant operation. Supplementation improves the prognosis in so many instances that I think the condition is best described as a CoQ_{10} deficiency.[4]

Generous doses of CoQ_{10} have helped a clear majority of my cardiomyopathy patients, and several of them, who were on the waiting list for a donor heart, found that their old heart would do just fine. My experience is by no means unique, as the abundant research documents.[5] In one study, 87 per cent of 126 cardiomyopathy patients displayed noticeable improvements in heart function, again without adverse effects, after taking 100 mg per day.[6]

The virtual absence of side effects could arguably be CoQ_{10}'s foremost advantage. Drugs merely mask symptoms; they don't solve the underlying problem, which for most heart disease is the continued presence of atherosclerotic plaque buildups that ultimately block blood vessels. Most cardiovascular drugs not only fail to deal with hardening of the arteries, but in many cases compound it, exposing people to even greater perils. CoQ_{10}, in contrast, deals effectively with most of the factors that cause atherosclerosis.

The heart is utterly dependent on CoQ_{10} to meet its constant energy needs; the muscle contains twice as much of the nutrient as any other organ or tissue in the body. People with heart disease have 25 per cent less CoQ_{10} than their healthy counterparts. Should the deficiency reach 75 percent, some experts have speculated, the heart would stop beating.[7]

Perhaps this explains why lovastatin and the other overprescribed cholesterol-lowering drugs have such a mediocre record for saving lives: one of their side effects is inhibiting the body's natural ability to make CoQ_{10}. One investigation documented six cases of cardiomyopathy that were caused by lovastatin. Cholesterol drugs are self-defeating in another CoQ_{10}-related way. The ubiquitous quinone actually is a good antioxidant, helping to prevent the oxidation of LDL cholesterol, considered to be the most artery-clogging substance of all.[8] Because CoQ_{10} migrates naturally to the heart, some researchers suggest that it may be the most important of all antioxidants for preventing atherosclerosis.[9]

High Blood Pressure Hypertension is a major risk factor for heart disease, but CoQ_{10}'s contribution to overcoming the disorder is worth mentioning separately. In no small part because of the nutrient, some 85 per cent of all people we treat for high blood pressure can end their reliance on antihypertension medications. More than a few studies confirm that dosages of

60–100 mg per day will significantly lower blood pressure readings.[10] This ability accounts for why I occasionally caution people with low blood pressure against taking CoQ_{10}: it might lower their blood pressure even more.

Diabetes Diabetes is arguably the most common metabolic cause of heart disease. Happily, a daily CoQ_{10} dose of 60 mg can help reduce high blood sugar within six months.[11] Because hardening of the arteries is a frequently encountered complication of diabetes, CoQ_{10} is doubly important.

Obesity Decades spent watching overweight people become slim and trim convince me that the Atkins diet, or another low-carbohydrate eating plan, is the surest way to shed excess weight. CoQ_{10} lends its weight to reducing yours, researchers think, by facilitating the use of stored fat as fuel. About half of the people with weight problems lack a sufficient amount of the energy nutrient, which may help explain why obese people are prone to both heart disease and diabetes.

CoQ_{10}'s value is plain to see in a study of overweight people following a low-calorie diet. Those who were deficient in the nutrient took a daily 100 mg supplement of the nutrient; the others received no additional nutritional support. After two months the supplement takers had lost 13.5 kilograms – considerably more than the 6 kilograms that their counterparts dropped.[12]

Cancer The presence of cancer correlates strongly with a reduced amount of CoQ_{10}. Complementary practitioners have long known this, and animal studies reinforce the link. The inverse of this relationship is becoming quite apparent, too, and I'm now convinced that CoQ_{10} should be a permanent fixture in cancer therapy. If the research conclusions are true for all people, we may have found something that can stop certain malignancies dead in their tracks.

Several years ago Danish researchers gave daily 390 mg in supplements (quite a hefty dose) to members of a group of women with metastatic breast cancer. After several months the cancer went into remission for four women. After eleven months one woman's cancer, which had spread from the breast to the liver, was completely gone, and doctors reported that her health was excellent.[13]

Dosage is apparently the key here. In an earlier trial, the Danish researchers gave 90 mg per day to a different group of breast cancer patients. That amount didn't reverse the malignant onslaught, although it probably helped to prolong the women's lives.[14]

Like most other complementary cancer therapies, CoQ_{10} seems to work by revitalizing the immune system, not by directly attacking a tumour. If that's true, we're all the more disadvantaged because of some convoluted regulations imposed on cancer investigators by the US National Cancer Institute. The NCI authorizes research into potentially therapeutic substances only if they are 'effective agents'. The institute defines 'effective' as the ability to kill tumour cells. If a substance opposes cancer in any other way, it doesn't qualify. CoQ_{10} (or any other harmless, nontoxic agent that helps our own cancer defences get the job done) is therefore deemed 'ineffective' and intrinsically worthless. This stipulation encourages scientists to work only with radiation therapy and chemotherapeutic drugs, both often futile and lethal treatments.

Other Illnesses The full therapeutic reach of CoQ_{10} is still largely unknown. It may not turn out to be a panacea, but many studies suggest a wide world of possibilities. Against Alzheimer's disease, to use one example, CoQ_{10} joined iron and vitamin B_6 in minimizing symptoms of dementia and slowing progressive memory loss. For some people in the study, symptoms actually improved enough that researchers diagnosed them as 'normal'.[15]

Other work suggests a role for the energy enzyme in preventing miscarriages and treating tinnitus, Ménière's disease, Bell's palsy, deafness, muscular dystrophy,[16] Huntington's disease,[17] ulcers and a low sperm count.[18] Seven different clinical trials demonstrated its ability to reverse periodontal disease.[19] Because it fortifies the immune system, CoQ_{10} also enriches my overall treatment of chronic fatigue syndrome. For the same reason, it even may help people infected with HIV.

Fatigue For an everyday advantage, I've saved the best for last. Partly because it's an antioxidant and partly because it helps turn food into energy, CoQ_{10} is a fatigue fighter par excellence. It is especially valuable for elite athletes, such as marathoners and triathlon participants, who must perform under prolonged aerobic conditions. This activity generates free radicals capable of damaging the mitochondria, the little energy-generating furnaces inside each of our cells. It is here that CoQ_{10} exerts much of its protective power. In all probability, athletes who 'burn out' prematurely and can no longer perform as they once did are, in fact, victims of a relative CoQ_{10} deficiency.

People with health problems will notice more of an improvement from using supplements than will elite athletes. When, for example, a group of people with chronic lung disease took 90 mg of CoQ_{10} for eight weeks, they showed significant normalization of their oxygen levels. In contrast, a similar group of sedentary but otherwise healthy young men gained only a moderate (3–12 per cent) improvement in pulmonary capacity.[20]

In those rare conditions where the mitochondria are the focus of illness, such as mitochondrial encephalomyopathy, CoQ_{10} administration produces a dramatic reversal of symptoms.[21]

SUPPLEMENT SUGGESTIONS

Our need for CoQ_{10} supplements can be pronounced, especially after the age of forty, when we begin to make less of the nutrients. The body's production peaks around the age of twenty, declining to some 60 per cent below that mark by the time we are eighty years old. Low-fat dieters probably have lower than average body stores of CoQ_{10} because our best food sources are organ meats (such as heart and kidney), other red meats, nuts and unprocessed vegetable oils. Cereal bran and dark green vegetables will provide a lesser amount. Consuming the nutrient with an oil or a fat improves our absorption, while our own internal production depends on the presence of a sufficient amount of the B-complex vitamins.

I take CoQ_{10} every day, and I prescribe it readily to anyone who has a health problem related to the heart, blood pressure, metabolism, energy level or cancer. That seems to be just about everyone I treat. In most instances 90 mg a day is the bare minimum required to get a therapeutic response. For cancer protection the usual dose is 200–400 mg a day.

Unpublished studies circulating within the vitamin industry suggest that much of the commercially available CoQ_{10} is poorly absorbed or assimilated. Products labeled 'hydrosoluble' are claimed to achieve significantly higher blood levels. If you find such a product, you may be able to get equivalent results with one-half the dose.

LIPOIC ACID: *Proven diabetic treatment*

Lipoic acid, alpha-lipoic acid or thioctic acid – whatever you want to call it, the fact remains that until a few years ago no one ever heard of it. Today, however, progressive health advocates recognize it as a universal antioxidant and a major treatment for diabetic neuropathy. If it lives up to what the research suggests, lipoic acid will become one of our most precious nutrients for helping stave off many of the repercussions of high blood sugar and perhaps even the aging process itself.

The crux of lipoic acid's power is its dual role in the body. Like the team member who can play both attack and defence, it can act as an antioxidant and as a protector of both water-soluble and fat-soluble antioxidants, including glutathione, vitamin C, vitamin E and coenzyme Q_{10}.[1] This is a feat no other nutrient can accomplish. Additionally, lipoic acid encourages the body to convert food into energy more efficiently, helps prevent what we eat from being deposited as fat, and participates in the cleanup of toxins and other by-products of fat metabolism.

The Diabetes Defence

Few compounds are of greater value to someone with diabetes, whether they have Type I or Type II, two quite different disorders. Basing my opinion on work done in Europe, where it's been used for some thirty years, I'm convinced that lipoic acid is destined to become our single most effective therapy for diabetic neuropathy. Especially since no other therapeutic help exists, it's an excellent example of a natural substance deserving, but not receiving, the ranking of treatment of choice; in this case diabetes' painful degeneration of nerves in the arms and legs.

In one study, a daily dosage of between 300 and 600 mg of lipoic acid decreased neuropathy pain within twelve weeks, although actual nerve function did not improve.[2] Long-lasting relief was brought about in another study with both oral and intravenous dosages of 600 mg.[3] In yet another experiment, researchers calculated an 80 per cent improvement in symptoms after 320 people hospitalized for neuropathy took a three-week course of the nutrient.[4]

Excess sugar in the bloodstream causes diabetic retinopathy's nerve damage. The process, called 'glycation', is one of the major forms of cellular destruction that scientists associate with aging. Anything that keeps a tighter rein on glucose levels, then, could slow, if not quite reverse, some of the consequences of growing older.

Lipoic acid fights insulin resistance and markedly stimulates our cells' uptake of glucose. For example, a 1,000 mg intravenous dose increased cellular glucose uptake by 50 per cent. The results of animal experiments demonstrate that lipoic acid also protects the pancreatic cells that manufacture insulin. The destruction of these cells leads to Type I diabetes and the consequent reliance on insulin injections. Theoretically lipoic acid should be useful as part of a treatment for the earliest stages of Type I, when not all insulin cells on the pancreas have been killed off. I've started to use it for that purpose, but I have not treated enough of these patients to report my conclusions.

Meeting Universal Needs

Anyone who is overweight or follows a high-carbohydrate diet risks developing an insulin disorder, so lipoic acid is potentially useful to most of us. Other common health perils also increase the need. The nutrient slows all forms of free radical oxidation, whether in the arteries or in the eyes. In the brain it may assist in curbing or preventing the cell damage of Alzheimer's disease.[5]

Animal research already has demonstrated its ability to enhance memory and cognitive function.

Lipoic acid is also a powerful protector of the liver, where it fends off alcohol's toxic effects, according to one study of wine drinkers.[6] It's also a vital component of any AIDS therapy because it inhibits HIV replication. It also might be useful as a chelating agent, especially to rid the body of excess copper.

SUPPLEMENT SUGGESTIONS

In the absence of any medical problems, a good daily lipoic acid dosage ranges from 100 to 300 mg. Take some vitamin B_1, too, as a supporting nutrient. For conditions that require a full antioxidant response to overcome metabolic resistance to losing weight, I prescribe between 300 and 600 mg per day. As part of a programme to treat diabetes, cancer or AIDS, I use 600–900 mg.

Except for rare skin reactions, lipoic acid has no adverse effects and no drug interactions. The only possible medicinal consequence would be the need for diabetics to reduce their dependence on insulin or other antidiabetic drug under the guidance of a doctor. But this, after all, should be one of your main objectives.

PHOSPHATIDYL SERINE: *The smart nutrient*

Of all the brain nutrients I use and recommend, phosphatidyl serine (PS) may be the most effective. By maximizing nerve transmission between brain cells and supplying them with this extremely valuable nutrient, PS may reverse, as one researcher concluded, more than a decade's worth of age-related mental decline.

I think of PS as a biological detergent for our brains. It keeps cell membranes fluid, fats soluble and brain neurons flexible. It can also actually increase the number of receptor sites on brain cells, giving us more docking points and circuits for neural communication. The combined impact improves memory, energizes thinking and counteracts stress-related neurological damage. Mental performance improves even for people with Alzheimer's disease or Parkinson's disease.

Age-Proofing Your Brain

Our brains are awash in essential fatty acids and phospholipids, one of which is phosphatidyl serine. About 60 per cent of our brain tissue is fat, and if enough isn't on hand, the brain just won't work right. The relationship between mental health and dietary fat is an important one. Without fats the brain can't produce and transmit electrical energy smoothly. A lack of phospholipids like PS also slows our mental processes, no matter what our age. As some two dozen studies show, replenishing the PS supply boosts brain power, mood and learning ability, with the most pronounced benefits seen among older people.

The therapeutic effect helps against serious mental and neurological problems, as we'll soon see, and against 'normal' age-related memory loss, as demonstrated in a study of 149 people over the age of fifty. Some of them took 300 mg of PS daily for twelve weeks, while the others took placebos. At the end of the experiment the PS users improved their scores on memory and learning tests by 15 per cent. The people who had the greatest impairment in their mental faculties improved the most. The benefits remained for up to four weeks after the subjects stopped taking the nutrient. One of the study's authors concluded that PS seems to reverse about twelve years of mental decline.[1]

Stress Damage Taking PS regularly can tame the body's production of cortisol, one of the hormones secreted in response to emotional or physical stress. Intense exercise and the mere process of aging also generate a larger output of cortisol. While the hormone is essential to our lives, too much takes quite a toll. An excess can prevent the brain from feeding on glucose, inhibit communication among brain cells, injure blood vessels, break down muscle tissue and weaken the immune system, to name but a few of its consequences.

Seasonal Depression I prescribe PS for all of the people I treat for depression. It's particularly useful for easing seasonal affective disorder, the wintertime blues caused by lack of exposure to natural light. Without causing any complications, the nutrient can be taken right along with antidepressant medications, although many of my patients tell me they no longer need those drugs when they're using PS.

Parkinson's Disease Changes in phospholipid levels are associated with a deficiency of dopamine, the neurotransmitter absent in the brains of people with Parkinson's disease. Medicine has been aware of this for more than two decades, yet it promotes drug therapy with L-dopa to treat this degenerative neurological disease. Supplements of PS, in doses of 300–500 mg daily for three to six months, have substantially increased brain activity, as measured with modern scanning techniques.[2]

Alzheimer's Disease People afflicted with an early onset of this memory-destroying condition show a dramatically greater use of energy by their brain cells with regular use of phosphatidyl serine. They recalled names better, remembered the locations of misplaced objects, recounted more details of recent events and displayed more intense concentration. This is front-page news, and all of us should be excited to know that nutrition, not drugs, holds the power to preserve or reverse the brain damage that occurs as we age.

Exercise Recovery High-intensity physical activity triggers the release of cortisol and other stress hormones that break down muscle tissue. In an attempt to limit the increased secretion, bodybuilders and other athletes are taking PS supplements.[3]

Alcoholic Influences You won't find this described in any research studies. Taken before a wine-tasting party or similar event, PS can make you noticeably more resistant to alcohol's inebriating effect. Even though you will still need to appoint a designated driver, you will be in considerably better control of your senses. PS will not protect your liver or your waistline from the effects of alcohol. I'm not encouraging drinking; I'm encouraging sobriety.

SUPPLEMENT SUGGESTIONS

PS is very safe and has no side effects. As with any brain-energizing nutrient, don't take it in the evening because it may keep you awake. It's best used as a brain awakener before breakfast. The usual dose is 300 mg per day for a month, after which you can take the maintenance dose of 100 mg per day. If you're depressed, suffer from seasonal affective disorder, or have Alzheimer's or Parkinson's, you may need to take 300–500 mg per day indefinitely. Because it's a fat, PS is vulnerable to free radical damage and should therefore be taken with some antioxidant support from vitamin E, vitamin C and selenium.

You can't boost your PS reserves through diet. It is present in nearly all foods, but only in trace amounts. That's why even though soya is used to make the PS products available in health food stores, you can't obtain it by taking lecithin, itself rich in other phospholipids. The body's production is also far from the optimal quantity needed.

For the past decade there has been considerable interest in taking 'smart drugs', the term applied to pharmaceuticals that enhance brain function. But now that vita-nutrients such as PS, acetylcarnitine and NADH are available over the counter, the benefit-to-risk ratio has escalated exponentially, and the pharmaceuticals are destined to play a smaller and smaller role.

DMSO: *The healing penetrant*

You might wonder why I've included a paint solvent in this book. DMSO (dimethyl sulfoxide) is an extraordinary natural curative. Whether used topically or intravenously, it promotes wound healing, eases pain, prevents cellular deterioration and ameliorates the symptoms of a wide variety of autoimmune diseases. From sprained ankles and arthritis discomfort to previously untreatable urinary dysfunction, the sheer number of health problems for which DMSO can be used seems too good to be true.

More than forty thousand studies have been done on DMSO, many of them concentrated on the health benefits for humans. The conclusions, while not unanimous, overwhelmingly reaffirm the solvent's value.[1] In exchange for its alleviating influence, however, users must tolerate an unusual side effect – a most unpleasant smell that emanates from their breath and body.

The aroma, reminiscent of garlic, is certainly one reason we don't use DMSO at the Atkins Center as regularly as it deserves to be used. When we do use it, an olfactory remnant stays in the building for days. Its unmistakable presence may, at least in part, explain why scientists haven't performed double-blind studies on DMSO. The absence of wide-scale use, I think, can be attributed more to its small profit potential than to its lack of safety or effectiveness.

THE SCENT OF SUCCESS

In America, the FDA has frequently obstructed research into DMSO, relenting only to authorize several narrowly defined uses: to preserve organs for transplant, to treat closed-head injuries and to relieve a painful bladder condition called interstitial cystitis. Yet DMSO can be used for so much more. Its biggest application may be pain relief, which it probably achieves by blocking conduction of the nerve fibres that transmit pain signals.[2] Still, the FDA seems reluctant to allow anyone to document this use. The irony (or, perhaps, the reason) is that DMSO would probably prove much safer and more effective than many of today's commonly prescribed medications. It often works when standard painkillers fail.[3]

Three other qualities compound DMSO's worth: it's an antioxidant, a skin penetrant and an anti-inflammatory. All together, it sounds tailor-made for people with *arthritis* – and it is. In this area I use it or its biological cousin, methyl sulfonyl methane (MSM), with good results. The dearth of published work in treating arthritis is therefore rather strange. Other applications are documented a little more fully.

Ulcers DMSO compares very favourably with the popular ulcer drug cimetidine. In one experiment, 220 people with a duodenal ulcer began to take 500 mg of DMSO orally every day. By the end of the study they had fewer than half of the ulcer recurrences experienced by people taking cimetidine alone.[4]

Scleroderma This usually fatal disorder, in which fibrous tissue grows through the skin and internal organs, wouldn't be considered untreatable if medicine looked a little closer at DMSO. It brought about remarkable results for twenty-six of forty-two scleroderma patients who participated in one small study.[5] In addition, the solvent apparently is the most effective treatment available for sparing the kidneys from secondary amyloidosis, in which sclerodermalike fibrillar growths occur in conjunction with certain chronic diseases.[6]

Interstitial Cystitis For years conventional medicine has ignored this curious bladder problem, discounting as unfounded the complaints of hundreds of sufferers, almost all of them women. No infection or other abnormality has ever been identified, yet the symptoms, including pain or a burning sensation upon urinating and an almost constant urge to void, are real. DMSO is one of the few substances that will relieve the agony. A majority of the women in one large study benefitted measurably from a DMSO cocktail that included steroids, heparin and bicarbonate injected into the bladder through the urethra.[7] The results were so consistently good that in America the FDA felt compelled to allow the solvent's use for this one condition. In so doing, it allowed tens of thousands of patients to demonstrate its safety for human use.

Absorption Problems When DMSO penetrates the skin, which it does quickly, it brings along whatever else is mixed with it, and this allows for some fascinating applications. Digestion problems, we know, impair nutrient absorption in older people, leaving them vulnerable to any number of health problems. In a study of macular degeneration, a group of older people improved their sight simply by rubbing on their skin a DMSO solution that contained nutrients known to reverse the course of this degenerative eye disease. The penetration proclivity, rivalled only by another natural substance, hyaluronic acid, also enhances an antifungal drug's effectiveness against toenail infections and alpha-interferon's work against genital herpes. It also dissolves certain hemorrhoids overnight.

Sprained Ankles One of DMSO's most widely used applications, especially by a number of professional sports teams, is the treatment of sprained ankles. Rubbing it directly on the injured joint relieves pain and reduces swelling within an hour. You may assume that the ankle is not the only site where DMSO-responsive sprains can take place.

SUPPLEMENT SUGGESTIONS

The quality of DMSO varies widely. I recommend a pharmaceutical-grade brand that is between 50 and 70 per cent pure dimethyl sulfoxide. You also should use it only under the supervision of a health care practitioner who is familiar with it. Because of the terrific absorbency, special care must be exercised. DMSO will draw into the bloodstream virtually anything that's on your skin. Thoroughly wash and rinse the area on which you will apply it. The same goes for your hands.

CALCIUM AEP (COLAMINE PHOSPHATE):
The most underrated nutrient; autoimmune saviour

For a nutrient with an almost priceless medicinal value, calcium AEP (colamine phosphate) is tragically underused and pitifully underresearched. It's the first mineral I turn to when treating multiple sclerosis, Type I diabetes and most other illnesses that stem from a self-destructive immune system disorder.

The calcium salt of 2 amino ethanol phosphate, or calcium AEP, is widely distributed throughout our bodies, yet we do not know its function. But the few doctors who work with it understand that it offers true therapeutic hope against autoimmune diseases, conditions where the immune system turns on the body's own cells, attacking joints or nerves or other tissues as if they were a virus or some other foreign substance.

Conventional medicine offers no effective therapy for autoimmune disorders other than prednisonelike steroids and drugs that suppress the immune system and thereby expose people to a variety of hazardous side effects. Calcium AEP doesn't do that. For an autoimmune condition like MS, it allows for real neurological improvements. And it doesn't work for just a handful of people; it works for a majority.

One doctor, Hans Nieper, MD, deserves all the credit for discovering the impressive benefits of calcium AEP over thirty-five years ago. The German oncologist and cardiologist has administered it with great results to more than four thousand people. I've treated more than one thousand or so of my own patients with it and can attest to Nieper's clinical findings.

The hardest part is notifying the rest of the world. Since the initial publications of Nieper's research in 1966–68, virtually no other researcher has bothered to experiment with this remarkable substance. Thus, sadly enough, it is invaluable but remains largely ignored.

NOT YOUR ORDINARY CALCIUM

Perhaps I should refer to calcium AEP by its other name, colamine phosphate. When I extol its virtues, a patient typically will say, 'But I'm already taking calcium. I don't need any more.' Well, this is not your average calcium supplement. AEP is the therapeutic workhorse in this compound. It transports minerals such as calcium, magnesium and potassium to positions along cell membranes, which serve to protect the cells from harm while allowing nutrients and biochemicals to enter. Based on these actions, Nieper calls calcium AEP 'membrane integrity factor', or vitamin M_i, for short.

The safeguard provided by AEP is ideally suited to treat any autoimmune disorder – including rheumatoid arthritis, lupus, scleroderma, Crohn's disease, colitis, pulmonary fibrosis and gastritis. Although I use colamine phosphate whenever a blood test reveals an increase in ANA, a biochemical associated with autoimmune malfunctions, the most astounding results appear in people with MS or early-stage Type I diabetes.

Multiple Sclerosis During the early stages of this autoimmune disorder, marked by the immune system's erosion of myelin, the protective covering that surrounds our nerves, colamine phosphate usually provides significant relief, if not a complete remission. People are more coordinated, feel less limb numbness, experience fewer muscle spasms and often have a dramatic increase in energy. The therapeutic help is not as consistently beneficial when the disease is far advanced. But my experience places it light-years ahead of any conventional therapies now used.

However, don't take my word for it. Ask people who have tried it. Some 63 per cent of Nieper's 151 American patients have said their MS improved with calcium AEP. Another 19 per cent reported that their MS had stabilized, a result considered equally remarkable in this progressively debilitating disease. Only 3 per cent reported that their health grew worse, the unfortunate fate of most people treated conventionally for MS. My patients' results are similar to Nieper's. Most of them say they experience less fatigue, improved bladder function, a steadier walking gait, more strength, better balance, improved coordination, less arm and leg numbness, and fewer muscle spasms.

Contrast these results with those of beta-interferon, the expensive, widely promoted, officially sanctioned drug treatment for MS. The medical community has marvelled at its so-called success, yet beta-interferon merely allows the disease to progress more slowly. When failure becomes the standard for success, the futility of mainstream offerings is made clear.

Insulin-Dependent Diabetes My most dramatic successes with calcium AEP have come with people in the initial stages of Type I diabetes. Here the immune system assaults the pancreatic cells that manufacture insulin. When a sufficient number of cells are destroyed, the body can no longer make enough insulin to help metabolize the sugars in food. Daily insulin injections must then compensate for loss of the hormone, and a lifelong struggle begins against blood sugar instability and its many undesirable consequences. However, regular calcium AEP injections can keep the disease away for years – provided we catch it soon enough, which is usually the snag. By the time a person is typically diagnosed with Type I, his or her insulin-making machinery has been irreparably damaged. Marie Speller, whom you learned about on page 19, is one of our AEP successes, but we have not yet been referred enough patients with early Type I diabetes to know how consistently we can forestall the destruction. Perhaps the awareness this book may provide will give the world a chance to bring this illness under control.

Cancer Curiously, few of Nieper's MS patients have developed cancer, which goes against the odds and suggests that calcium AEP might somehow prevent the disease. He feels confident that further research will confirm some role for calcium AEP in decreasing the risk of cancer. Let's hope he's right. The idea of calcium attached to a molecule that transports it to its target means calcium AEP would help restore bone loss from osteoporosis or bone cancer. Nieper's experience in both has led him to tell me it is his treatment of choice.

SUPPLEMENT SUGGESTIONS

Injectable calcium AEP isn't available to the average supplement user and you will need to find a doctor who is familiar with it or who will at least agree to administer it to you. For the full therapeutic punch, it must be injected intravenously but never intramuscularly. The most commonly used dosage is 400 mg from a 10 cc vial, injected three times a week.

Oral forms, either calcium AEP or a mixture of calcium, magnesium and potassium salts of AEP, are available by mail order. I give them to my patients to enhance the effects of the injections, but on their own they simply do not possess the effectiveness of intravenous calcium AEP.

CREATINE: *What muscles are made of*

Creatine is one of the most plentiful and important protein substances in the body. It is the major substrate for phosphocreatine, which fuels our muscle contractions, so it is logical that competitive athletes are now trying it.

Most of us carry about 120–140 grams of creatine in our muscles, but the nutrient is not essential to our diet. Vegetarians take in essentially no creatine, yet they are rarely deficient, manufacturing it from the dietary amino acids arginine, glycine and methionine.

A Proven Performance Enhancer

The value of creatine seems to be in enhancing short-term athletic performance, such as sprints, bursts of cycling and weight lifting. Doses of 20–25 grams have been used in most studies.[1,2] Creatine appears to work by helping to keep our supplies of immediate energy high. It also prevents plasma levels of ammonia from climbing, which otherwise would slow athletic performance. There is no evidence that creatine improves our long-term stamina. But it does allow weight lifters to increase muscle mass by about 1.8 kilograms, according to a Swedish sports physiologist.[3]

Its Medical Value

Therapeutically, creatine appears to be useful in treating and preventing disturbances in the heart's rhythm. For fifty people who were undergoing an operation to replace a heart valve, supplementation reduced arrhythmias by 75 per cent.[4] People with chronic heart failure have also used the supplement, in a daily dosage of 20 grams, to increase their exercise capacity.[5] Other research suggests it may have some anticancer activity.[6]

Supplement Suggestions

The effective dosage for creatine appears to be about 20 grams per day, which can be expensive. It's not clear that smaller doses are of any benefit. Its full use, then, may be limited to elite athletes, heavy-duty weight trainers and people with certain heart conditions. The 20 gram dosage appears to be very safe and without side effects. A dose in that range is best taken in powder form (sold at health food stores). Four teaspoons (that's 20 grams) are recommended as a dose before a workout.

OCTACOSANOL: *Reliable brain fuel*

In the early days of my nutritional career, I was fortunate enough to work side by side with Dr Carlton Fredericks, one of the true greats in nutritional medicine. With tube feedings of octacosanol, he helped dozens of people emerge from comas that had left conventional doctors scratching their heads. The cases were so numerous and the results so dramatic that no one familiar with them could conclude anything but that octacosanol is a miraculously effective brain nutrient. But though the results are impressive, few medical studies have examined or attempted to explain its powers. The sad truth is this: no studies means no mainstream acceptance. So people in a coma will continue to miss the opportunity to benefit from octacosanol.

I began my own therapeutic use of octacosanol by prescribing it to patients complaining of a general lack of energy. Impressed by their improvements, I turned my attention to a group of people whose fatigue was associated with brain damage – multiple sclerosis (a lack of stamina is one of the autoimmune disorder's most prevalent symptoms). Hundreds of them have since gone on to live fuller, more active lives. I'd estimate that some 90 per cent of my MS patients have reported that our programme, which always included octacosanol, reduced their feelings of fatigue. Even when the treatment's benefits were not apparent neurologically, these people said they could do more than before and felt better doing it.

Octacosanol's value was first demonstrated by Thomas Cureton, PhD, a pioneer in the field of exercise physiology. Supplements of wheat germ oil, from which octacosanol is extracted, can increase an athlete's endurance and oxygen consumption at a high altitude, Cureton demonstrated.[1] Scientists later identified octacosanol as the most potent ingredient of wheat germ oil, although other components (including triacontanol, tetracosanol and hexacosanol) may also contribute to its effectiveness, as Dr Fredericks believed.

Neurological Disorders

The sparse number of scientific studies published tends to confirm that octacosanol's best therapeutic application is against certain degenerative neurological diseases.[2] Taking 5 mg per day, one small experiment showed, improved muscular coordination for people with Parkinson's disease. A larger dose, I've found, is even more effective.[3] People with Lou Gehrig's disease (ALS) have noticed some slight improvement in their symptoms after taking 40 mg per day,[4] although the changes are not dramatic. Octacosanol might also help people who have muscular dystrophy, other research suggests,[5] although the benefit here might come from other compounds in wheat germ oil.

Supplement Suggestions

Therapeutically, a natural extract of wheat germ oil works better than synthetic octacosanol. In the small number of published studies, dosages ranged from 40 to 80 mg per day, although the average adult can easily tolerate up to 150 mg. I usually give my MS patients 15–30 mg a day. That's also a good amount for anyone who wants additional nourishment for the central nervous system. Higher amounts can be somewhat expensive but are definitely worthwhile and apparently safe.

GAMMA-ORYZANOL: *The ulcer healer*

I hope you will share my enthusiasm for gamma-oryzanol, an extract from rice bran oil whose healing powers against gastric and cardiovascular ailments have been investigated for the past two decades, especially in the Far East. Japanese scientists lead the field in research of the compound. Some two dozen studies, many of them involving hospital patients, attest to its medicinal power against ulcers, gastritis and irritable bowel syndrome, as well as high cholesterol and symptoms of menopause.

Digestive Problems Supplements of gamma-oryzanol help promote relief in gastrointestinal problems in just a few weeks.

One of the widest-based studies in all of nutritional medicine compared taking 300–600 mg of gamma-oryzanol daily against orthodox treatments for gastrointestinal ailments. The study was conducted at 375 Japanese hospitals with thousands of patients. After three weeks more than 90 per cent of the gamma-oryzanol users had achieved better recoveries than the patients who used conventional medications.[1]

Heart Disease A considerable drop in high triglycerides and LDL cholesterol typically accompanies gamma-oryzanol supplementation.[2] HDL levels also may increase moderately. Doses of 300–600 mg a day apparently achieves this improvement by blocking the absorption of cholesterol and speeding its conversion to bile.

Menopause Hot flushes, night sweats and other menopausal symptoms diminish for many women who use gamma-oryzanol regularly. Depending on the study, up to 85 per cent of the supplement takers noticed a benefit.[3] In those studies effective dosages ranged from as little as 30 mg per day to as much as 300 mg.

Other Conditions Preliminary results from other research suggests possible roles for gamma-oryzanol in treating depression and helping weight lifters to build muscle tissue.[4] Some patients find that it eases symptoms associated with prostate disorders. In Japan gamma-oryzanol is in widespread use. This rather varied list of clinical uses may be just the tip of a therapeutic iceberg.

SUPPLEMENT SUGGESTIONS

For gastrointestinal diseases and severe cholesterol disturbances, I usually prescribe 450–600 mg of gamma-oryzanol per day. When those problems are secondary to another ailment or when treating menopause, I normally reduce the dosage to between 150 and 450 mg daily. The higher amounts don't carry any risk. I simply find that the lower range is just as therapeutic.

DMG (DIMETHYLGLYCINE):

Fatigue fighter, autism conqueror

For average, run-of-the-mill fatigue, DMG (dimethylglycine) is almost the ideal quick pick-me-up, an entirely safe energy booster that lasts for most of the day. I had prescribed the nutrient before it became one of the hottest supplements of the 1970s (mistakenly billed as 'vitamin B_{15}'). I continue to dispense it today as a nonspecific treatment for fatigue.

DMG is poised to be much more than a natural pep pill. Because it's one of the so-called methyl donors, the body uses it for myriad health-promoting biochemical reactions by adding a single extra carbon cluster, thus converting one chemical into another, neutralizing toxins and protecting our genes. DMG's success with my patients convinced me that a good number of us are walking around with a relative shortage of the methyl-donating nutrients. Published DMG research is scarce, but we can glean some indication of its other therapeutic abilities from the personal experience of the practitioners who use it.

Immune Function DMG quadrupled the immune responses of people who took 120 mg daily for ten weeks, according to the results of one study.[1] The researchers concluded that DMG strengthens the body's defences on a cellular and hormonal level. It also helps cells to use oxygen more efficiently.

Athletic Endurance DMG's reputation was muddied because of its confusion with a similar compound, pangamic acid, that was first studied in Russia. Researchers there showed that pangamic acid improved athletic endurance by preventing a buildup of lactic acid in the body. DMG was also thought to possibly contribute to athletic performance, but the question remains open today, with few studies showing that it offers any athletic benefit. However, one of the positive experiments concluded that taking 5 mg per day enables an athlete to exercise longer before becoming physically exhausted. In another series of experiments, a dosage of 1.6 mg per kilogram of body weight gave horses some additional stamina and reduced lactic acid.[2]

Seizure Frequency Although animal studies suggest that DMG may reduce the frequency of epileptic seizures,[3] the small clinical trials involving people have failed to find a benefit. On the other hand, anecdotal evidence from doctors who use it is far different. According to case reports, the number of seizures dropped significantly when people with epilepsy took 180 mg of DMG daily. When they stopped taking the supplement, they experienced considerably more episodes.[4]

Autism Therapy The foremost proponent of nutrient-based medicine for autism, Bernard Rimland, PhD, presents case reports showing that DMG can lengthen autistic children's attention spans, brighten their moods, and reduce their tantrums and their obsessive-compulsive behaviour.[5] In several instances, mute autistic children began to speak overnight. No formal studies have been done, but the absence of documented research in no way undermines the firsthand evidence. Personal clinical experiences can be very convincing and contribute immensely to a doctor's education. Rimland's patients report a large degree of success among children exhibiting obsessive-compulsive symptoms.

Antioxidant Action Gary Price Todd, MD, a leading nutritional ophthalmologist, has reported that daily 250 mg doses of DMG reversed early cataract growth in some of his patients.[6] Again, no supporting research exists, but Todd's reports do lend credence to a conclusion in the immune study that DMG displays antioxidant capabilities.

Supplement Suggestions

Personal clinical experience is often one of my best guides, so the lack of hard research evidence means little. I believe DMG has many therapeutic uses, and we need more research and more practical hands-on observations to pinpoint them. Until then I'll continue to trust my own eyes and recommend the supplement on a try-it-and-see basis as a fatigue remedy. If a patient notices an increase in energy or stamina, I'll make it a regular prescription. Conventional medicine often endorses such speculation with prescription drugs, even when the medications carry detrimental side effects. Whatever else may or may not be claimed of DMG, at least it is entirely safe, based on all clinical evidence.

Pure DMG tablets containing 125 mg each are the only form of the supplement available. Placed under your tongue, the pill is absorbed within seconds, so if it's going to lift that lethargy, you'll notice within a few minutes.

TRIMETHYLGLYCINE (BETAINE):
Methyl donor, homocysteine fighter

If two methyl groups are beneficial, then three must be better. Many scientists believe this is true, and I tend to agree. Trimethylglycine, also known as betaine, may not be an immediately recognizable nutrient, but it's readily available (in the form of betaine hydrochloride) as a digestive aid. For the millions of people who lack a sufficient amount of stomach acids, it's a truly useful supplement (see page 263 on HCl).

Of late, interest in betaine, apart from the hydrochloride, which releases hydrochloric acid, has been rekindled because it reduces blood levels of homocysteine, a toxic amino acid and a dangerous independent risk factor for heart disease, among other illnesses.[1] There's little need to avail ourselves of betaine specifically for homocysteine control, because folic acid, B_6 and B_{12} do the job quite well.

Its real value, though, is in its generous methyl donation, which comes courtesy of that third methyl group. Betaine neutralizes homocysteine through this reaction, converting it into the amino acid methionine. The process could also be linked to protection from cancer, based on some animal research, liver disorders and the very act of grow-ing old.

The research in this direction is still too early and too fragmented to know how this concept will play out, but I suspect that it will prove more valuable than DMG. The dosage used most often is 125 mg three to four times daily.

NADH: *The cell energizer*

Anyone who understands the biochemistry of energy metabolism knows the pivotal role that NAD (nicotinamide adenine dinucleotide) plays in producing energy for our bodies. When it is in its usual oxidized form, it serves as a vehicle for just about every energy reaction taking place in our body's cells. In its reduced form (that is, after it has added an extra hydrogen) it is ready to deliver energy by giving up that hydrogen. It may take a biochemist to understand this reaction, but one thing is clear: the reduced NAD, called NADH or coenzyme 1, is the specific way in which all our cells get their energy. That would make NADH the quintessential energy-giving vita-nutrient, but there was one catch. In the past, no one could deliver this highly active molecule in a form stable enough to exist in an oral prescription. Fortunately European scientists have now succeeded in making coenzyme 1 available in supplement form.

When people afflicted with Parkinson's disease have taken this form of vitamin B_3 (which takes its name from the nicotinamide part of the molecule), their hands have stopped trembling and they've regained a steady gait. People with Alzheimer's disease improved in memory. Anyone else who uses the supplement can expect a pronounced surge of energy that helps athletic performance, depression, heart problems and other ailments.

Not everyone will enjoy such a pronounced turnaround after using coenzyme 1, but most of its failures are due to giving doses too low, since not everyone is able to afford the cost when high doses are necessary. Found naturally in the heart and brain, NADH extends antioxidant protection to our cell's power source, the mitochondria. The body normally makes its own NADH from niacinamide, but aging and disease slow the conversion.

Parkinson's Disease When one of my NADH-treated Parkinson's patients returns with a measurable improvement in his or her symptoms, I'm left with few words to describe the satisfaction I feel. The difference can be remarkable in older people, who seem to derive a greater benefit than my younger patients. I'll let the research speak for itself:

Of some nine hundred people with Parkinson's who took NADH supplements regularly, 80 per cent showed moderate to excellent relief from hand tremors, head wobbling, limb stiffness, slow gait, fatigue and other symptoms of the disease. With years of regular use, it also appears to slow the deterioration of their nervous systems.[1]

In the brain, NADH helps neurons make dopamine, a neurotransmitter that is relatively deficient in people with Parkinson's. Conventional medicine treats the disease with L-dopa, a prescription dopamine replacement that, over the long term, further impairs the brain's ability to make the neurotransmitter. For these reasons, Jorg Birkmayer, MD, the Austrian researcher who developed the product and did most of the original work with NADH, recommends that doctors allow their Parkinson's patients to take a smaller dose of L-dopa while trying NADH therapy. L-dopa causes the release of free radicals, which can damage brain cells, whereas NADH is one of the brain's most powerful antioxidants. Thus NADH usually provides the same benefits as L-dopa but without the side effects.[2]

Alzheimer's Disease I've used NADH on people with all degrees of memory loss, and a surprisingly high percentage of them regained at least some short-term memory. Birkmayer tested the supplement on seventeen people with Alzheimer's, which shares many biochemical similarities with Parkinson's disease. All of his patients significantly improved their performance on standard memory tests. The progression of brain deterioration, presently an inevitable occurrence with the disease, was also slowed.[3]

Depression The third condition Birkmayer studied formally was depression. Ninety-three per cent of 205 depressed subjects were benefitted, although many received an injectible form of NADH.[4]

Heart Disease Although researchers are beginning to explore its possible uses elsewhere, NADH already seems to be of significant value against heart disease. It has already saved the lives of ten people with terminal heart failure. When doctors administered 15 mg of the nutrient intravenously in this small experiment, their patients weren't expected to live longer than two days. But they beat the odds and ended up living far beyond their doctors' expectations.

My guess is that combining NADH with other standard cardiovascular nutrients, such as coenzyme Q_{10} and carnitine, will serve people with many types of heart ailments. In other research it shows signs of lowering elevated cholesterol and blood pressure readings.

Chronic Fatigue Although there are many causes of this debilitating and misunderstood syndrome, preliminary results with NADH are encouraging, and clinical trials are now under way.

Energy Enhancement Encouraged by successful European studies on athletic performance, American studies are now in progress. In the one study reported upon, seventeen athletes age to eighteen to thirty-five achieved quicker reaction times and better overall performance after four weeks of taking 5 mg of NADH.

SUPPLEMENT SUGGESTIONS

If you take too much, NADH may stimulate you too much; used late in the day, it can prevent you from falling asleep. It should be taken before eating anything, first thing in the morning. If you take it with a meal, digestive juices will break down the coating.

Your best source for obtaining NADH may be a complementary doctor, because an effective form could be hard to find. Health food stores might carry something called NAD, but that would be ineffective. In this book I have not been making product recommendations by brand name, but at this writing I have found only one effective form of NADH – the NADH made with Dr Birkmayer's process.

Precise dosages must be individualized, because each person will react differently. It is easy to find your ideal dose because too much of it will overstimulate you, so start with 2.5 mg every morning and add a 2.5 mg-increment increase each week until you find the optimal blend of energy and ability to sleep restfully. For Alzheimer's and Parkinson's diseases, the effective therapeutic range may extend upward to some 20 mg per day or more.

CHAPTER 11

CARTILAGE-BUILDING NUTRIENTS

SHARK AND BOVINE CARTILAGE:

Arthritis therapy, cancer hope

Cartilage therapy has fomented a lot of debate, not only from its critics, but among its competing advocates, too. Though it almost certainly helps treat inflammatory conditions such as arthritis, it fans the flames of controversy as a cancer therapy.

Proponents of alternative medicine generally consider cartilage to be at least somewhat useful and occasionally essential. Among truly dedicated advocates of the treatment, a more hotly contested issue is which of the two kinds is better, bovine cartilage or shark cartilage. Each has a different story.

Bovine Cartilage The first cartilage product that was used clinically, based on the work of John Prudden, MD, bovine cartilage initially demonstrated its medical worthiness by improving wound healing for people who were taking the drug cortisone. It strengthened the quality of newly forming tissue and speeded up the healing process.[1] He found that bovine cartilage extract applied directly to a surgical wound was a potent accelerator of its healing.[2] Dry socket, a painful complication that sometimes occurs following a tooth extraction, is one condition that bovine cartilage helps dramatically.

Next Prudden discovered that bovine cartilage was a powerful anti-inflammatory with a certain value in alleviating pain from both osteoarthritis and rheumatoid arthritis. The treatment decreased pain and increased joint mobility.[3] In 90 per cent of seven hundred people involved in one of his studies, 60 per cent considered the overall results to be excellent.

Critics, however, want independent studies to confirm Prudden's claims that bovine cartilage, in doses of 9 grams a day, can completely cure cancer of the prostate and pancreas. He also has reported good results against lung, renal and colon cancer, as well as a form of brain cancer called glioblastoma. According to one of his studies, bovine cartilage benefited nearly all of the thirty-one cancer patients who took it, with 35 per cent reportedly cured.[4]

Shark Cartilage Although better known and publicized than its bovine competitor, shark cartilage also lacks independent confirmation of its reputed anticancer capability. Its foremost advocate, William Lane, PhD, claims that his research, done in Cuba and Mexico, proves its effectiveness. However, I have not seen any reports of a high percentage of long-term successes. In a few instances tumours have shrunk in size, according to lab evidence that, Lane says, came from Cuba. Of perhaps greater interest, though, are Lane's slides that show sheets of fibrous tissue invading the tumour. This is a typical bodily effort to control an illness. Though the tumour remained, this fibrous scar tissue had replaced the cancer, rendering it unable to grow.

As a tool for healing inflammatory conditions, both cartilage preparations – in fact, any cartilage product – have impressive credentials. After all, they are major sources of chondroitin sulfate and glycosaminoglycans and therefore share their capabilities for success in arthritis and myriad other inflammatory conditions. Unpublished reports of dramatic successes of patients with the autoimmune skin-tightening disease scleroderma suggest that an extract of shark cartilage may prove to be its most effective therapy.

SUPPLEMENT SUGGESTIONS

I can't pick a winner between the two cartilage competitors. Each seems to work impressively about 20 per cent of the time, I'd estimate, based on my own observations with Atkins Center cancer patients. Because I treat cancer with twenty or more biological substances almost simultaneously, isolating the impact of one can be difficult. I'd like to see comparative analyses done, but I'm not willing to hold back any effective treatment for a patient in order to learn something.

Treatments like cartilage – bovine or shark, both readily available in health food stores – make a major contribution to the overall quality of our fight by helping us achieve a goal generally rejected in mainstream circles: fighting cancer to a prolonged stalemate without even trying to cure it. Many practitioners say that bovine cartilage works better, although I believe shark cartilage may have the edge. We often make the decision based on how easy it is to administer and how much it costs. For fighting cancer or scleroderma, my personal favorite is frozen shark cartilage extract. All you need to do is place 1 teaspoon a day under your tongue. Shark cartilage powder requires a very large daily dose – at least 1 gram for every 900 grams of body weight, consumed orally or inserted rectally. Bovine's effective dose, per Dr Prudden, is 9 grams per day, whether inflammatory or malignant disease is the problem.

GLUCOSAMINE: *Osteoarthritis's best treatment*

Progress towards my goal – making natural healing mainstream – is made when a book achieves enough popularity to create demand for a specific treatment. I must confess that I hope this book will do that.

The next two nutrients I will describe to you are examples of just how that can happen.

Glucosamine sulfate is considered by complementary doctors to be the treatment of choice for osteoarthritis not only because we have all had long successions of satisfied patients, but because it can boast an array of impressive clinical studies attesting to its effectiveness.

But virtually no mainstream rheumatologist prescribed it until they were inundated by their own patients asking for it and demanding them to read a best-selling book by Dr Jason Theodosakis, *The Arthritis Cure*.

Glucosamine works because it provides the building blocks for new cartilage, the protective joint padding that prevents bones from scraping against each other as we move but gets worn away by this common form of degenerative (wear-and-tear) arthritis.[1] It enables us to treat this illness effectively, possibly for the first time in history.[2]

For the seven million or so Britons with osteoarthritis, medicine's preferred treatment is long-term use of short-term painkilling medications. These nonsteroidal anti-inflammatory drugs (NSAIDs) don't heal osteoarthritic joint damage. Many of them, including aspirin, accelerate the deterioration and stop the growth of cartilage.

Though NSAIDs can be used for temporary relief, habitual use is ruinous, for these drugs kill more than pain.[3] Every year thousands of people die from using NSAIDs. Hundreds of thousands of others develop bleeding ulcers and liver damage, to name two of the drugs' notorious side effects. Some people end up on kidney dialysis.

JOINT RESOLUTION

Healthy joints make their own glucosamine, an essential building block for cartilage. The body manufactures cartilage, but only if glucosamine is plentiful. When production of the nutrient falters, joints begin to lose cartilage, bones erode as they grind against each other, and osteoarthritis sets in. As the painful condition progresses, glucosamine output may cease entirely.

According to head-to-head research comparisons, taking supplements (which appear to trigger the joints' own production of the nutrient) will dampen osteoarthritic pain and increase joint mobility better than taking pharmaceutical pain relievers.[4] The nutrient therapy also displays some anti-inflammatory action.

Glucosamine's relief and rejuvenation aren't immediate. Although some people with osteoarthritis do notice an improvement within a few weeks, some of my patients had to take it for as long as six months to feel an effect. But the relief is definitely worth the wait. In an eight-week study that pitted glucosamine against ibuprofen, a common painkiller for osteoarthritis, participants reported that they initially felt greater relief with ibuprofen. But by the end of the experiment the glucosamine users felt far better. Cell samples from their joints offered visible proof: the degenerating joints were in fact healing – something never before observed in ibuprofen users.[5]

SUPPLEMENT SUGGESTIONS

Different glucosamine formulations are available, and while all of them are helpful, some debate exists over which works the best. Glucosamine sulfate, backed by more than twenty solidly conducted studies on people, is probably the best for osteoarthritis relief. It is now ubiquitous in health food stores. Glucosamine hydrochloride, shown to heal cartilage in animal studies, is the least expensive. N-acetyl glucosamine, yet another formulation, will not deliver as much of the active ingredient to joints as its two competitors.

Whichever preparation you select, the usual dose is 500 mg three times per day. It's safe and, except for some minor digestive upset, free of side effects. However, I see no reason not to give 3,000 mg daily or more – safety is not an issue. To enhance its medicinal power, I combine it with chondroitin sulfate (see below), fish oils, bovine or shark cartilage, sea cucumber, cetyl myristoleate, and the antioxidants. Anyone over forty years of age may want to use it preventively against osteoarthritis, which most of us will develop, to some degree, as we age. Taking 500 mg twice daily may delay what could otherwise be inevitable.

CHONDROITIN SULFATE: *How joints get well*

We feed our dogs bones because we want these loyal family members to have strong bones. The same logic tells us that if we want to rebuild our cartilage, as we must if osteoarthritis is taking its toll, then perhaps we should feed ourselves cartilage.

Well, for decades scientists in the know have been demonstrating the effectiveness of the principal unique constituent of cartilage, chondroitin sulfate. Although not a single chemical entity, but rather a class of related substances, chondroitin has a surprisingly wide range of activities. Its activity comes from its content of a group of complex sugar molecules called glycosaminoglycans, which can offer anti-inflammmatory effects and activity against heart disease as a bonus to their ability to help us re-form cartilage.

Though found primarily in bones, cartilage and connective tissue, chondroitin sulfate extends its curative influence throughout the body by easing pain, helping wounds to heal and improving cardiovascular health.

THE OTHER 'ARTHRITIS CURE'

Osteoarthritic aches diminished for a group of two hundred people who participated in one chondroitin sulfate study. The anti-inflammatory effect also allowed them to bend their knees, elbows and other joints more freely and with none of the complications of standard arthritis medications.[1] People with gout may also enjoy some pain relief, because supplements reduce high uric acid levels.[2]

CHONDROITIN'S OTHER VIRTUES

In the cardiovascular system, chondroitin sulfate works on several levels. It stimulates fat metabolism, lowers cholesterol,[3] reduces blood clotting, inhibits plaque accumulation and improves circulation. Surgical incisions heal faster when they're coated with a chondroitin sulfate concentrate. Normal cells may become cancerous more readily, animal research suggests, in the face of a chondroitin sulfate deficiency,[4] while other lab experiments hint at some direct action against HIV.[5]

SUPPLEMENT SUGGESTIONS

For arthritis or blood lipid imbalances, take between 250 mg and 1 gram of chondroitin sulfate a day. When given in conjunction with glucosamine sulfate for osteoarthritis, as is now done on a wide scale, its dose in milligrams is usually 60–80 per cent that of the glucosamine. Doctors have administered dosages as high as 10 grams daily for six years without noting side effects, so this substance is unquestionably safe. Although its glycosaminoglycans are complex sugar molecules, it doesn't work like sugar and won't create a problem for anyone with diabetes or a related insulin disorder. If you can't find a product plainly labeled 'chondroitin sulfate', get bovine or any form of cartilage. It's another good source.

SEA CUCUMBER: *Joint reliever*

The sea cucumber is a living creature, not an ocean vegetable. It earned its name from its looks, but don't expect to get a pickle out of it. More likely it will get you out of a pickle, the one caused by arthritis.

Sea cucumber (*bêche-de-mer*) is one of the most useful arthritis treatments I've ever dispensed. Without any side effects, it significantly relieves joint aches and stiffness, particularly when combined with the essential oils, glucosamine sulfate, cetyl myristoleate and other nutrients in my arthritis therapy. The Chinese have known of its therapeutic might for thousands of years. Modern medicine still hasn't quite caught on, although Australia's equivalent of the FDA designated sea cucumber an official arthritis treatment in 1992.

The creature, a relative of the starfish, hails from the waters of Australia's Great Barrier Reef. Long-term studies have yet to be done, but informal clinical experiments show that supplements considerably reduce arthritis pain and expand joint mobility for about 60 per cent of the people who take them. I have been using it in patient care for years, and to me the 60 per cent improvement figure seems a bit understated. Sea cucumber provides glycosaminoglycans, making it an alternative to chondroitin. I suspect it has other active principles as well, and since it has no negative side effects, I'm inclined to prescribe both.

SUPPLEMENT SUGGESTIONS

The extent of the relief depends on the size of the dosage. I tend to start new arthritis patients on three or four 500 mg capsules per day, tapering the dosage down to two capsules a day once the effects are noticed.

CHAPTER 12

HORMONES AND GLANDULARS

Hormones are not nutrients: they're drugs. As such, they should be prescribed by a doctor. But events have taken a curious, albeit encouraging, turn, for a certain few hormones are now available over-the-counter, sold as vita-nutrients at pharmacies, supermarkets, and health food stores. Thus it is important to know about them – not only because they're there, but because they are potent controllers of many body functions.

Although these prescription-free supplements can satisfy some of the body's most fundamental needs, they are among the substances that your doctor is least likely to recommend. In many respects, figuring out which hormones are right for you may be of greater importance than determining the right doses of vitamins and minerals. Let's face it: hormones are much stronger modulators of health than nutrients. While having this kind of increased power within easy reach is exciting, it also means that you must be more responsible in using them.

As we proceed, keep in mind the one important difference between over-the-counter hormones and other supplements. Vitamin C, vitamin E and almost all other nutrients are safe for virtually everyone in a vast dosage range. We cannot be so cavalier with hormones. They require specific, individualized dosages, based on 'before' and 'after' blood measurements. Even though they are relatively free of risk, their safest use requires the expert guidance of a doctor – one familiar with their benefits, indications and dosages, as well as with your particular needs. I offer my own guidelines only because such practitioners are not in plentiful supply.

The three readily available hormones – DHEA, pregnenolone and melatonin – share one noteworthy feature: their natural levels in your body peak during your early twenties, then drop steadily and dramatically as you grow older. Their decline is closely associated with a number of the health-related changes that occur as we age. Indeed, some of these changes might be reversed by restoring the hormones to what I call their 'prime levels' – the amounts your body generated during your prime, which is about the age of thirty. Careful, measured supplementation may achieve this; megadoses will not.

DHEA: *The mother hormone*

If an antidote to aging exists, it may well be DHEA. Improved sex drive, enhanced immune function, renewed energy and stamina, brighter mood, keener memory – all have been attributed to replenishing a dwindling blood level of the 'mother hormone', so named because it is the source of all other sex and steroid hormones. The body makes DHEA (dehydroepiandrosterone) from cholesterol, that infamous blood lipid so valued by me and so reviled by mainstream medicine. DHEA's very presence is yet another example of our undeniable need for dietary cholesterol. Without an adequate amount, DHEA and its hormonal offspring would be in short supply.

When DHEA levels are less than optimal, health is less than optimal. By the time we're seventy years old, we have just 10 per cent of what we had at twenty-five. As a truly remarkable body of research shows, it's no coincidence that good health is associated with youth and a strong blood concentration of DHEA. I began to prescribe the hormone several years ago, and now more than half of my older patients take it.

The initial inspiration came from a University of California study, headed by Samuel Yen, MD Every day for three months he gave either 50 mg of DHEA or a placebo to a small group of men and women who ranged in age from forty to seventy. Then, over the next three months, the groups were switched.[1]

As it turned out, during the period of DHEA use, more than three-quarters of the men and women said they felt an extraordinary increase in general physical and psychological well-being. Arthritis discomfort improved, sleep was more restful and energy levels rose dramatically. Only 10 per cent felt better when taking what turned out to be the dummy supplements. In this sort of study, such statistical results involving the question of simply 'feeling better' are almost unprecedented.

Since I began to measure my patients' DHEA levels, I've noticed several interesting correlations. One in particular stands out: my sickest patients, regardless of their afflictions, almost invariably had the lowest DHEA readings. Even younger patients who don't respond well to specific therapies typically run a DHEA level far below what I expect for their age. Most important, though, the majority of all patients, young and old, begin to feel much better once supplementation restores DHEA to an optimal level.

Although the hormone elevates overall health and well-being, the medical literature and my own clinical patients' outcomes point to several specific benefits, including the following.

Fatigue One of the most common reasons doctors prescribe the mother hormone is to overcome fatigue. Our adrenal glands, increasingly overworked and exhausted as we age, secrete diminishing amounts of their hormones, including DHEA. Supplements, especially for people older than fifty, can revive energy levels in just a few days to a few weeks.[2]

Immune Weakness In lab experiments, researchers see that DHEA protects the immune system from some of the damage inflicted by stress and the stress-triggered release of cortisone and other glucocorticoids.[3] It also bolsters certain components of the body's natural self-defence system, including natural killer cells and T cells. What does this mean in practice? Well, for many of my patients with chronic fatigue syndrome, AIDS and other immune-crippling illnesses, DHEA readings are often very low before taking supplements, and correcting the deficit will, with similar consistency, strengthen immune function, relieve depression, boost energy and sharpen thinking.

Autoimmune Diseases DHEA may regulate our internal defences in another way – when the immune system turns against the very body tissues it should protect. A six-month course of DHEA, in a daily dosage of 200 mg, markedly diminished symptoms of lupus for a small number of women involved in a study of the hormone. Because of the improvements, researchers were able to reduce the women's medication dosages (always an objective because of the side effects from these immune-suppressing drugs).[4]

Rheumatoid arthritis is another autoimmune ailment for which I prescribe DHEA. Most people who contend with the degenerative joint disease have lower than usual readings of the hormone.[5]

Cancer Little human research has been published on DHEA's anticancer potential, but a lot of work is in progress, including studies in which up to 3,000 mg daily are given to patients with active cancer. People in their sixties face a cancer risk ten times higher than a twenty-year-old, and the decline in DHEA may be one of the explanations. Blood concentrations are lower in people with bladder cancer than in their cancer-free counterparts.[6] Thus it would seem that DHEA is a good safeguard against many types of malignancies.

There is, however, one major exception: prostate cancer. DHEA can stimulate testosterone production, and the male hormone feeds prostatic tumours. Any man with prostate cancer or who has a high risk of prostate cancer should take DHEA supplements – but only when prescribed by a doctor who 1) understands the risks and benefits, and 2) is willing to frequently monitor PSA blood levels (which measure prostate cancer risk).

Heart Disease Cutting down on cholesterol consumption probably won't reduce blood cholesterol, but it may inhibit DHEA production. Taking supplements of DHEA, though, may reduce a high cholesterol level.[7] That's just one way the hormone helps to prevent heart disease. It also thwarts blood clot formation[8] and may encourage blood vessels to relax, which could lower high blood pressure. In men who have had a fatal heart attack, DHEA levels are notably depressed, as they are in men with narrowed arteries.

Weight Loss Much of the excitement over DHEA in magazine and newspaper articles centres on its supposed ability to burn off body fat. Experiments on lab animals do show a drop in fat – but only if very high doses are taken. In my practice, DHEA's performance in aiding weight loss has been unimpressive.

Low Libido Although we still need clinical verification, the anecdotal evidence is in. DHEA rejuvenates sex drive in older adults, both men and women. Men with a decidedly low natural level seem to benefit the most, probably because the body uses DHEA to make testosterone. Perhaps more valuable in this regard is a metabolite of DHEA called andristeriedione, which serves as the immediate precursor of testosterone. It is able to raise blood levels of male hormone.

Mental Disturbances As demonstrated by a four-week study of older adults who took 75 mg supplements daily, DHEA improves memory and brightens mood.[9] It may also guard the brain against Alzheimer's disease, but that research is so far inconclusive.

Blood Sugar Instability Studies of people (not lab animals) are also sparse in this area. If the results of animal experiments apply to humans, supplements may improve the body's sensitivity to insulin, which would help keep blood sugar in line.

PREGNENOLONE: *The grandmother hormone*

If DHEA is the 'mother hormone', then pregnenolone is the 'grandmother hormone', the substance from which the body makes DHEA and almost all other sex steroid hormones, including testosterone, oestrogen, cortisol, and aldosterone. However, pregnenolone, unlike DHEA, can lead to progesterone production, making it an especially vital supplement to women by creating a balance with oestrogen to reduce the risk of certain cancers that develop in women.

Interest in pregnenolone dates back to the 1940s, when Dr Hans Selye, the father of the 'fight or flight' theory of stress, studied its usefulness against anxiety and fatigue. In 1950 his contemporaries studied it against rheumatoid arthritis. Pregnenolone controlled pain, swelling and other symptoms of the disease as well as the body's other adrenal steroid hormones, but with an important difference: it was the only hormone tested that did not cause metabolic side effects.

Unfortunately the medical profession abandoned pregnenolone, perhaps because the corporations could not patent this natural substance, and turned their research attention to one of its offspring, cortisol and its synthetic derivatives. Doctors soon heralded cortisol derivatives as 'miracle drugs' for relief from rheumatoid arthritis and other inflammatory or autoimmune ailments. True, pregnenolone wasn't quite as powerful as prednisone, prednisolone or similar medications. But it caused none of the horrendous adverse effects for which corticosteroids are so well known – including water retention, high blood pressure, susceptibility to infections, weight gain, greater risk of diabetes and that ballooning facial puffiness known as 'moon face'.

These days, many doctors hesitate to keep patients on corticosteroid drugs, recognizing that the treatment may be worse than the disease. 'If only there were an alternative,' I'm sure they say to themselves. There is. I was awestruck upon learning pregnenolone's history, and we're now rediscovering its exciting possibilities. Atkins Center doctors are now using the hormone supplement to treat any condition for which prednisone would be prescribed – arthritis, multiple sclerosis, asthma, temporal arthritis and lupus, to name a few.

Combined with DHEA, pregnenolone proves to be very useful for relieving depression. Finally, if results from some newer animal research hold true for humans, the grandmother hormone may become one of the most powerful substances yet found to enhance memory.[1]

Because of its biochemical bias towards progesterone, pregnenolone could become the treatment of choice for several oestrogen-related health problems. In a woman's body, progesterone accomplishes more than just rounding out the monthly menstrual cycle. It curbs the tendency of certain forms of oestrogen to overstimulate breast and uterine cells. Unless checked by progesterone, this overstimulation can lead to breast cancer, uterine fibroids and fibrocystic breast disease.

MELATONIN: *The mystery of the pineal*

Besides its classification as a hormone and the fact that our levels decline as we age, melatonin shares little with DHEA, pregnenolone or any other adrenal secretion. As a therapy and maybe as a preventive, it could become widely used for everything from relieving insomnia to protecting us from cancer.

The more we learn about melatonin, the active hormone of the pineal gland, the more it distinguishes itself as a world-class antioxidant. By stimulating our number one antioxidant enzyme[1], it protects us from two of the most dangerous free radicals, hydroxyl and peroxyl. Thus, in an optimal amount, melatonin may shield us against cataracts, heart disease, neurological disorders, and, perhaps, cancer.[2] I should begin, though, with its most popular use.

Insomnia Our pineal gland, by releasing melatonin, keeps our wake-sleep cycle in perfect synch with day and night. For almost anyone who can't drift off when at rest, melatonin is the best, most physiologically active sleeping pill available.

Especially for older people, it's a well-established solution to insomnia. Simply taking a mere 0.3 mg of melatonin at bedtime (I use ten times that amount), one study demonstrated, markedly improves sleep patterns among elderly people who had problems falling asleep and remaining asleep for the remainder of the night.[3] Most supplement takers say that their rest is longer and sounder and that they awaken feeling refreshed and rejuvenated.

With Swiss precision, melatonin resets our internal clocks, making it the perfect potion for shift workers and travellers. Its value in overcoming jet lag symptoms has been confirmed.[4] Short-term use, in this regard, is safe for virtually any adult. A dose of between 1 and 3 mg every evening for a week acclimatizes you quickly to a new sleep schedule, restoring sound slumber (in the dark) with a minimum amount of fatigue upon awakening (when it's light).[5]

Timed-released formulas, in dosages as low as a single milligram, may be more advantageous.[6] They prevent the hormone's level from peaking too soon, which will awaken you too early.

Cancer Whether for prevention or treatment, melatonin could become an important weapon against certain cancers, notably those of the breast, skin and prostate. The list will lengthen, I'm sure, as this research field expands. The hormone rejuvenates several components of our natural defence system, and their strength combines to create a more powerful immunity. One way in which melatonin might fight cancer is by stimulating the immune system's natural killer cells.[7] Other studies confirm that the hormone sends white blood cells a signal to protect the body[8], and animal research points to its ability to bolster overall immunity.[9] Some scientists speculate that this immune impact might be targeted against AIDS.[10]

I've been telling the majority of the Atkins Center's cancer patients to take between 12 and 20 mg of melatonin every night. In some research, people with metastatic cancer have lived longer by taking at least that amount.[11] Even daily dosages of 200 mg, according to European investigators, are safe.

Heart Disease In the not-too-distant future, cardiologists may take a melatonin reading to assess your risk of heart disease. As the body's melatonin concentration falls, research affirms, the likelihood of heart disease rises. A deficiency is also associated with elevated blood levels of cholesterol and triglycerides.[12]

Headache I found a promising pilot study suggesting that melatonin (10 g) could prevent cluster headaches (throbbers that come in bunches) from taking place.[13] If this is replicated, millions of sufferers could benefit.

Alzheimer's Disease A melatonin deficiency commonly appears in people with this mind-destroying disease. The implication, of course, is that supplements may play a preventive or remedial role. Alzheimer's-affected brain cells are also damaged by hydroxyl, one of the free radical molecules that melatonin controls so effectively.

Another possible application: Italian doctors have reported dramatic early success after giving daily 20 mg doses of melatonin to two people with sarcoidosis.[14]

SUPPLEMENT SUGGESTIONS

Hormone restoration isn't a do-it-yourself project. Everyone's needs are different. You'll require the help of a doctor who can gauge your existing levels and continue to monitor them as you take supplements. I measure blood levels of each and prescribe accordingly, adjusting dosages based on subsequent tests. Experience, though, teaches that lab results aren't the only determinants. In one person a small dose may increase the blood's concentration dramatically; in another person a large amount may have only a minimal impact.

DHEA and pregnenolone seem to play off each other's strengths and weaknesses, so I normally establish their dosages together. For these purposes, though, I'll address each of the three hormones individually.

DHEA The quality and absorbability of DHEA supplements will vary from brand to brand, and I'm not at all certain that everything labelled 'DHEA' truly is the real thing. Some products contain dioscorea, also known as 'Mexican yam', which manufacturers claim is either actual DHEA or one of its natural precursors. Don't be duped. No metabolic pathway exists for converting this plant extract into DHEA.

Ask a knowledgeable doctor for the name of a reputable brand, or go to a compounding pharmacist, a rare breed of apothecary who is specially trained to fill custom-made prescriptions and obtain hard-to-get drugs. (You can also get pregnenolone and melatonin of unquestionable quality from this source.)

The average twenty-year-old human body makes between 20 and 30 mg of DHEA per day; perhaps one-tenth of that is made at the age of seventy. Many adults, therefore, take between 5 and 25 mg a day. However, scientists have not clearly determined if the body absorbs everything in each supplement, so higher doses may be needed to replenish your blood level.

As a rule of thumb, I try to get blood measurements of DHEA-S (DHEA sulfate, the form it becomes when metabolized) into a range of 400–600 µg/dL for men and 300–500 µg/dL for women. Everyone's thumb is unique, though, and a few points either way can make a big difference. If you don't work with your health care practitioner to establish the optimum dosage, you will put yourself at quite a disadvantage.

When secreted during youthful years, DHEA peaks in the morning hours. To mimic the natural ebb and flow, take your supplements upon waking. Side effects are relatively minor and can be corrected by adjusting the dosage. DHEA may increase natural testosterone levels slightly, so women and men occasionally develop a little acne. Women may also notice the growth of a little facial hair. The nice thing about DHEA, however, is that you will know if it helps you; you should feel a tremendous difference in a short time. And if DHEA enables you to live longer, you can enjoy the extra years with more vibrant health.

Pregnenolone The grandmother hormone has not been studied as extensively as DHEA, so we have fewer guidelines for its use. We do know that cholesterol is the basic building block of pregnenolone, which could mean that a determined effort to lower your cholesterol, either by modifying your diet or by taking drugs, might create a pregnenolone deficiency.

Food, as we know, often doesn't provide us with enough of our natural health promoters, be they nutrients or the building blocks of hormones. Thus a typical seventy-five-year-old person will have about 60 per cent less pregnenolone than will someone who is thirty-five years old. Depending on the results of blood tests, I might start a patient on a daily dosage of between 20 and 40 mg, taken in the morning. After two months or so and another blood test, I might gradually increase this amount. Symptoms suggesting the dose is too high are bloating and fluid retention, reminiscent of the premenstrual syndrome – a time when progesterone is at its highest.

Capsules are commonly available in dosages of between 5 and 100 mg per pill. Sublingual tablets and oral sprays are sold, too. For most purposes, don't take more than 60 mg per day without a doctor's evaluation. When I try to replace prednisone as a treatment for rheumatoid arthritis or another condition, I could conceivably prescribe as much as 200 mg per day, even if blood tests suggest a much lower dosage. Usually, though, I will prescribe 60–100 mg, plus twice that amount of DHEA.

Melatonin A variety of factors may suppress our natural production of the hormone, including alcohol consumption, lack of sleep and insufficient exposure to darkness. Electromagnetic radiation, such as that emitted by an electric blanket or waterbed heater, also may reduce the pineal gland's output.

To give your body its best chance of making melatonin on its own, don't drink alcohol, give yourself enough time for rest, and don't fall asleep with the lights on. Certain nutrients also support its production, including protein, niacinamide, vitamin B_6, vitamin B_{12} and acetyl carnitine.

Supplements won't work for all insomniacs, however. A variety of factors, both physiological and psychological, influence sleep, and not all of them are subject to the hormone's control. Its best applications are for correcting a deficiency, which becomes more probable as we age, and for occasionally readjusting the wake-sleep cycle.

Some people may experience unwanted side effects from melatonin, such as an occasional vivid or unpleasant dream. In my own use and in my practice, however, I rarely encounter these adverse effects.

Blood tests for melatonin aren't generally available, so I usually begin with a low daily dose, maybe 2 mg and perhaps as little as .5 milligram. Increase the amount somewhat if you don't notice an effect after several days. As much as 200 mg per day can be taken safely without upsetting the body's natural hormonal balance, although I heartily encourage you to find a nutritionally oriented doctor to help you fine-tune your own programme.

GLANDULAR EXTRACTS
(PROTOMORPHOGENS): *Can the organ do the job?*

Eating liver is good for your liver. That makes perfect sense, because the organ meat is loaded with nutrients that your liver needs. It doesn't necessarily follow, though, that eating a thyroid gland or taking an adrenal extract delivers anything of value to the corresponding gland in your body. Even though research offers little documented support for taking these supplements, some of them, I know, do promote and restore health, and some of them play a big role in my patient treatment strategy.

A gland's greatest therapeutic assets are its hormones. Some evidence suggests that if properly processed, certain proteins from the glands of animals may survive the digestive process and be absorbed intact.[1] Research into the usefulness of these protomorphogens, as they're called, is still in its earliest stages, but thousands of practitioners have chalked up a good record of success with them.

Thymus Glandulars The thymus gland is the organ of immunity, and as such, its output is vitally necessary to managing every patient whose immune response needs support. Yet it is rarely a part of mainstream prescribing. Even after being stripped of its hormonal content and processed into a supplement, thymus extract still retains some biological activity that can help support your own thymus. High-quality supplements (I prefer those made in Germany) have been found to augment immune function, especially against hepatitis.[2] I'll also prescribe them, in a daily 2 gram dose, for the entire spectrum of immune problems, including recurrent infections, yeast overgrowth, cancer and AIDS.

But two new breakthroughs promise to make thymus therapy

more valuable than ever. A brand-new extraction process may improve the overall quality of glandulars and reduce their cost, another factor that limits wider use. I have been using these supplements in recent years. The new extraction process is based on the live-cell therapy of Paul Niehans, MD, the renowned Swiss doctor who treated Churchill, De Gaulle and other celebrated twentieth-century figures. Niehans injected patients with an animal extract from a specific organ; those cells then migrated to the recipient's corresponding organ, after which the organ's function often improved. In the new extraction process, a frozen extract from animal thymus is used. After the thawed liquid is dissolved under the tongue, it is presumably absorbed intact.

The second breakthrough is based in a new procedure in which thymus cells are perpetuated by growing them on cell culture; they produce a protein called thymic protein A, which strengthens immune function.[3] I have used it to produce some impressive changes in my patients' T cell counts.

Adrenal Extracts Persistent fatigue and a seemingly inexplicable lack of vitality often signals adrenal exhaustion. Stress easily drains our adrenal glands, which control blood sugar balance, mental alertness and a host of other bodily functions. Although adrenal extracts probably do not contain a significant amount of hormones, thousands of doctors attest to the dramatic turnaround in energy their patients have experienced after using the supplements. Ovarian, testicular, pituitary, thyroid and other hormonal extracts have all been used by practitioners enthused about this therapeutic strategy.

SUPPLEMENT SUGGESTIONS

Because glandular therapy presents more questions than answers, don't try to take advantage of it on your own. Proceed with the guidance of an experienced practitioner. He or she can determine the best ways to address your individual needs and can recommend high-quality extracts from organically fed animals.

CHAPTER 13

Herbs

Nature's Pharmacy

At first glance, herbs might not seem appropriate for a book on nutrient therapy. However, many of them are, in fact, foods, such as mushrooms, cranberries, garlic, ginger and cayenne pepper. In reviewing my treatment plans for various illnesses, I couldn't ignore the fact that herbs are an inseparable part of nutritional medicine.

If the distinction between herbs and nutrients seems blurry, take a moment to consider the distinction between herbs and drugs. About one-third of our prescription medications – digitalis, antispasmodics, painkillers and certain chemotherapeutic agents, to cite a few examples – are derived from plants. Thus it's ironic that mainstream medicine generally tends to look down upon herbal treatments. This attitude didn't always exist. Until the 1920s or so, medical schools taught students to recognize the therapeutic value of plants through the study of pharmacognosy, and pharmacies stocked their shelves with herbs that doctors prescribed regularly. But somewhere along the way, the emphasis shifted to pharmaceuticals, and the profession was denied access to this wonderful knowledge.

Although pharmaceutical companies never lost sight of the medicinal potential of herbs, they've always sought more buck than the natural bang could provide. Because plant extracts and natural substances cannot be patented, the surest path to bigger profits is lost. Drug researchers, therefore, began to look for individual active ingredients within each therapeutic herb, chemically dissecting the herbs in search of something they could duplicate artificially and patent. In so doing, they concentrated on plant chemicals that possessed significant adverse effects, ignoring the considerable health-bestowing power of naturally balanced whole herbs and whole extracts.

Today's rediscovery of a more natural plant pharmacology occurred largely through the work of researchers in Europe, where herbal medications are a routine part of mainstream medicine, manufactured to the same exacting standards as pharmaceuticals. Some of the world's most esteemed laboratories make and promote herbal medicines. For example, in Germany doctors write millions of prescriptions every year for a pharmaceutical-grade herbal extract of *Ginkgo biloba*. Here in America, even though we have access to ginkgo of the same quality, mainstream medicine still refuses to recognize its medicinal roles.

In this chapter I've divided the most commonly used herbs into several categories, according to how I most frequently use them. These classifications may seem arbitrary, but that's because of the very nature of our medicinal herbs. Most of them defy classification because they work simultaneously on different levels. The same herb that I give to one patient as a cold cure, for instance, can also help another patient recover from cancer. In many cases even the herbs with specific purposes can advance our health in other ways, and fortunately most of these natural extracts are available over-the-counter.

MULTIPURPOSE HERBS

GINKGO BILOBA

Derived from the world's oldest living species of tree, *Ginkgo biloba* is the most important plant-based medicine available. An important part of mainstream medicine in Europe, with sales accounting for more than 1 per cent of all pharmaceutical purchases, it's widely heralded as a mental and vascular stimulant and a powerful protector of the brain, liver, eyes and circulatory system.[1]

As more than three hundred studies demonstrate, ginkgo facilitates better blood flow throughout the body, notably the brain, where it both protects and promotes memory and mental function, even for people with Alzheimer's disease.[2] The greater flow of blood also can stabilize an irregular heart rhythm, help men to sustain erections and ease the numbness and pain of intermittent claudication, a circulatory disorder of the legs. Taking the extract also can be helpful in treating cataracts, retinopathy, macular degeneration, tinnitus, dizziness, asthma, headaches, premenstrual syndrome and depression.

Almost all of the ginkgo research tested an extract standardized to contain a 24 per cent concentration of flavonglycosides, the plant's active chemical ingredients. Weaker preparations might be beneficial, but I'd stick with using those products whose label specifies the 24 per cent concentration. No one with a serious mental or vascular problem should give in to drug therapy, I believe, without first trying ginkgo in a therapeutic range of 240–360 mg per day. For general mental acuity, anyone forty years old or older should take 120–160 mg every day. As a matter of fact, ginkgo's wide range of benefits, combined with its virtual complete safety, makes it worth trying for just about anyone.

GINSENG

Ginseng is known as an 'adaptogen', meaning that it helps the body to adapt. To what? Well, to just about any physiological stress. This root, prized for millennia, seems to display the rare ability to restore equilibrium to the body, either stimulating or dampening certain biochemical processes that are thrown out of synch by a variety of stressors. Obviously this is an extremely accommodating natural remedy.

The two main varieties of ginseng have somewhat different effects. Depending upon the condition, you can use either *Eleutherococcus senticosus,* commonly referred to as 'Siberian ginseng', or the potentially more powerful panax, better known as Chinese or Korean ginseng. *Panax quinquefolium*, called 'American ginseng', is another well-regarded panax variety.

Siberian Ginseng This form plays special roles in strengthening the immune system and stabilizing blood sugar. For people with either Type I or Type II diabetes, a daily 200 mg dose of the standardized extract reduced high blood sugar, improved mood and enhanced overall physical endurance.[3] Many of my dieters are convinced it helped them lose weight. You needn't have a metabolic problem to enjoy Siberian ginseng's mental and physical stimulation. Studies show that it can allow you to work better under stress.[4] People with cancer or AIDS benefit from the herb's immune system reinforcement, which can be measured in lab tests.

Panax Ginseng For mental and physical stamina, panax is more potent than eleutherococcus. Such strong stimulation is ideally suited for people with cancer, who need its greater invigorating powers.[5] Chinese or Korean ginseng might be too potent, in fact; some users have complained of irritability, anxiety and insomnia.[6] That's why I prefer to use *Panax quinquefolium*. Its stimulatory effect is mellower, but the immune system revitalization remains excellent. The combination, a European bestseller under the trade name of Ginsana, in placebo controlled studies was a significant benefactor for both the common cold and the influenza virus.[7]

Whichever variety of ginseng you choose, remember that its effects won't be felt immediately. You may take supplements for weeks or months before feeling more energetic or alert. Some products contain a powdered form of the root, but I prefer a pill or liquid ginseng extract whose concentration is standardized and consistent. In cities and towns with Asian enclaves, you will find shops where the whole root can be purchased. Ginseng experts can judge which individual root is more potent simply by examining them. Translating this piece-to-piece variability into milligram recommendations would be doing a disservice. You'll do better by trying a few capsules each day and judging the effect yourself.

CAT'S CLAW

Many people, including me, harbour a fanciful yet plausible belief that nature has indeed created a botanical cure-all buried in the depths of some rain forest and still untouched by civilization. One day, perhaps, we will discover this mythical plant. Until then we have cat's claw, touted by many as the closest thing yet to an herbal panacea.

Harvested in the Peruvian rain forest, cat's claw is one of my most widely prescribed herbs. South American herbalists have dispensed it for centuries, and I use it to treat many of the same ailments: digestive problems, ulcers, arthritis and inflammatory ailments. Since the 1970s European researchers have been establishing a sound scientific foundation for these applications and others. The herb can lower blood pressure and cholesterol and, as animal studies suggest, may help to deter blood from clotting.[8] It also contains a number of compounds that, among other effects, may enhance the immune system and inhibit cancer.

Not all varieties of cat's claw offer the same therapeutic benefit. The *Uncaria tomentosa* type possesses the most health-promoting qualities. A similar variety, *Uncaria guianesis,* is helpful but lacks tomentosa's most medically important compound, called isopterodine. Brewed teas and diluted extracts, known as tinctures, are probably the best ways to absorb the active ingredients in cat's claw, although capsules seem to work just as well if they contain a standardized extract. Avoid supplements of ground cat's claw bark. The bark is indigestible and, therefore, probably of no benefit.

I have found an unacceptably wide variety of potencies between one distributor's products and another. This makes dosage recommendations difficult. For instance, the cat's claw I prescribe for my patients is effective in three to six capsules of 500 mg each. An experienced herbal practitioner should be able to advise you.

ALOE VERA

This popular plant represents true home-grown health care. If aloe vera didn't require light, I'd recommend potting it right inside your medicine cabinet. A living, growing plant (kept on a sunny windowsill, of course) is the best source of aloe vera's healing energy. Commercial ointments are beneficial and convenient, but nothing beats the effectiveness or the economy of fresh aloe resin from a just broken leaf.

Most people use the 'the plant of immortality', as the Egyptians called it, to speed the healing of minor burns, cuts and scrapes, but it's also a soothing salve for sunburn, cellulitis, minor electrical shocks and frostbite. Apply the gel as soon as possible, and try to keep the wound covered for at least twenty-four hours, which, at least when treating a burn, will minimize scarring. Although animal studies hint at aloe vera's role in treating diabetic skin ulcers, don't rely on it to mend deep wounds or more serious skin injuries. In these cases it can actually impede healing.

Some of the more recent aloe research points to the plant's additional capabilities against immune weakness, viral infections and, perhaps, cancer. Stronger preparations are necessary here, but they may not always be practical because of the high dosages involved. Oral supplements are frequently prescribed against intestinal toxins, and research shows they can contribute to ulcer therapy.[9] Other research holds out some hope for people with asthma[10] and Type II diabetes.[11]

Don't eat aloe leaves in an attempt to tap their therapeutic potential, and don't let the plant's reputation sway you to use any aloe products billed as 'natural laxatives'. While the plant's skin contains a bitter substance that does exert a laxative effect, relief comes at the cost of gripping intestinal pains. Fortunately most commercial manufacturers remove the noxious compound from their products.

Other active ingredients in aloe might reinforce the immune system enough to affect the course of viral infections and cancer, but not enough research has been done to prove this definitively. We do know, however, that the best known of these compounds, acemannan, is an approved veterinary treatment for feline leukaemia, believed to be caused by a virus similar in action to HIV. Acemannan's benefits can be quite dramatic, according to reports I've heard from colleagues. In a few small clinical trials, the supplement improved certain indicators of immune system activity in people with AIDS.[12]

Acemannan's availability and high cost present two major practical obstacles to further clinical and personal experimentation. The effective daily dosage is at least 800 mg – the equivalent of drinking 1.75 litres of aloe juice every day. While that may be feasible for some people, especially when cancer or AIDS is the motivation, we can't be sure that the juice contains acemannan, which is chemically unstable. The alternative is to convince a veterinarian that you are indeed the family cat. For skin conditions, simply apply the leaf's contents over the affected area. For intestinal conditions, the effective daily dosage is 1 tablespoon three times a day.

LIQUORICE (GLYCYRRHIZIN)

Long before it became a staple at the sweet counter, liquorice was a favourite herb among native American Indians, Chinese medical practitioners and ancient Greeks. The dramatic anti-inflammatory action of its main chemical constituent, glycyrrhizin, slows the deterioration of the body's own inflammation-fighting adrenal steroids and magnifies the power of other herbs. Research backs its use in treating rheumatoid arthritis, allergies, bronchial disorders, viruses, mouth sores (boil some liquorice root in water and use it as a mouthwash), chronic fatigue, blood sugar imbalances and several skin afflictions, including eczema, dermatitis and impetigo.

Science has known since the early 1960s that liquorice can curb a cough just as well as codeine. The extract enhances the heartburn-soothing action of antacids by some 80 per cent, cuts in half the ulcer-forming potential of aspirin and may even minimize dental plaque. It also may prevent HIV from developing into full-blown AIDS and inhibit the growth of other viruses, including hepatitis B and Epstein-Barr.[13]

Taken in high doses for a lengthy period, glycyrrhizin can elevate blood pressure and cause fluid retention – side effects that are reminiscent of corticosteroid drugs; that's because it prevents the breakdown of our body's natural adrenal steroids.[14] To avoid such problems, most herbalists use the whole herb or a glycyrrhizin-free extract, even though they are less potent than the pure extract. Deglycyrrhizinated liquorice is the one most widely used, and it's a treatment of choice for peptic ulcer disease and other gastrointestinal disorders. In one head-to-head comparison, it prevented ulcers more effectively than the best-selling ulcer drug, cimetidine.[15]

Don't go to the sweet shop to fill your prescription. The junk food treat bearing the herb's name contains sugar and artificial flavourings and little or no liquorice. I generally prescribe three to six capsules containing 300–600 mg for my patients with ulcer, allergy or inflammatory conditions.

GARLIC

This pungent bulb deserves four chapters, not four paragraphs. One of the best-studied plants in the world, garlic is a veritable panacea, whether eaten as a food or used as a medicinal extract. Its array of benefits is staggering. For starters, it boosts immune function, favourably modifying the course of almost any infectious disease. It lowers high blood sugar and might increase the body's metabolism enough to promote weight loss.[16] Big doses of the extract may even help to prevent cancer.[17]

Garlic's most exciting use, I think, is in cutting back the risk of heart disease. It lowers cholesterol, prevents blood fats from sticking to artery walls and reduces high blood pressure.[18] It also inhibits the body's release of thromboxane B_2, a substance that constricts blood vessels and bronchial passages.[19]

What's the best way to get your garlic? Any way that's convenient. If you don't like the taste or can't eat it every day, try an extract of aged garlic, either in a capsule or as a liquid. Odourless and tasteless, it's the form that researchers have studied most extensively. Because the herb's healing strength increases proportionately with the dose, supplements are the better therapeutic choice. I recommend taking 2,400–3,200 mg every day.

Beware of products that promote their allicin content. Allicin is a short-lived substance formed by crushing fresh garlic. It is not absorbed by the digestive tract – and for good reason: it damages red blood cells and irritates body tissues, lab studies report.

GINGER

You may know it from Chinese cooking, gingerbread or from soft drink ginger ale, but ginger first earned a reputation in herbal medicine. It prevents blood from clotting just as effectively as aspirin, but without aspirin's stomach irritation or other side effects. The spice also reduces cholesterol, strengthens the heart's overall functioning and is a very effective anti-inflammatory agent that helps rheumatoid arthritis.[20]

Ginger's traditional use in quelling an upset stomach has been fully validated by science. Supplements, as one study demonstrated, counteract motion sickness and dizziness better than dimenhydrinate.[21] Ginger can also relieve morning sickness in pregnant women[22] and cut down the need for antivomiting medications in a variety of situations.[23] It even soothed seasick Danish sailors who were observed out on high, heavy ocean waters.[24]

TURMERIC

Although added to curry powders for its yellow colouring rather than its taste, which is rather bland, turmeric certainly spices up an antioxidant programme. A dose of curcumin, its active compound, as low as 20 mg considerably hampers the cell-damaging ability of free radical molecules. It also reduces cigarette smoke's cancerous threat and, when applied directly, helps improve the treatment of skin cancer.

Because curcumin eases inflamed tissues, it is an essential ally against arthritis, irritable bowel syndrome, asthma and any other inflammatory ailment.[25] By stimulating bile secretion in the liver, it improves digestion. The extract also improves sugar metabolism, opposes cholesterol increases and deters blood clotting. According to some lab experiments, it also shows an ability to inhibit the HIV virus.[26] It was shown recently to reverse precancerous mouth lesions by enhancing the antioxidant activity of the healthy cells.[27]

I usually recommend between 400 and 1,200 mg of curcumin every day, although I often double the dosage for better results against arthritis and similar inflammatory problems. Don't rely on the whole spice for therapeutic assistance. Turmeric itself contains only 1 per cent curcumin; capsules with a consistent concentration of the extract contain 95 per cent.

IMMUNE-ENHANCING HERBS

Medicinal Mushrooms

Don't be fooled by the 'medicinal' designation. Although they constitute a major part of cancer therapy in Japan and China, the most potent medicinal mushrooms are also among the best tasting. Each has a different flavour, both gustatorily and therapeutically, but they share the ability to build stamina, reinforce the immune system and promote general health. Different mushrooms are used by different complementary practitioners throughout the world, but four warrant special attention.

Shiitake   Because it is a mainstay of the Japanese diet, this mushroom holds the longest track record for health care, showing promise in treating cancer and, perhaps, HIV. Lentinan, shiitake's strongest active ingredient, is usually administered intravenously because some doubt exists over whether it is absorbed well orally. One study, however, did find some benefit against stomach cancer when ingested.[1]

While you certainly need to consult a complementary doctor for lentinan injections, you should make these delectable mushrooms a part of your diet. Perhaps their other therapeutic constituents, the most important of which is polysaccharide KS-2, are absorbed better. Any well-stocked supermarket or Asian grocery should carry them. Shiitake supplements are another alternative. Search your health food store for a brand that's standardized for its KS-2 content.

Reishi   This mushroom is my burnout tonic, a good restorative for workaholics, type A's and other hyperactive people who never seem able to slow down. Like all of the great mushrooms, reishi increases overall well-being, but it has more specific purposes, such as treating allergies and controlling blood clotting and high blood pressure. Some of its active components energize the immune system, while others fight tumours.

To make a refreshing reishi tonic, mix 1 dropperful of the liquid extract you can find in better health food stores into a glass of water. Three or four capsules of the standardized extract provide a similar amount. For a therapeutic anticancer tonic, amounts three times greater are beneficial yet safe.

Maitake The mushroom I prescribe most frequently, almost routinely, to cancer patients, is maitake. Supplements of its active ingredient, called the 'D fraction', have prevented the spread of malignant tumours. Unfortunately, none of the maitake research has been done on humans, but many doctors are using it successfully. Clinical trials, when finally completed, promise to confirm this experience.

Although the mushroom usually has been given intravenously in the animal experiments, we give the liquid extract by mouth to our cancer patients, normally in a dosage of 50–80 drops per day. When cancer prevention rather than treatment is the objective, I may prescribe half that amount.

PSK Fortunately, one of the most exciting mushroom-derived adjuvant cancer therapies to surface in a long time may soon be within our grasp. Polysaccharide K (PSK) was on the verge of availability as this book went to press. I haven't used it personally, but its reputation is well established. In Japan PSK is used in routine postoperative treatments, and annual sales there reach into the hundreds of millions of dollars.

An extract of a fungus called corioulus versicolour, PSK more than doubles the long-term survival rates of lung cancer patients, even if they are otherwise treated conventionally.[2] Another study revealed that those colon cancer patients who received PSK remained healthier and survived significantly longer than those who did not receive it.[3] When the medicinal herb was administered to people with stomach cancer, the five-year survival rate jumped from 59 to 70 per cent.[4] Unlike conventional cancer therapies, PSK showed no side effects.

We're not entirely certain how PSK interrupts tumour growth, but animal studies indicate that it revitalizes two components of the immune system, natural killer cells and T cells. It also enhances the therapeutic strength of other cancer treatments, generates a greater production of the natural antioxidant enzyme SOD, and protects chromosomes from malignant harm.[5] The icing on the cake is that PSK is completely nontoxic and can be taken by mouth. All in all, it stands ready to become a supplement of enormous significance.

MISTLETOE

Aside from correcting a deficiency of kisses at Christmastime, mistletoe (*Viscum album*) has been ingested for centuries to treat everything from epilepsy to high blood pressure. Its most established use is fortifying the immune system. As my patients' test results so frequently show, the blood tests demonstrating a cancer's extent, called tumour markers, drop dramatically following a series of twice weekly mistletoe injections. Quality of life, something that standard chemotherapeutic drugs rarely improve, also seems better after taking the herb, as shown in a recent human study.[6]

Like any other therapy that rebuilds the immune system, mistletoe works best in a body that has not been damaged by chemotherapy or radiation. That's why it's so crucial to find a practitioner willing to administer the extract as soon as possible after a cancer is discovered. Mistletoe comes in several varieties and, although it can be taken orally, it requires considerable experience by a practitioner to use it effectively, since the injectable form is much more effective.

ASTRAGALUS

Of the many plants that refresh a lethargic immune system, astragalus is one of my favourites. It's a wonderful long-term tonic for anyone, especially cancer patients and elderly people who need extra infection protection during the winter. In one study the herb quadrupled natural killer cell activity, a measurement of the immune system's vigour, among people afflicted with viral myocarditis.[7] Other research suggests that it might reduce blood pressure, boost energy and increase sperm motility enough to overcome infertility.[8]

Tincture of astragalus works best, in my experience. Squirt 1–2 droppersful into a glass of water, stir and drink up.

PAU D'ARCO

The reddish bark of a tropical South American tree, pau d'arco possesses strong antibacterial, antiviral and antifungal properties, but its higher medicinal calling seems to be cancer therapy. In 1968 scientists at the US National Cancer Institute learned that lapachol, the bark's most active chemical constituent, has remarkable anticancer abilities, yet by 1973 the research was discontinued, a rejection that happens all too often with promising nontoxic compounds. Animal studies later supported the initial findings, which alone justified human clinical trials. I'm not willing to forfeit the herb's contributions, so I continue to prescribe it, often blending 2 droppersful of the tincture with other herbs into a tea.

Look for a printed guarantee that a pau d'arco extract does, in fact, contain the bark's active components. In 1987 a chemical analysis of a dozen commonly available Canadian supplements disclosed that they contained no more than a trace of lapachol.[9] It is readily available in health food stores.

INFECTION FIGHTERS

ECHINACEA

Many gardeners love to grow the purple coneflower but are unaware of its medicinal benefits. German researchers put this beautiful plant and its magenta-coloured leaves on the herbal therapy map. Through their exhaustive research, we've come to learn, as the Plains Indians first understood and as over three hundred studies have confirmed, that echinacea reinforces our natural defences in a number of ways.[1]

By targeting viral and bacterial invaders, echinacea can

prevent and treat upper respiratory infections[2] and vaginal yeast infections.[3] It also speeds recovery time from an infection without causing any of the side effects typical of pharmaceutical antibiotics, especially the overgrowth of intestinal yeast responsible for a great deal of chronic illness.

The liquid extract, echinacea tea and freshly pressed juice are fine preparations, but freeze-dried echinacea powder achieves the best results. As a cold and flu preventive, take two or three capsules containing 760–1,040 mg every day. To treat an infection, I suggest somewhat more, usually six to eight of these capsules a day.

GOLDENSEAL

Before modern science developed antibiotics, Native American Indians had their own exceptionally good therapy. Goldenseal (*Hydrastis canadensis*) gave them an excellent source of berberine, a substance that blocks bacterial growths, the *Candida albicans* yeast and even some parasites.[4] The herb seems to work best against urinary, respiratory and sinus infections, as well as others that settle in the body's mucus membranes. It also works well against forms of infectious diarrhoea.[5] In addition to elevating white blood cell numbers, a sign of a healthier immune system, goldenseal assists in lowering blood sugar and blood pressure. It also helps to control disturbances in heart rhythm.

Because of several notable adverse reactions, don't use goldenseal or any other berberine-containing plant for any length of time. They overstimulate the nervous system, cause intestinal problems and can even induce abortion. As a short-term treatment I prefer the tincture, standardized to contain 5 per cent hydrastine, another of the active chemicals. A good dosage range is 750–1,500 mg per day, in capsules you will find in any health food store. Combined with echinacea, it's a great cold and flu remedy.

OLIVE LEAF

One of the hottest new infection fighters isn't new at all – doctors used olive leaf as long ago as 1927 to knock out malaria.

Calcium enolate, the leaf's most active ingredient, is an extraordinarily effective killer of viruses and bacteria. It also keeps latent viruses from emerging.[6]

The leaf offers at least some relief, if not complete recovery, from the entire rogues' gallery of microbial ailments – pneumonia, gonorrhoea, tuberculosis, influenza, viral encephalitis, viral meningitis, hepatitis B, shingles, herpes and Epstein-Barr. It's also a worthwhile treatment for urinary infections, surgical infections and any sort of bacterial infection. But olive leaf also destroys yeast infections at the same time.

Olive leaf grabbed my attention because of its ability to produce a side effect. It is, however, a beneficial side effect that mirrors its value. While the extract is entirely nontoxic, taking too much too soon can make you sicker before you get better. This temporary side effect apparently stems from the so-called die-off reaction, which is normally a concern only when antimicrobial agents are extremely effective. Killing larger microorganisms, such as yeast, on a massive scale inundates the body with toxins from the dying organisms, and the liver can't dispense with them fast enough. Symptoms vary, depending upon the infection, but at first you may feel worse, particularly with respect to fatigue. Once the reaction passes, shortly after you scale down the dose, your ailment usually disappears, too. And that's what impresses me about olive leaf. After all, antibiotics do not kill both bacteria and yeast.

I've been able to minimize the risk of die-off by keeping the initial doses of olive leaf small, usually a single 500 mg capsule a day. Over the course of the week I increase the amount until my patient is taking 2,000 mg per day, which is usually all that is necessary. Once the infectious illness begins to abate, I taper down the dose to one or two capsules a day. There are several manufacturers, but most seem to provide 500 mg capsules.

Oil of Oregano

The oils extracted from spices, such as thyme, cloves, rosemary and oregano, are often good fungus and virus fighters. Oregano oil is probably the champ. Ever since my introduction to it, when a single dose quickly relieved a bad wintertime cold I had contracted, I've used oregano for many patients. Now I've come to depend upon it to treat almost any infection, including yeast overgrowth, for which it is one of the very best treatments.

Two antioxidants in oregano, thymol and carvacrol, probably account for its antimicrobial ability. Whole oregano leaves contain enough of the two compounds to stave off certain foodborne fungi and prevent fresh meat from spoiling. To change the course of an infection, however, you'll need to take an extract, in a dosage of 2–4 drops. It also works topically. For relief from a toothache, put 1–2 drops on a cotton wool ball and rub it inside your mouth. An oil of oregano liniment, made by mixing one part of the extract with three parts of oil, soothes sprains and rheumatic limbs very nicely.

However, there's another rub, and one that's not so nice: the aroma. Oil of oregano is so strong that a single drop imbues a room with the smell of an oregano factory. If you don't notice the scent, you don't have true oil of oregano. The acrid essence, which lingers for a day or two, needn't go to waste. A few whiffs will help clear a sinus infection.

My only precaution against oil of oregano is directed to expectant mothers. Don't use this or any other herbal oil during your pregnancy. Oils can be potent, and we simply don't know enough about their safety or their effect on the unborn baby.

Tea Tree Oil

If you are planning a family camping trip and can take along only one topical first-aid remedy, your choice should be tea tree oil (melaleuca). Its antibacterial, antifungal and antiseptic properties are ideal as a general disinfectant and as a treatment for acne, fungal infections, athlete's foot and cold sores. The oil, obtained from a tree native to Australia, matches the effectiveness of standard antifungal medications, as demonstrated by a study of 117 people who had toenail infections.[7] Minor cuts also heal more effectively and with fewer infections.

Just a drop or two contains all the antiseptic power you need. However, my caution against using an herbal oil also applies here. It's otherwise safe for any external use but shouldn't be ingested. Be prepared not only for its sting when applied to an open wound, but also for its strong aroma. Finally, watch where you put the oil. It stains clothing.

CARDIOVASCULAR HERBS

HAWTHORN

I call this herb 'the wise man's digitalis' in tribute to the excellent medicine, derived from the foxglove plant, that cardiologists once used to strengthen the heart and reduce how rapidly it beats. To our great disservice, pharmaceutical companies extracted but a single one of foxglove's constituents and created a different drug, digoxin, whose side effects include heart blockages and rhythm disturbances.

Hawthorn extract works just as well as digoxin and its predecessor, with virtually no side effects or long-term risks. In my opinion, the herb (*Crataegus oxyacantha*) should be prescribed as a matter of course to every person with a cardiovascular problem.

In many gentle ways, hawthorn impressively addresses almost every major factor involved in heart disease. By keeping blood vessels relaxed, it reduces blood pressure and permits a freer flow of blood to the heart muscle.[1] Better blood flow, in turn, increases the heart's oxygen supply, allowing the muscle to pump more efficiently and with less strain.[2] Additionally, through its influence on inflammation and allergic reactions, the herb brings some therapeutic relief from chest pains (angina), an unusually fast heartbeat (tachycardia), shortness of breath and hypertension.

The extract is quite potent. The usual dosage is 240–480 mg daily. If you need heart medication, use it only under a doctor's guidance. Because it functions much the same way as heart medications, it may make the medications excessive, and the doctor will probably have to lower the dosages of some medications.

COLEUS FORSKOHLII

Though few people may be familiar with *Coleus forskohlii*, I sense that this ayurvedic herb, thanks to the active compound forskolin, is destined for a famous future. A flurry of research during the last several years has established that forskolin can lower blood pressure, increase the heart's strength and relieve congestive heart failure.[3] The extract has been shown to benefit asthmatics[4] and may alleviate psoriasis as well. Some researchers see a role in weight loss, because forskolin stimulates the release of thyroid hormone and helps the body metabolize it.[5] For cardiovascular purposes, take 50 mg of the extract two to four times a day.

BROMELAIN

While I often prescribe it to minimize blood clotting, bromelain gained its reputation from its widespread use in sports medicine and trauma treatment. An enzyme found in pineapple stems, it cools inflammation and promotes healing in injured muscles and joints. The anti-inflammatory influence also comes into play in relieving discomfort from asthma, arthritis, colitis and inflammatory bowel disorders.[6]

Some European cardiologists use bromelain to reverse the symptoms of coronary heart disease. I have seen people benefit from it. It may do more for the heart than its known effect of keeping our blood platelets from sticking to each other, a process known to be involved in plaque formation.

Only high-quality supplements are capable of such therapeutic effects. Look for a tablet or capsule rated at 2,000 GDU. A dosage of 600 mg per day seems to work well against inflammation. Take it on an empty stomach, or it will serve more as a digestive aid than as an anti-inflammatory.

CAPSAICIN

I use capsaicin, the powerful extract of cayenne pepper, fairly routinely in treating heart patients, often combined with hawthorn. I also rely on it as a topical painkiller. As an herbal heart medication, capsaicin (*Capsicum annum*) can cut cholesterol, lower high blood pressure, thin the blood and help combat fatigue. These actions make it suitable as a general cardiovascular supplement and as a treatment for specific heart ailments, including chest pains and rhythm disturbances.

Elsewhere in the body, capsaicin is as effective a topical painkiller as any we have seen. Knowing a good thing when they see it, the drug companies now use it as the active ingredient in their high-priced, heavily advertised pain preparations. Originally sold only by prescription, but now available over-the-counter, the salves tout capsaicin's ability to relieve everything from run-of-the-mill achy muscles to pain from a mastectomy. As the ads say, it's the pain reliever that most doctors recommend. Just don't count on them to mention that you can get the same stuff, often at a more reasonable price, at a health food store.

Cayenne's nerve-numbing, desensitizing effect, according to the research, eases arthritis, herpes zoster (shingles),[7] psoriasis, asthma, incontinence and inflammatory bowel disease. It can also relieve pain from diabetic neuropathy and fibromyalgia.[8] The liquid extract, massaged on the gums, will dampen toothache pain. Rubbed inside your nose, it'll relieve a cluster headache; on the vagina it will clear up a painful case of vulvar vestibulitis.[9] And while the spice was once thought to cause ulcers, we now know that it actually may prevent them.

As an alternative to buying a capsaicin cream, you might mix up a home-made salve, blending some cayenne powder into a base of cocoa butter. You can also eat foods peppered with cayenne, although I suggest starting with a mere sprinkle if you're not accustomed to hot spices.

In capsule form, cayenne's strength is measured not in milligrams, but in units of a 'heat index'. The higher number of heat units, the more of the active ingredient it contains. Use the real scorchers, the supplements that contain 100,000 heat units.

GUGGULIPID

An extract from an Indian gum called 'guggul', guggulipid is another natural ally in the fight against high blood triglycerides and a poor HDL-LDL ratio.[10] By helping to reduce the viscosity of blood, it also gives us extra protection against blood clots. Widely available in health food stores, a typical dose is 50–100 mg twice a day.

Cactus (Night-Blooming Cereus)

In 1921, years before the pharmaceutical industry and consensus panels assumed control of the medical profession, a leading distributor of herbal medicines surveyed doctors to learn which herbs they prescribed most frequently. One of the favourites turned out to be night-blooming cereus, which may be more familiar as cactus.

In today's average doctor's surgery, cactus is more likely to be found on a windowsill than in the dispensary, and just about every heart patient in the country is worse off as a result. Cactus is an effective herbal enhancer of the heart, capable of substantially reducing the need for risky, costly heart medications.

If cactus were a patentable drug instead of an inexpensive herb, its impressive range of benefits would probably make it a top-selling medication. Although it can strengthen the heart muscle in virtually every form of cardiovascular disease, it gives its best performance in treating cardiac rhythm disorders and mitral valve prolapse, which involves a weakness in a heart valve.[11]

When cactus is taken with hawthorn, magnesium, coenzyme Q_{10}, taurine and L-carnitine, among other heart nutrients, the therapeutic effect can be surprising. The wonderful thing about cactus is that the longer you use it, the better it works. It won't weaken the heart, as do many cardiac medications. In fact, regular use often greatly reduces the need for such drugs.

The value of cactus is therapeutic, not preventive, so only people diagnosed with heart disease should use it, preferably as a tincture available in health food stores. A daily 1/2 teaspoon is a typical dosage. As with hawthorn, anticipate a less dire need for heart medications. However, reduce the dosage only under a doctor's supervision.

METABOLIC HERBS

Milk Thistle

Unquestionably the most potent of all herbal detoxifiers, milk thistle (*Silybum marianum*) is a must-have supplement for anyone concerned about blood sugar, liver health, pollution, chemical allergies or cancer. In a dosage of 600 mg per day, it enabled people with liver cirrhosis due to diabetes to decrease the amount of insulin they needed.[1] As a liver medication, milk thistle slashed the death rate from cirrhosis by an astounding 50 per cent and improved the outcome of hepatitis treatments.[2] Daily supplements of 150–300 mg encourage the liver to make glutathione, one of the body's best antioxidants. Doses of 400–800 mg are required for treating liver diseases.

FENUGREEK

Tea brewed from this herb (*Trigonella foenumgraecum*) breaks up congestion and loosens phlegm when you have a cold, but the true medicinal talent of fenugreek rests in its seeds. In very large amounts (between 25 and 100 grams per day), pulverized seeds impressively reduce high blood fats and blood sugar for people with Type I and Type II diabetes.[3] The studies used defatted seeds that were incorporated into recipes. Supplements work well, too, but may be difficult to find in the necessary quantity. Taking smaller amounts, though, does provide some improvement in blood lipid measurements.

GYMNEMA SYLVESTRE

Only a few experiments, all of them done in India, have tested the therapeutic ability of this herb, but I hope other scientists investigate the extract and find a similar potential. *Gymnema sylvestre,* according to reports, enables some people with Type I diabetes to cut their insulin needs almost in half.[4] For people with the Type II form of the disease, the herbal extract may decrease the dosage requirements of their oral glucose drugs.[5] I'm currently giving 100 mg thrice daily to many of my Type II patients.

HERBS FOR MEN

SAW PALMETTO (*SERENOA REPENS*)

More than twenty studies conducted according to the strictest of scientific standards have established that this herb is superior to Proscar, some urologists' favourite pharmaceutical for treating benign prostate enlargement.[1] They would help more people by using herbs. The drug doesn't help more than 60 per cent of the men who take it, according to comparative studies, while the extract of saw palmetto (*Serenoa repens*) helps about 90 per cent. Within just a month it relieves such symptoms as constricted urinary flow and need for frequent nighttime trips to the bathroom. It works by blocking the enzyme that seems to cause the prostate to enlarge.[2]

Science is less certain about another of saw palmetto's reputed qualities – sexual rejuvenation. The herb, actually a bush native to Florida, has been heralded for centuries as an aphrodisiac. Research doesn't corroborate the claim, although some of my patients say it helps.

Saw palmetto extract should contain an 85 per cent concentration of active sterols, the plant's medicinal ingredients. Widely available in health food stores, you may take 160 mg capsules twice daily with meals.

PYGEUM AFRICANUM

Derived from the bark of a tropical evergreen, pygeum is another excellent herbal tonic for the prostate. The standardized extract dependably relieves urinary problems, such as constricted flow, and other symptoms of prostate infections and benign prostate enlargement, according to European research.[3] Most men, as far as I can determine, don't mind the mild aphrodisiac effect it imparts.

I normally recommend a daily 100 mg dose of pygeum extract, along with saw palmetto and several other nutrients, including zinc and the essential fatty acids. Each of the herbs is well proven on its own, but their synergistic effect is better.

YOHIMBE

The yohimbe story is very basic: nearly half of the men who use its pharmaceutical derivative will regain some measure of erectile ability.[4] But the whole herb, and the yohimbe supplements billed as sexual tonics, display little of this power. Only the prescription drug yohimbine contains enough of the active ingredient to offer even some hope.

Although the concentration might be a little higher in some over-the-counter liquid extracts, no form of yohimbe should be considered a first-choice solution to erection problems. Nor should it be used as a weight-loss aid, even though it might be mildly effective in this regard. Yohimbine can raise blood pressure, among other side effects, even in healthy men. It should be used with great caution if you have hypertension, heart disease, diabetes, a thyroid disorder, a kidney disease or a mental illness.

Circulatory and heart-related disorders often underlie erection failure in men. The process, after all, is a matter of blood hydraulics. Instead of looking for direct therapeutic help from yohimbe and similar supplements, focus on controlling diabetes or on reducing high blood pressure (and thereby getting off medications) and high blood lipids. But tell your doctor that you want to explore nutritional medicine before resorting to drugs. The medications prescribed to address high blood pressure and other heart problems are notorious for causing erectile difficulties.

HERBS FOR WOMEN

BLACK COHOSH

The effect of the active ingredients in black cohosh (*Cimicifuga racemosa*) strongly resembles oestrogen's influence in the body.[1] The herb is therefore very useful for alleviating menstrual cramps and menopausal problems such as hot flushes and night sweats. A daily 16 mg tablet or capsule usually diminishes symptoms within two weeks.

Black cohosh is also an excellent nervous system tonic for

both women and men, and it brings desperately sought relief from the unexplained muscle pains of fibromyalgia.

Mexican Yam (Dioscorea)

Supplements of this vegetable have been hailed far and wide as a natural sex hormone. Don't be duped.

Mexican yam extracts have been pitched to men as a natural muscle-building, erection-raising supplement and to women as an alternative to oestrogen replacement therapy. According to the advertised claims, the body converts the extract's active ingredient, called diosgenin, into either progesterone, testosterone or DHEA – precisely which depends on the targeted audience.

In the real world, the body doesn't turn diosgenin into anything, at least not anything that resembles either gender's sex hormones. To accomplish the feat, you may start with dioscorea, but you also need a laboratory, knowledge of a complicated chemical procedure and a supply of sulfuric acid.

Be that as it may, I and thousands of my patients find that supplements, and especially creams, containing Mexican yam have minimized their menopausal and premenstrual maladies and allowed many of them to stop taking oestrogen. Dioscorea, however, does not deserve all of the credit. The most effective of these products have been spiked with synthetic versions of natural progesterone or contain other natural substances, such as pregnenolone and vitamin A, that help the body generate a little more of its own female hormones.

Vitex (*Vitex agnus castus*)

This wonderful plant, called the chaste berry because of its reputation for suppressing a woman's libido, has been used for centuries as a tonic for general female health. It seems to nourish the pituitary gland, a control centre for balancing hormonal activity. If a 175 mg capsule is taken once every morning, the extract can curb premenstrual tension and various symptoms of menopause.[2] Don't expect immediate results. Sometimes three to six months may pass before you notice Vitex's influence.

BRAIN STIMULANTS

ST-JOHN'S-WORT (HYPERICUM)

St-John's-wort is another example of a natural substance that could be awarded treatment of choice status – in this case, as an antidepressant. Its key ingredient, hypericin, elevates the spirits of people with mild to moderate depression. Scientists researching the herb administered 300–1,000 mg in eight different controlled studies, along with standard antidepressants. However, the drugs caused 2.67 times the number of side effects. Moreover, fifteen other controlled studies have demonstrated hypericum's efficacy. I prescribe it frequently for depression, and most of my patients feel a discernible improvement in mood after taking the equivalent dosage of 30 drops or so of the extract twice a day. Health food stores also provide capsules of 300 mg, often taken three times daily.

In addition, St-John's-wort fights influenza and Epstein-Barr, among other viruses.[1] Preliminary research suggests a role in treating AIDS (it knocks out the virus in test tube studies),[2] although clinical trials of people with HIV have, by and large, been disappointing. Our group of AIDS patients seems to have responded when we administered it intravenously; at the very least, it helped to lift the spirits of those who were depressed.

EPHEDRA (MA HUANG)

This supplement offers a most important lesson about herbal medicine. A good number of drugs, as I have explained, are extracted or otherwise derived from plants. Many plants, however, have a pharmaceutical effect in their natural state. Ephedra, or ma huang, as it's also known, may be freely sold as an herb, but it really is a drug. As such, we should avoid it with the respectful caution we normally reserve for pharmaceuticals.

Ephedra is nature's source of ephedrine, an adrenalinelike drug that suppresses appetite, dilates bronchial passages and stimulates metabolism, among other actions. Health food stores have crammed their shelves in recent years with 'natural' diet aids and mental stimulants that contain the herb. It's all a ruse, in my opinion, to sucker people into taking amphetaminelike medications under the false assumption that they've tapped into the wonders of herbal medicine. This widespread cavalier use also hands those who regulate these things a perfect pretext for interfering with the availability of natural supplements. There is ample reason to be concerned with the agency's actions against safe and effective supplements.

Ephedra will indeed encourage weight loss, partly by suppressing your desire to eat and partly by revving up the metabolism. The advantages, however, are temporary and illusory. After you stop taking the herb, your appetite comes back stronger than before, and your once accelerated metabolism slows to its previous rate. You then gain weight, often more than you lost. As many dieters regrettably discover, ephedra is useless and counterproductive in the long haul, and controlling obesity is a very long haul.

As a central nervous system stimulant, the herb is also potentially harmful, specifically for anyone with high blood pressure, diabetes or heart disease. All of these illnesses, by the way, are common among overweight people. Ephedra heightens anxiety, interferes with sleep and makes you sweat profusely. It also may irritate the prostate gland, perhaps enough to trigger benign enlargement. The only positive treatment role is as a bronchodilator. Some over-the-counter asthma medications contain ephedrine as an active ingredient, but they should be used only occasionally, if at all. Other herbs and nutrients, such as magnesium, fish oils, vitamin C and pantethine, are much safer.

GOTU KOLA

This remarkable Asian plant (*Centella asiatica*) suffers from a little therapeutic typecasting, to which I suppose I am contributing. It works so well as a brain energizer or mental pick-me-up that the public tends to overlook its other health-promoting features.

Because of an apparent ability to nurture skin and connective tissue, the herb gives us both cosmetic and clinical support in treating skin-related problems. It accelerates wound healing[3] and improves cellulite. Centella is probably the herb of choice in treating varicose veins and phlebitis. It speeds up healing, improves circulation and reduces ankle swelling.[4] People with scleroderma, a serious internal overgrowth of connective tissue throughout the body, might benefit as well.

There is also some evidence that gotu kola energizes the brain. Some experts have speculated that it prompts the body to manufacture choline, which might explain why it can enhance brain function in mentally retarded children.[5] The standard dose of gotu kola for the indications I have discussed is 60–120 mg daily of the titrated extract of *Centella asiatica*.

MENTAL RELAXANTS

KAVA

A single herb with a single job that it does very well, kava is a model of efficiency. As a natural tranquillizer, it lifts anxiety without causing drowsiness.[1] At the same time, remarkably, it enhances your ability to think and elevates mood. The pleasant feeling it induces works on several levels, making the herb an ideal substitute for pharmaceutical 'nerve pills', coffee and even alcohol.

Allowing body and mind to relax, I believe, facilitates healing, so I consider kava important to the treatment of cancer, AIDS or any other life-threatening condition.[2] Research suggests that it could also be used as a muscle relaxant, an anticonvulsant, a local anesthetic and a painkiller. The current debate over whether to allow the medicinal use of marijuana serves to emphasize how desperately some cancer patients need pain relief that does not wreak havoc on bowel function, as most pain drugs do. Kava's ability to potentiate pain relief from milder drugs has been the answer for many of my patients.

Teas and tinctures are equally good ways to take kava. So are capsules with a standardized concentration of the active ingredients, called kavalactones. A daily dose of 100–200 kavalactones normally is sufficient, although a larger amount might be necessary to help you fall asleep. Taking it during the day won't make you drowsy, just calmer and, yes, happier.

VALERIAN

If you feel anxious or have trouble sleeping, valerian may be for you. Swallowing a few capsules of the herb just before going to bed helps many people fall asleep without causing any of the side effects so common to sleep medications.[3] Most forms of the herb, standardized or not, seem to be helpful in this regard. Many of my patients drink 1 cup of valerian tea before bed; others take 150–450 mg of the capsules.

In other treatment possibilities, the *officinalis* variation of valerian relieved acute viral gastroenteritis infections better than standard antibiotics in one study. German researchers, meanwhile, have been exploring the anticancer properties of certain valerian extracts called 'valepotriates'. According to this work, these compounds seem to render tumour cells less malignant.[4]

SINGLE-PURPOSE HERBS

CRANBERRY

Only relatively recently has conventional medicine studied the time-honoured wisdom of drinking cranberry juice to treat or prevent a urinary tract infection.[1] Bioflavonoids in the tart-tasting berry interfere with the *E. coli* bacteria's attempts to cling to the bladder's interior lining. Some evidence also suggests that cranberries might prevent or deter kidney stones by discouraging calcium excretion.[2]

Many of my patients swear by cranberry therapy as an effective treatment for recurrent bladder infections. I normally recommend taking 6,000–9,000 mg of cranberry extract (four to six capsules), not drinking cranberry juice. The juice usually contains too much sugar, which suppresses the immune system and can encourage a stronger infection. If a patient prefers to use the juice, I insist that it be unsweetened.

FEVERFEW

Migraines are difficult to treat, and I cannot promise that a natural remedy will always be helpful. Nevertheless, feverfew is pleasingly reliable. Take a daily 100–200 mg dosage of the extract in capsules, which should have a guaranteed concentration of parthenolides, the herb's active compounds. Don't be impatient. You may not notice a decrease in the number of migraines for several months.

BILBERRY

The military upholds many traditions, sometimes out of habit, sometimes for thoroughly practical reasons. One practice with a purpose is the use of bilberry extract. As long ago as the Second World War and as recently as the Persian Gulf War, American pilots relied on it to enhance night vision.

Bioflavonoids in bilberry, a European relative of the American huckleberry (*Vaccinium myrtillus*), have an affinity for the retina at the back of the eye. They mend normal wear and tear on this light-sensitive tissue and generate the production of rhodopsin, an eye protein needed for night sight. Exposure to bright light, high-contrast light and computer screens depletes the eyes' supply of rhodopsin.

Research, done mostly in Italy, has also uncovered bilberry's potential for treating retinal problems stemming from poor blood circulation, diabetes-caused glaucoma and day blindness. The extract, along with vitamin E, halted cataract formation in 97 per cent of the people who participated in one study.[3] In another experiment, bilberry alone markedly improved nearsightedness for 75 per cent of the people who took it as a supplement.[4]

The berry's flavonoids, called anthocyanosides, are antioxidants, so they're called for when faced with any vascular ailment. They limit calcium deposits and blood clots inside arteries, help dilate blood vessels, relieve circulatory-caused leg swelling and numbness and diminish varicose veins and postpartum haemorrhoids. For people with arthritis, the supplement cools inflamed joints and may help to prevent the deterioration of joint collagen.

The better bilberry extracts are standardized to contain 25 per cent anthocyanosides. At this concentration, an effective dose would be between 250 and 500 mg per day.

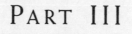

PART III

TARGETED VITA-NUTRIENT THERAPY

CHAPTER 14

APPLYING THE PROGRAMME

TREATING YOUR HEALTH PROBLEMS WITH VITA-NUTRIENTS

When leafing through this book for the first time, you might understandably start with this section. Why? Because it provides the solution to those health problems that are of greatest concern to you and your family. Indeed, this is the most essential service I can offer you.

At the Atkins Center, my staff and I help our patients use vita-nutrients to accomplish their health goals, and this is what I would like to do for you in this section.

Can You Manage Your Own Case? In the following pages I will provide you with individualized vita-nutrient treatment 'protocols', the unique approaches that I teach my professional staff and doctors in training. As a layperson, you are not likely to have the medical knowledge and experience necessary to treat your own illnesses. Therefore you should work with your primary care doctor to evaluate what may be causing any problems you are experiencing and the state of your health in general. (Pinpointing the cause of your health problems, after all, is the basic principle of complementary medicine and of prescribing appropriate vita-nutrients.)

Will Your Doctor Help? Given the state of resistance to nutritional medicine, you should make certain that your doctor shares your desire to maximize nutrition therapy, resorting to drugs and medications only for emergencies and for cases where the nutrition fails to optimize your health. If he or she resists this approach, you might present the parts of this book that pertain to your particular health problems. Its bibliography alone might convince dedicated doctors who want to treat their patients with scientifically based methods. If this fails, sadly, you may still need to change doctors. If a recalcitrant physician has been assigned to you through a managed care organization, you should complain to the administrators of your plan. If they hear enough similar complaints, they will be forced to incorporate nutritional medicine.

The very idea that my suggestions may lead you to abandon standard medical care in favour of a nutritional approach to your health care may cause mainstream practitioners to choke on their breakfast cereals. And if I were recommending over-the-counter medications or herbs with druglike effects, I, too, would feel that I was subjecting my readers to unnecessary risks. But I'm dealing with nutritional substances with a safety margin so great that as long as you observe a few necessary caveats, you will not subject yourself to risk. That's why when I say a nutrient is worth trying, you can assume that the worst thing that could happen is nothing.

Because the nutrients covered in this book have all been researched and tested, it is safe to assume that as long as you observe a few necessary caveats, they are risk-free. However, taking prescribed medications with vita-nutrients could be a whole different story. Make sure your doctor is completely familiar with the effectiveness of the vita-nutrients you will be using. Nutrients can do the same things as drugs and in certain circumstances can turn drugs into an overdose. Should that happen, the wiser strategy would be to decrease the pharmaceutical dosage.

Nutrients are not only safer than drugs; they are natural to the body. Our bodies are geared to handle nutrients because they belong there. However, they are not always equipped to handle newly invented chemical synthetics. Modern-day illnesses such as heart disease and diabetes are really diet-related disorders, and part of their treatment involves correcting deficiencies – of antioxidants, minerals such as magnesium and chromium, and other vita-nutrients such as coenzyme Q_{10} and carnitine. There can be no deficiency of beta-blockers or antidiabetic drugs.

THE NATURAL VS SYNTHETIC CONTROVERSY

Before we get into the specifics of individualizing your vita-nutrient program, you may want to know how I feel about two of nutrition's greatest controversies: 1) Are you better off seeking nutrients from food or from supplements? and 2) Should you consume natural or synthesized nutrients? My position is that natural sources of nutrients are generally superior to synthetic or unnatural sources, although the magnitude of this advantage varies from vitamin to vitamin. However, the cost of extracting vitamins from natural sources makes them so prohibitively expensive compared to the synthesized varieties that they have all but disappeared from the marketplace. In fact, virtually every convincing scientific study done establishing the proven benefits of nutrients used nonfood source nutrients. Thus it would seem that synthetic supplements not only work, but work very well.

But when synthetic beta-carotene failed to match the cancer-preventing capabilities of its natural counterparts in several recent studies, scientists were reminded that sometimes natural vita-nutrient sources are the most effective. Indeed, many scientific papers by nutrition pioneer Royal Lee, DDS, and others writing in the 1930s through 1950s showed that entire nutrient complexes were significantly more effective than synthetic vitamins.

Many times I have been tempted to devise diets in which natural foods provide all necessary nutrients. But in practice I found that the quantities of nutrients my patients could derive from those sources were less than optimal. Worse yet, those with weight problems had to take in more carbohydrate to accomplish the nutrient goal, and this led to further weight gain.

The Atkins Center's solution to this dilemma was to create the widest breadth of supplementation possible. Rather than providing a small number of inexpensively produced chemicals that supply the central constituent of a vitamin complex, we provided the entire complex. For example, we recommended all the tocopherols, not just one, when using vitamin E. Then we made certain we used as many *different* nutrient complexes as the body might need. With such a basic formula providing the backdrop for further nutrient prescriptions, we reduced the likelihood of running into built-in difficulties of single dosages of vitamins. A good multiple vitamin and mineral formulation would contain at least forty different nutrients. This form of 'group therapy' allows vitamins to be given safely in high dosages, thus strengthening the therapeutic effect.

An important part of this concept is that those vita-nutrients not on the usual list of vitamins and essential minerals can have a tremendous impact. Nutrients like glutathione, coenzyme Q_{10}, taurine, pycnogenol, lipoic acid and many others described in this book clearly add synergistic elements to the nutritional chain. This team approach packs a much stronger therapeutic punch than administering only a handful of isolated vitamins in the manner in which the early research was conducted.

Even more important is the principle of getting the maximum nutritional value from the food we eat. Eggs, meat and other animal products contain a wide spectrum of vita-nutrients. Nuts and seeds are extraordinarily good sources, and certain fats and oils – such as flaxseed, borage and evening primrose oil – can be among the most valuable nutrients of all. Specific vegetables, particularly those high in the C and E complexes, are also vital. But empty calories, which come from sweets, refined foods and foods designed to have long shelf life, have an antinutrient effect. Our celebrated food pyramid, which has been redesigned to be based on grain products, fails to distinguish empty calorie food from nutritionally dense food. Thus it can no longer be relied upon to prevent nutrient deficiency, let alone provide optimum nutrition.

The phytochemicals – which, as the name suggests, are the chemicals found in plants – play particularly important nutritional roles. Genistein from soyabeans, lycopene from tomatoes and sulforaphane from broccoli are among the most well-known of these substances. In all likelihood they provide many of the missing links between the moderate benefit provided by individual tableted vitamins and the greater benefit of the food containing those vitamins. (I had thought of including a section on these nutrients in this book, but because our medical knowledge of them is in its infancy, I decided it would be better to write about them after I have acquired my own clinical experience with a high phytochemical diet.)

For now, the message is to choose your foods wisely. Certain proteins, such as eggs and roe, are better than others. Certain fats, such as flaxseed oil and salmon oil, are better than others. As for plant-derived carbohydrates, those which are eaten directly after picking or harvesting will contain their full complement of phytochemicals and vita-nutrients, while those subjected to refining are likely to be nutritionally barren.)

Even people following a low-carbohydrate diet can, by choosing about 40 grams a day of phytonutrient-dense carbohydrates derived mainly from fresh, low-starch vegetables, take in more phytonutrition, not counting supplements, than the average American or Briton, who generally consumes seven times the amount of carbohydrates. I'm sure I do just that.

By the same token, vegetarians and people following low-fat and low-protein diets must choose wisely to ensure they consume sufficient levels of nutritionally essential fatty acids and amino acids. Egg substitutes and margarine just don't cut it. Ultra-low-fat diets followed at the austerity level recommended by some Pritikin followers may make adequate fatty acid intake impossible, thus, potentially causing a range of related ailments linked to this nutritional inadequacy.

The third logical solution to the dilemma is to include foods that are, in themselves, nutritionally complete. The two old standbys, brewer's yeast and liver extract, have become problematic since their heyday in the thirties. Brewer's yeast is poorly tolerated by the millions of people struggling with a candida epidemic; liver sources are increasingly contaminated by pesticide residues. But the spirulinas and the other algae, the propolis and royal jelly (which I have written about in this book), all serve to provide the accessory nutritional factors we are seeking.

If and when a technology develops to administer natural sources of nutrition at a cost comparable to the forms we are now using, it could prove to be a significant advance. But the programme we use at the Atkins Center – featuring off-the-shelf vitamins, selected in effective dosages, given with a broad spectrum of other nutrients, and with wisely chosen nutrient-rich foods – has achieved an enviable record of success.

Words of Caution In order to use this section safely and effectively, you must fully understand and follow this warning:

In treating any illness, do not take any vita-nutrient in doses beyond the basic, all-purpose recommendation without reading and thoroughly understanding the chapter dedicated to that nutrient. In particular, be sure to watch for statements like 'must be used with caution if on certain medications' or 'should be taken under medical supervision'. If you do not follow these caveats, a safe vita-nutrient could become dangerous.

Targeting Your Nutrition

In the wake of my overwhelming success with vitamin therapy, it soon became apparent that I would need to develop a formal system of selecting vitamins for my patients. This programme would be able to provide both the nutrients that everyone needs and the effective dosages of the nutrients that correct a person's specific problems.

Not surprisingly, these two requisites often called for a large number of supplements. Therefore in order to create a supplement programme targeted for your specific health goals, you'll need to determine which are most important to you. (For example, if you decide you want to control cholesterol, improve sleep and prevent osteoporosis, you might need to cut down supplementation in another arena.)

And that is exactly what you will have to do. To establish this kind of programme, follow these ten steps:

Step One: Establish the basics

Select a basic vitamin and mineral formula of good quality and great breadth. (It is the breadth of this combination of vita-nutrients that will prove most important, because your greatest need in a basic formula is to make sure that no essential nutrient is missing.) Your goal is to make sure your nutrient intake heeds Roger Williams's dictum: 'A nutritional programme is only as good as the weakest link in the chain.' Check to make sure that all of the trace minerals and B-complex constituents (as described in part two) are present.

Another part of the basic requisite is an essential fatty acid formula. I am mentioning them separately because the mechanics of vitamin manufacturing keeps them separate. In their physical states they exist as an oil, whereas most other vita-nutrients are dried powders. It is particularly important to keep these oils in mind, as an essential fatty acid deficiency could be the most significant type of nutritional shortfall.

I am tempted to add one other ingredient to your list of basic requirements – a nutrient-dense, phytochemical-rich natural source of undiscovered nutrient. By this I mean algae, brewer's yeast, bee pollen and the like. If your diet contains a liberal assortment of a variety of fresh vegetables, you are probably meeting that need. A superfood supplement, though, would still be a nice addition to the mix. As you read the superfood chapter (page 269), see if one or more of the featured performers sounds particularly attuned to your needs.

Step Two: Identify the specific vita-nutrients that are appropriate for you

First of all, identify any medical problems that you need to deal with.

• *Are you taking medications, or have you been prescribed them?*

I believe that unnecessary medications, in general, pose the greatest health risk of all. I have learned that nutrients can replace drugs for treating chronic illness more than four times out of five, and this is the vita-nutrient solution's greatest achievement.

• *Have you been diagnosed with any illness?*

Here is where your levels of cholesterol, triglycerides, blood sugar, blood pressure and the like enter the picture. Here, too, is where it is important to consider your family history or other genetic factors. Vita-nutrients are ideally suited for improving risk factors. A bona fide diagnosis is usually, but not always, a call for treatment. Where there is no effective treatment in mainstream medicine, none is offered, nor should it be. The treatment could be worse than the disease. I know of no examples where that statement applies to nutritional therapies.

• *Identify any symptoms that need to be dealt with.*

In reviewing your medical history, it is important to consider everyday symptoms that you may take for granted. Are you tired, cranky, subject to mood swings or forgetful? Are you achy, stiff, subject to colds and viruses? Do you get drowsy or have trouble sleeping? How about your bowel function, your appetite, your stamina, your temperament? All these and more are eminently approachable with vita-nutrition.

• *Are there any physical life stresses you may have to overcome?*

Is your work schedule too gruelling? Do you get enough sleep? Are your home and workplace properly ventilated? Do you frequently encounter odours you cannot tolerate? Is your community blanketed with smog or pollution?

If so, antioxidants are particularly important in your basic vita-nutrient formula.

Step Three: Create a list of all of the areas discovered in the foregoing that you feel apply specifically to you

If your list is a long one, divide it into primary and secondary needs.

Step Four: Pinpoint the specific vita-nutrients that address the problems you have listed in step three

Although this process can be rather time-consuming, it is in fact the most direct way in which this book can help you. Start by looking through the vita-nutrient treatment section (page 373) and locating those examples that are similar to your specific problems. If you can't find any matching descriptions, look in the index (the discussion may be located under the named condition or perhaps under a cause of your symptom or illness). And, of course, if you have further questions or feel unsure about the correct vita-nutrient therapy, you may wish to contact a nutritional or medical counsellor. The Atkins Center also provides nutrition counselling service; see the appendix for details.

Step Five: List all the nutrients that address the conditions or symptoms you wish to deal with

This step is easier than it may first appear because there are now targeted vita-nutrient formulations for specific conditions. And these formulations, pioneered by the Atkins Center, are becoming increasingly available nationwide. Therefore you should be able to find the formulations that combine as many vita-nutrient building blocks into a single capsule or tablet as are available.

Step Six: Use as many appropriate building block formulas as possible

Write down all of the formulations and individual nutrients that are appropriate to you, along with the dosage range. Then note the number of tablets/capsules that most closely approximates the dosage range suggested. Here, you may find some variation in quantities if you use building block formulations, but come as close as you can. If a nutrient appears on your list more than once, it is likely to be extremely valuable to you; therefore keep such nutrients at the high end of the dosage range.

Step Seven: Add up the actual number of vita-nutrient formulations and pills you would have to swallow every day to achieve the goals denoted in step six

If the total number seems manageable, proceed to step nine. If not, go to step eight.

Step Eight: Estimate the number of listed vita-nutrients in step seven that you could take comfortably with each of your three meals

Divide that number by the total in step six and determine the percentage of the vita-nutrients that you would be comfortable taking. Multiply the enire list by that fraction to get your complete programme. Another option is to omit vita-nutrients related to therapeutic objectives of lesser importance to you.

Step Nine: You now have your personalized, targeted vita-nutrient solution

If you are not accustomed to taking supplements, start slowly. Begin at one-third to one-half the total vita-nutrient supplements and increase the number each day. That way you may find you can eventually build up to the total indicated in step six.

Step Ten: Taper down your vita-nutrient dosage

Once you notice the maximum benefit from your vita-nutrient programme, you may decrease the quantities you take. And as your particular health problems become controllable, you will also be able to reduce the nutrients pertinent to those problems. The reason is, in part, that it takes higher doses of vita-nutrients to overcome a long-term deficiency than it does to maintain an optimum level after the gross deficiency is corrected.

These ten steps should enable you to do for yourself, with some homework, what I do for my patients every day. If the process at first seems daunting, rest assured: as you gather more experience using vita-nutrients, targeted therapy will become much easier.

How to Use the Vita-Nutrient Treatments

The Basic Formula Because the diets of so many adults lack so many essential nutrients, everyone should build their vita-nutrient programmes around certain nutritional basics. These general multivitamin formulas provide a foundation that specific vita-nutrients can enhance. In addition, increasing ordinary intake will in almost every instance bring the nutrient level closer to the optimal range. The result is an individualized health programme targeted for particular purposes.

Let's start with a prototypical formula, similar to the one I developed for my Atkins Center patients and which is now available to my readers through my website or by contacting the Atkins Center (details on page 479). The basics for everyone include that extra-broad multiple vitamin and mineral combination, plus the essential (and virtually essential) fatty acid capsules. You may also choose one of the hundreds of other basic formulas; just make sure the one you end up with is similar to this formula, both in breadth and dosages. In the United States some provision must be made to compensate for the government regulation that limits the folic acid content of a multiple vitamin to a dangerously low level. For most people, extra folic acid should be included.

BASIC NUTRITION VITAMIN/MINERAL FORMULA
Daily Intake–Individual Doses

Natural beta-carotene	3,000–6,000 IU
Vitamin A	1,500–3,000 IU
Vitamin B_1	30–60 mg
Vitamin B_2	24–48 mg
Niacin	15–30 mg
Niacinamide	30–60 mg
Pantothenic acid	75–150 mg
Pantethine	75–150 mg
Vitamin B_6	30–60 mg
Folic acid	2,000–4,000 mcg*
Pyridoxal-5-phosphate	6–12 mg
Biotin	225–450 mcg
Vitamin B_{12}	180–240 mcg
Vitamin C	500–1,000 mg
Vitamin D_2	90–180 IU
Vitamin E	150–300 IU

BASIC NUTRITION VITAMIN/MINERAL FORMULA
Daily Intake–Individual Doses
(CONTINUED)

Copper	600–1,200 mcg
Magnesium	50–100 mg
Calcium	200–400 mg†
Choline	300–600 mg
Inositol	240–480 mg
PABA	300–600 mg
Manganese	12–24 mg
Zinc	24–48 mg
Citrus bioflavonoids	450–600 mg
Chromium	150–300 mcg
Selenium	120–240 mcg
N-acetyl cysteine	60–120 mg
Molybdenum	30–60 mcg
Vanadyl sulfate	45–90 mcg
Octacosanol	450–900 mcg
Reduced glutathione	15–30 mg

* Unless you are a woman who needs to shrink uterine fibroids, prevent breast cancer recurrences or deal with endometriosis or fibrocystic breasts, you should supplement your basic formula with enough folic acid to provide at least 3,000 mcg (3 mg). This means taking four tablets of 800 mcg each. If the above conditions need your attention, keep your supplemental folic acid below 600 mcg.
† Note that for the purpose of making basic formulas less bulky, many manufacturers provide less than a minimum daily requirement for calcium, as does this example. If you select such a formula and your dietary calcium intake is low, you should include a 500 mg calcium tablet, such as calcium carbonate, as part of your basic programme.

The other basic requirement for optimal health is the oil-based essential fats formula. For most of my patients I prescribe a combination of the three oils with the highest concentrations of the most needed essential fats. It was developed for the Targeted Nutrition product line and provides an equal mixture of borage oil (the richest source of the fatty acid GLA), fish oils (concentrated for EPA/DHA content) and flaxseed oil (a source for the essential fatty acids linoleic and alpha-linolenic acid). Each capsule contains 1,200 mg of the combination (400 mg of each), and I recommend at least three of them daily, even for healthy adults. As you read through the targeted protocols, you will see this referred to as the 'essential oils formula'.

Several Other Descriptions

• For beneficial bacteria supplements, I recommend an equal mixture of acidophilus and bifidobacterium, the two most important good bacteria for promoting digestive health. Bulgaricum may also be part of the mix in such a supplement. I generally recommend 1/4–1/2 teaspoon of such a powder in most applications. Should you not want to use a powder, you can use three to six capsules of a similarly blended formula. However, I find that the powdered versions are more effective.

• A mixed fibre supplement refers to a blend of beneficial fibres such as oat bran, psyllium and rice bran. Remember that to maximize fibre benefits, you should consume a blend of fibres, not one single form.

• Keep in mind that most pantethine supplements contain an equal mixture of pantethine and its relative pantothenic acid. When I suggest a certain amount of pantethine in a given treatment, this refers to the amount of both nutrients, assuming that half is pantethine.

• The protocols that follow were created with the assumption that you will already be taking a basic multivitamin formula similar to the one I've just given. Nutrients found in the basic formulation are important for treating every ailment. Therefore, be sure that the following protocols are usually just an addition – not a replacement – to the basic formula you should already be taking. However, you should note that there are higher doses in the protocols than in the basic formula, so simply augment your intake to reach the higher doses for a nutrient. In other words, simply add the difference between the amount in your basic formula and the total listed for the condition.

B Complex There are as many different B-complex formulas as there are all-purpose multivitamins, and I often prescribe them as a unit. Note that this will be listed simply as 'B complex' and will be referred to as '50 mg strength', even though not all constituents are 50 mg (the body needs more of certain B vitamins than others; a perfectly 'balanced' formula is inappropriate). Following is a typical example of a B-complex formula found in most pharmacies or health food stores.

B_1	50 mg
B_2	25 mg
Niacin	25 mg
Niacinamide	50 mg
B_6	50 mg
Pyridoxal-5-phosphate	2 mg
Pantothenic acid	50 mg
Folic acid	400 mcg*
B_{12}	100 mcg
Biotin	100 mcg
PABA	50 mg†
Choline	50 mg†
Inositol	50 mg†

* Inappropriately low essential nutrient. Needs to be supplemented to 2–3 mg daily. However, women who need to shrink uterine fibroids, prevent breast cancer recurrences, or deal with endometriosis or fibrocystic breasts should keep supplemental folic acid below 600 mcg.

† The usual dose that is included, but inappropriately low.

CHAPTER 15

THE VITA-NUTRIENT SOLUTIONS

I have explained the value of targeting your vita-nutrient supplement programme to specific conditions that you and your doctor consider to be the most important to you; now I would like to provide the specifics.

Your first task is to identify which of the following list of nutritionally treatable conditions best apply to you. I have grouped them into cardiovascular categories and metabolic conditions, nervous system problems, gastrointestinal problems, fatigue, infections, allergy, lung conditions, cancer, gender-specific problems and, finally, arthritis, immune diseases, and skin, gum and eye problems. Please leaf through these next pages and try to locate any conditions of concern to you. If you do not find them, use the index to help locate them. Sometimes the information you need will be mentioned in the discussion of individual vita-nutrients.

In these next pages you will see an extremely brief discussion of the major types of conditions that respond well to nutritional therapy (the list is incomplete, by necessity), followed by listings of vita-nutrients I use in treating and preventing them. In most lists you will see a subdivision of two groupings, the most essential and those that are moderately valuable and therefore worth trying. These groupings were created to make sure, first, that you do not omit the most valuable nutrients for your condition and, second, to help you select others should more help be needed. I have tried to keep the lists in descending order of importance.

In all cases I will assume that you will be taking all the basic nutrients described on pages 369–70. The dosage range indicated in the following lists represents your new *total* daily dose (including the dosages in the basic programme). They should be evenly divided (unless otherwise specified) into three or more approximately equal doses so that they can be taken with meals (or before them, when so specified). The low end of the range applies to adults weighing less than 59 kilograms or to those with less severe illnesses. The upper end of the range applies to people weighing over 109 kilograms or to those in great need of effective therapy. Now I'll present the treatments themselves.

CARDIOVASCULAR CONDITIONS

It is certainly logical that we begin with the heart, the organ most responsible for determining our life span. Cardiovascular disease is one of the most glaring examples of mismanaged health problems in medicine today. While cardiologists possess excellent diagnostic skills, many show an ignorance of nutritional medicine, which can easily lead to second-rate health care. Coronary heart disease – more specifically, the clogging of arteries that leads to heart attacks and heart muscle deterioration – was extremely rare a hundred years ago. (In fact, the symptom complex of crushing chest pain and sudden death had not even been described by medical writers until the early part of the twentieth century). One hundred years ago, people ate considerably less sugar and refined starches. They also derived a larger percentage of dietary fat from animal sources, a fact that should cause you to question the official warnings to avoid such fats.

Anyone (myself included) who claims that his is the only diet that will prevent heart disease must be at least partially wrong. There are several relatively diverse paths to heart disease, and no one diet would stave off the condition for everyone. The trick is to find the specific abnormalities, if any, that serve as metabolic risk factors and eradicate them as dramatically as you can. The most common of these abnormalities is not, as previously thought, a problem of high cholesterol. But rather, it involves a defect in our insulin's activity against glucose. This can be detected by abnormal glucose and insulin levels during a glucose tolerance test or whenever the critically important (yet rarely stressed) triglyceride-to-HDL ratio is greater than two to one. (You can calculate it yourself from the numbers in your lipid profile.) Other abnormalities involve elevated homocysteine levels and a variety of lipid disturbances such as elevated levels of oxidized LDL cholesterol or of lipoprotein(a). Each is best corrected by a different programme.

Certain generalities apply. Eat a diet extremely low in sugar, corn syrup or other natural sweeteners. Avoid margarine or any other similar fat that provides a source of unnatural *trans*-fatty acids. Try to eat at least three servings of fatty cold-water fish per week (salmon, sardines, mackerel and the like) or else take fish oil supplements. Use flaxseed oil and olive oil on your food, and keep away from foods with antinutrient effects, such as white flour and cornflour. Nuts and seeds rich in essential fatty acids should be included as additional snacks.

Heart disease may also be prevented by taking in enough antioxidants (such as vitamins C and E) and minerals (such as magnesium, zinc, copper, chromium and selenium). This short nutrient list is also valuable in helping to treat established heart disease. Heart-energizing nutrients such as carnitine and CoQ_{10} are major players, as are herbs like hawthorn and garlic. And let's not forget folic acid and vitamin B_6, which are crucial for preventing homocysteine from damaging the coronary arteries.

My general programme for maximizing heart health is listed below (note that it does not include multivitamins).

Heart and Vascular Health

Most Important	Moderately Important
Magnesium 400–800 mg	Garlic, 1,600–3,200 mg
CoQ_{10} 60–120 mg	Bromelain 200–400 mg
L-carnitine 1,000–2,000 mg	Gamma-oryzanol 300–600 mg
Taurine 500–1,000 mg	Acetyl L-carnitine 500–1,000 mg
Vitamin E 400–800 IU	Selenium 150–300 mcg
Vitamin C 1–3 grams	Vitamin B_6 100–200 mg
Essential oils formula 3,600–7,200 mg	Folic acid 3–6 mg*
Mixed tocotrienols 100–200 mg	Quercetin 300–600 mg
Chromium 200–400 mcg	Lipoic acid 100–300 mg
Pantethine 450–900 mg†	Fibre 7.5–15 grams
Natural-source beta-carotene 25,000 IU	Grape seed/pycnogenol 150–300 mg
Ginkgo biloba extract 240–360 mg	Calcium 600–1,200 mg
Hawthorn 240–480 mg	Cayenne (three pills)
B complex 50 mg	Coleus forskohlii 50–100 mg

*Women who need to shrink uterine fibroids, prevent breast cancer recurrences or deal with endometriosis or fibrocystic breasts should keep supplemental folic acid below 600 mcg.

† See the discussion of pantethine supplements on page 371.

Angina Pectoris The words mean 'chest pain', and this is the most characteristic symptom of a narrowing or spasm of the coronary vessels – the ones that supply the heart's life blood. Because the chest pain can herald an impending heart attack, I recommend doses beyond those in the general cardiovascular protocol, as the following will show. Note that the list is headed by arginine, which, along with a remarkable non-nutritional complementary practice called chelation therapy, is my treatment of choice for angina.

Most Important	Moderately Important
Arginine 2–4 tsp (8–16 grams total)	Essential oils formula 3,600–7,200 mg
L-carnitine 1,500–3,000 mg	Garlic 2,000–4,000 mg
CoQ$_{10}$ 100–200 mg	Hawthorn 360–720 mg
Vitamin E 800–1,600 IU	Pantethine up to 900 mg*
Magnesium 800–1,200 mg	Natural-source beta-carotene 25,000–50,000 IU
Bromelain 450–600 mg	N-acetyl cysteine 1,500–3,000 mg

* See the discussion of pantethine supplements on page 371.

Arrhythmia and Mitral Valve Prolapse An irregular heartbeat poses a different threat from that of angina. Although the worst-case scenario is sudden death, the more usual occurrence is simply the disturbing symptom of palpitations. Mitral valve prolapse, a billowing out of an undamaged valve, can lead to rhythm abnormalities and is also included here. The higher dosages of heart rhythm benefactor nutrients are these:

Most Important	Moderately Important
Magnesium 600–1,000 mg	Inositol 500–1,500 mg
Potassium 600–1,200 mg	Bromelain 400–800 mg
Hawthorn 240–480 mg	Manganese 30–60 mg
Taurine 2,000–3,000 mg	Cactus (alcohol tincture) 8–16 drops
L-carnitine 1,250–2,500 mg	Chromium 300–600 mcg
CoQ$_{10}$ 100–200 mg	

Cardiomyopathy and Congestive Heart Failure Heart failure is the result of the organ's inability to maintain the effectiveness of its blood-pumping activity. This leads to fluid buildup in the lungs and in the legs. Cardiomyopathy refers to a variety of conditions impairing the heart's pumping ability, which are fairly common causes of heart failure. Increased doses of the following nutrients are helpful in counteracting this dangerous condition:

Most Important	Moderately Important
Taurine, 2,000–4,000 mg	Copper sebacate 2–4 mg
CoQ$_{10}$ 200–400 mg	Pantethine 600–1,200 mg*
L-carnitine 2,000–4,000 mg	Vitamin E 600–1,200 IU
Hawthorn 300–480 mg	Cactus (alcohol tincture) 5–10 drops
Magnesium 600–1,200 mg	Essential oils formula 4,800–9,600 mg
B$_1$ 150–300 mg	B complex 100 mg

* See the discussion of pantethine supplements on page 371.

Blood Lipid Elevations

Elevated levels of blood lipids, such as cholesterol and triglycerides, are one of the most widespread causes of heart attacks, strokes and clogging of the arteries in general. Remember, despite all the publicity, high cholesterol is not a disease. Rather, it and other lipid abnormalities are simply predictive factors for a hardening of the arteries. Therefore, changing lipid levels without changing the reason they are elevated may neither prevent nor reverse the illness. However, by consistently bringing these blood markers for heart and artery health under control, diet and nutrient therapy, will, at the very least, allow you to avoid side effect-laden cholesterol drugs. Some people get the best results by restricting saturated fats, while others do better if they eliminate all sugar from their diet and reduce consumption of carbohydrates. You must learn which works best for you. In either case, your lipid levels should improve if you add the nutrients that correspond to your particular need.

High Cholesterol

Most Important	Moderately Important
Pantethine 600–1,200 mg*	Copper sebacate 2–4 mg
Inositol hexanicotinate 500–1,500 mg	Vitamin E 400–800 IU
Chromium 300–600 mcg	Taurine 1–2 grams
Essential oils formula 7,200 mg	Ginger 2–3 capsules
Vitamin C 1–5 grams	Fenugreek 1–4 capsules
	Selenium 200–400 mcg

(CONTINUED)

Most Important	Moderately Important
Mixed fibre supplement 10 grams	Folic acid 3–6 mg†
Lecithin granules 2–3 tbs	Arginine 6–12 grams
Guggulipid 100–200 mg	Inositol 500–1,000 mg
GLA (borage oil) 1,200–3,600 mg	Chlorella 1/4–1/2 tsp
Garlic 2,400–4,000 mg	Royal jelly 1/4–1/2 tsp
Gamma-oryzanol 300–600 mg	DHEA 20–40 mg
Mixed tocotrienols 200–400 mg	Chondroitin sulfates 250–500 mg
Beta-carotene 25,000–50,000 IU	

* See the discussion of pantethine supplements on page 371.
† Women who need to shrink uterine fibroids, prevent breast cancer recurrences or deal with endometriosis or fibrocystic breasts should keep supplemental folic acid below 600 mcg.

High Triglycerides and Low HDL Cholesterol High triglycerides and low HDL levels are the two lipid abnormalities that are clearly and unequivocally linked both to insulin resistance and to the intake of carbohydrates. People who are resistant to insulin should avoid excess carbohydrates or even 'average' levels of carbohydrate, because their body chemistry turns the carbohydrates into triglycerides, which in turn seem to inhibit the formation of HDL, or the 'good' cholesterol. The Atkins Center experience is that people whose trigylceride levels are more than double their HDL levels (in mg/ml) do better on carbohydrate restriction, so you must be sure to avoid sugar in all its forms, even fruit and fruit juices, and you should keep your intake of starches to a minimum. In treating for high triglycerides, you should follow the regime for 'High Cholesterol' (page 378), but increase the dosage for the following nutrients to the indicated levels:

L-carnitine 1,500–3,000 mg
EPA/DHA (from fish oil) 1,200–2,400 mg
Chromium 400–800 mcg
Vanadyl sulfate 15–30 mg

High Lipoprotein(a) This protein, to which lipids attach, is a risk factor for heart disease with great predictive ability. Elevations are not lowered by the usual cholesterol-modifying approaches. However, the following nutrients may prove valuable and should be raised to the following levels:

N-acetyl cysteine 2–4 grams
Vitamin C 4–8 grams
Inositol hexanicotinate 1,500–3,000 mg
Gamma-oryzanol 300–1,200 mg
Lysine 600–1,200 mg
Proline 600–1,200 mg

Hypertension Hypertension (or high blood pressure) is an important risk factor for stroke. While scientists debate what actually causes hypertension, one thing is clear: it is very responsive to nutrient and diet therapy. At the Atkins Center we routinely see blood pressure return to normal when the Atkins diet is used along with the right nutrients. A low-carbohydrate diet is important, because this helps bring down the elevated insulin response that appears to be one of the major causes of hypertension. To that we add the following nutrients:

Most Important	*Moderately Important*
Taurine 1,500–3,000 mg	Vitamin C 1–3 grams
Magnesium 500–1,000 mg	N-acetyl cysteine 1–2 grams
Hawthorn 240–480 mg	GABA 2,000–4,000 mg
Potassium aspartate 400–800 mg	Arginine 2–5 grams
Vitamin B_6 100–200 mg	Inositol 500–1,500 mg
Essential oils formula 3,600–7,200 mg	Kava 100–200 mg
Garlic 2,400–3,200 mg	Reishi extract 2–4 capsules
CoQ_{10} 100–200 mg	Choline 1,000–1,500 mg
Carnitine 500–1,000 mg	Calcium 750–1,500 mg
Chromium 300–600 mcg	

One caveat for hypertensives: introduce vitamin E slowly if you have not taken it before, because at first it may slightly increase high blood pressure. This is best done under the supervision of a doctor.

BLOOD SUGAR IMBALANCES: DIABETES AND HYPOGLYCEMIA

I consider blood sugar imbalances to be the most important nutrition-based conditions in the Western world. Diabetes is both a major disease in its own right and a major risk factor for coronary heart disease.

The term 'diabetes' really applies to two very different illnesses. Type I is an acquired autoimmune illness in which the pancreas's insulin-making capacity is destroyed; insulin must be provided for the victim to survive. Type II, the more prevalent form, is characterized by blood sugar elevations due mainly to the body's inability to use insulin effectively (insulin resistance). Most Type II diabetics have elevated insulin levels, and providing more insulin, a frequent medical practice, simply accelerates the cardiovascular complications. As many as 40 per cent of those who eat a Western diet have some characteristics for this condition; the most common are high insulin output, insulin resistance, tendency to gain weight and 'hypoglycemia', the unstable blood sugar syndrome. Many of the same nutrients can be helpful for all of these conditions. Why? Because the treatment goal is basically the same: to keep your blood sugar within normal ranges by helping the body metabolize it more effectively.

Here are the nutrients that by keeping the blood sugar in balance will ameliorate or prevent early Type II diabetes, prediabetes and hypoglycemia:

Most Important	*Moderately Important*
Chromium 200–600 mcg	Vitamin C 1–2 grams
Zinc 50–100 mg	Vitamin E 300–600 IU
Magnesium 300–600 mg	Carnitine 500–1,000 mg
Lipoic acid 150–300 mg	Vitamin A 10,000–20,000 IU
CoQ$_{10}$ 45–90 mg	Siberian ginseng 100–200 mg
Biotin 2–4 mg	Manganese 25–50 mg
Essential oils formula 7,200 mg	Mixed fibre blend 10–15 grams
Selenium 100–200 mcg	Calcium 1,000 mg
B$_6$ 75–150 mg	Liquorice 1–3 capsules
	Curcuminoids 400–1,200 mg
	Copper sebacate 2–4 mg

When your objective is to bring elevated blood sugar to normal levels or reduce your dosage of antidiabetes medications, the following list should prove helpful:

Most Important	Moderately Important
Chromium 500–1,000 mcg	Gymnema sylvestre 200–400 mg
Vanadyl sulfate 30–60 mg	Fenugreek 100–200 mg
Lipoic acid 300–600 mg	Taurine 1,500–3,000 mg
CoQ_{10} 90–180 mg	Folic acid 2–4 mg*
Biotin 7.5–15 mg	Beneficial bacteria 1/2–1 tsp
Inositol 800–1,600 mg	Lysine 400–800 mg
Zinc 90–180 mg	Milk thistle 400–800 mg
Niacinamide 300–600 mg	Garlic 2,400–4,800 mg
DHEA 20–40 mg	Calcium AEP (see note below)

* Women who need to shrink uterine fibroids, prevent breast cancer recurrences or deal with endometriosis or fibrocystic breasts should keep supplemental folic acid below 600 mcg.

Niacinamide will be the most beneficial to Type I diabetics. DHEA doses should ideally be taken after testing for blood levels, and more than the recommended amount should be taken if blood levels still remain low. Calcium AEP should be taken during the early onset of Type I diabetes (usually intravenously) under a doctor's supervision. Also, remember that with diabetes, niacin and fish oil supplements should be used only with a doctor's guidance, as they may cause elevation of blood sugar in some diabetics. Ideally vanadium should also be used with doctor supervision.

OVERWEIGHT AND OBESITY

Severe weight gain, America's most prevalent metabolic disturbance, and an increasing problem in the United Kingdom, is actually a manifestation of insulin resistance. To counteract this problem, I strongly recommend the strategy presented in *Dr Atkins' New Diet Revolution*. It has proved powerful in the management of weight problems, and I believe any deviations from it will reduce the chances of success. However, many nutrients can facilitate the weight-loss process by opening up blocked metabolic pathways. Here are some of the nutrients I have found valuable:

Most Important	*Moderately Important*
Chromium 400–800 mcg	BMOV vanadium 2–4 mg
L-carnitine 1,000–2,000 mg	Vanadyl sulfate 10–20 mg
CoQ$_{10}$ 75–150 mg	Taurine 1,000–2,000 mg
Glutamine 2–4 grams	Pantethine 600–2,000 mg*
Phenylalanine 750–1,500 mg	Vitamin C 3–6 grams
Choline 750–1,500 mg	Zinc 40–80 mg
Inositol 1,000–2,000 mg	Acetyl L-tyrosine 500–1,000 mg
Methionine 400–800 mg	Fibre 8–16 grams
Lipoic acid 100–300 mg	Biotin 5–10 mg
Siberian ginseng 1–2 grams	Selenium 200 mcg with iodine
Conjugated linoleic acid 2–4 g†	150 mcg

* See the discussion of pantethine supplements on page 371.
† Not mentioned in text. I am just starting to use it. It is safe and effective.

NERVOUS SYSTEM DISORDERS

The coming of the new millennium has fostered widespread interest in ways to improve and maintain brain function with vita-nutrients. Convincing scientific evidence has shown that nutrients are better than drugs at preserving our nerve cells. Clinical tests have also proved their inability to prevent memory loss and overcome Alzheimer's, Parkinson's or mood and psychiatric disorders. Even better, optimal nutrition can improve your memory, concentration, mood and judgment, and will promote the maximum life span of your brain and nerves.

Nutrients for maximizing brain function in general should include the following:

B complex	50–150 mg
Ginkgo biloba extract	60–120 mg
B$_6$	100–200 mg
Folic acid*	3–5 mg

(CONTINUED)

B$_{12}$	1,000–2,000 mcg
B$_1$	100–200 mg
Octacosanol	6–12 mg

* Women who need to shrink uterine fibroids, prevent breast cancer recurrences or deal with endometriosis or fibrocystic breasts should keep supplemental folic acid below 600 mcg.

For those with Alzheimer's and Parkinson's diseases, the following additional treatment programme is recommended:

Most Important	*Moderately Important*
Vitamin E 1,000–2,000 IU	Glutathione 250–1,000 mg
NADH 2.5–10 mg	B$_1$ 250–1,000 mg
Acetyl L-carnitine 1,500–3,000 mg	Lipoic acid 500–1,000 mg
Phosphatidyl serine 300–500 mg	B$_6$ 100–200 mg
Ginkgo biloba extract 160–320 mg	Vitamin C 5–10 grams
CoQ$_{10}$ 100–300 mg	Selenium 400–600 mcg
N-acetyl cysteine 1,000–2,000 mg	Grape seed/pycnogenol 100–200 mg
B$_{12}$ 5,000–10,000 mg	Zinc 60–120 mg
Phosphatidylcholine 2–4 grams	Magnesium 400–800 mg
	Methionine 3–6 grams

Note: Self-prescribed doses of brain nutrients and antioxidants should never be higher than those listed here without being monitored by a doctor. Although we are dealing with the management of illnesses that are otherwise untreatable, overstimulating the brain could lead to adverse effects. If you are currently taking L-dopa alone, do not take B$_6$ or a B-complex multivitamin that contains B$_6$ without discussing it with the doctor who signs your prescription.

Anxiety We all know the anxiety that is precipitated by life stress and the insecurities that come with it. But, surprisingly, a significant amount of anxiety is related to diet and nutrition. Unstable blood sugar, individual food intolerances and overgrowth of the yeast organism *Candida albicans* tend to increase one's anxiety level.

The vita-nutrients I recommend for anxiety are the following:

Inositol 1,000–2,000 mg
GABA 1,500–3,000 mg
Tryptophan 1.5–3 grams or 5-hydroxy-tryptophan 200–400 mg
Kava extract 100–200 mg
Calcium 400–800 mg
Niacinamide 250–500 mg
Magnesium 300–600 mg
B complex 1–3 capsules
Valerian 2–4 capsules
B_6 100–200 mg
B_{12} 2–4 mg at bedtime

Depression In the treatment of depression, the major goal is to build up the neurotransmitters that keep our moods upbeat. One of these is serotonin, which combats our tendency to develop an agitated, anxiety-laden form of depression. Another is a group of adrenalinelike compounds, called 'catecholamines', which keep us from feeling lethargic, apathetic and depressed. If we provide our bodies with the building blocks for these neurotransmitters, our bodies will make them, and voilà – no more depression.

To combat this illness, I recommend the anxiety prevention regime described previously, plus the following nutrients and herbs. Add each of these supplements to your regimen singly every week, so that you can determine which are helping you:

L-tryptophan 1,500–3,000 mg or 5-hydroxy-tryptophan 200–400 mg
N-acetyl tyrosine 500–1,000 mg
B_{12} 1,000–3,000 mcg
Methionine 1,200–2,400 mg
B_1 150–300 mg
St-John's-wort 100–200 mg
Acetyl L-carnitine 500–1,000 mg
Phosphatidyl serine 300–600 mg
B_6 100–200 mg
Folic acid 30–60 mg (women who need to shrink uterine fibroids,
    prevent breast cancer recurrences or deal with endometriosis or fibro-
    cystic breasts should keep supplemental folic acid below 600 mcg)

Attention Deficit/Hyperactivity Disorder (ADHD) If there is a single condition that is purely diet related and not recognized as such, it would be hyperactivity and decreased attention span in children. This problem has become so widespread that sales of the drug Ritalin, supposedly the cure for this disorder, seem to double every three or four years.

The diet connection is usually found in the child's inability to keep blood sugar levels stable after consuming sweets, a dietary staple of too many of our children. Other sources include allergies to specific foods (often milk or grains) and yeast overgrowth, often the consequence of too many thoughtless antibiotic treatments for recurrent ear infections.

Nutrients I have found helpful in treating hyperactivity and attention deficit disorder are as follows:

Most Important	*Moderately Important*
B complex 50–100 mg	Niacinamide 200–400 mg
Phosphatidyl serine 300–600 mg	Essential oils formula 3,600–7,200 mg
GABA 1,200–2,400 mg	Beneficial bacteria 1/2–1 tsp
Phenylalanine 500–1,000 mg	Magnesium 250–500 mg
Zinc 50–100 mg	Manganese 10–20 mg
5-hydroxy-tryptophan 200–400 mg	Selenium 50–100 mcg
B_6 75–150 mg	Calcium 750–1,500 mg
Inositol 750–1,500 mg	B_1 50–100 mg
Chromium 200–400 mcg	B_{12} 500–1,000 mcg

Note: To adjust the dosages for children, divide the child's weight by 70 kilograms and multiply the indicated dosage range by the fraction obtained. (Example: The zinc dosage for a 35-kilogram child would be 35/70, or 50 percent, × 50–100 mg, or 25–50 mg.)

Headaches As I've mentioned, determining the cause of various illnesses is a vital part of vita-nutrient therapy. The proper treatment of a headache is to prevent it. This is accomplished by determining its cause and steering clear of it. In general, a good strategy is to check for food allergies, avoid sugar and caffeine, and eliminate the foods to which you may be allergic. You should also try to avoid proinflammatory fats, such as safflower, sunflower and corn oil, and check for toxic metals and high copper, both of which can cause headaches. Remember, though, that painful recurring headaches require medical supervision to rule out serious health problems.

Nutritional supplements I have found helpful for eliminating headaches are the following:

Most Important	Moderately Important
Magnesium 500–1,000 mg	Vitamin E 200–400 IU
Beneficial bacteria 1/2–1 tsp	Molybdenum 500–750 mcg
B complex 50–100 mg	Bromelain 100–200 mg
Vitamin C 1–3 grams	Ginger 1–2 capsules
Essential oils formula 4,800–7,200 mg	Curcuminoids 200–400 mg
Ginkgo biloba extract 240–480 mg	Milk thistle extract 100–200 mg
Feverfew 100–200 mg	Thiamine pyrophosphate 100–200 mg
	Kava 100–200 mg

DIGESTIVE HEALTH

The health of the digestive tract is crucial for the overall health of the body. If you cannot digest your food and eliminate toxins well, you do not stand a good chance of being optimally healthy. In addition, virtually every chronic condition will be exacerbated if the intestinal tract accumulates toxic by-products.

For those with poor digestive function, supplements of hydrochloric acid and digestive enzymes can also be helpful. Still, it is best to work with a health care practitioner to determine whether these supplements will help your specific problem. You especially do not want to take hydrochloric acid if you don't need it, as it may cause gastric upset.

For maximum digestive function, these supplements are recommended:

Most Important	Moderately Important
Beneficial bacteria 1/2–1 tsp	Taurine 1–3 gram granules
Fibre 7.5–15 grams	Lecithin 1–2 tbsp
Zinc 25–50 mg	Royal jelly 1/4–1/2 tsp
	Curcuminoids 400–800 mg

Candida Overgrowth The overgrowth of the yeast organism *Candida albicans,* which normally resides peacefully in our intestinal tract, is one of our most significant new epidemics. The result of sugar gorging and overuse of antibiotics, candida overgrowth plays a contributing role in the larger disease picture of chronic fatigue syndrome, immune system weakness, 'brain fog', irritable bowel syndrome and food intolerances. A sugar-free diet, which also eliminates fermented foods, is the starting point. Next come these nutritional therapies:

Most Important	Moderately Important
Beneficial bacteria 1–3 tsp	Molybdenum 500–1,500 mcg
Undecenylic acid* 2–4 capsules	Goldenseal† 1–3 capsules
Caprylic acid* 2–4 capsules	Cat's claw extract 2–4 capsules
Ergotransferrin* 2–4 capsules	FOS 1/4–1/2 tsp
Oil of oregano 2–4 drops	Pau d'arco 1–3 droppers
Olive leaf extract – start with	Vitamin B₆ 100–200 mg
1 capsule, build up to 3–4 capsules	Echinacea 3–5 tsp
Vitamin C 1–3 grams	Vitamin E 400–800 IU
Pantethine‡	Pyroxidal-5-phosphate
600–1,200 gm	95–150 mg
Garlic 75–1,500 mg	Arginine 1,500–4,000 mg
Essential oils formula 3,600–7,200 mg	Propolis 1/2 dropper of tincture
Biotin 7.5–15 mg	in water
Mixed fibre blend 8–16 grams	Chlorella 1/2–1 tsp
	Copper sebacate 2–4 mg

* These three compounds are not mentioned in part two of the book. However, they are natural substances and work by interfering with the nutrition of the yeast organism. Clinical experience has found them to be effective treatments for the candida syndrome and well tolerated.

† Short term only. Not to be used during pregnancy.

‡ See the discussion of pantethine supplements on page 371.

Constipation and Diverticulitis Problems like constipation and diverticulitis, the painful condition where the mucus membranes of the large intestine become inflamed, are unknown in cultures that consume diets low in sugar and high in fibre. Yet these problems, once present, need more than a sugar-free diet to be treated effectively. For constipation I recommend the foregoing fibre and beneficial bacteria regime, plus the following:

Most Important	*Moderately Important*
Beneficial bacteria 1–3 tsp	Flaxseed oil 1 tbsp
Magnesium oxide 250–1,000 mg	Pantethine* 600–900 mg
Psyllium husks 1–2 tbsp,	Vitamin C 3–6 grams
taken with 350 ml of water	Bentonite powder 2–4 tsp in
	250 ml water

* See the discussion of pantethine supplements on page 371.

Those with constipation should also exercise regularly and have their thyroid functions checked. Drinking eight 250-ml glasses of water a day is also important. Finally, make sure to check for an overgrowth of candida, which can often cause constipation.

Heartburn (Esophageal Reflux) I have rarely seen a case of heartburn (gastroesophageal reflux disorder [GERD] is the medical term for the condition) that did not improve when simple sugars – sweets, fruit and milk – were removed from the diet. Fibre and beneficial bacteria can also be helpful in treating this condition. Sometimes heartburn is caused by a lack of stomach acid and can be relieved with betaine (this treatment should not be started unless a doctor's test confirms the absence of gastric acid). In addition to the basics of fibre, zinc and beneficial bacteria, I have found the following treatment programme useful for heartburn and reflux:

Most Important	Moderately Important
Vitamin U 120–240 mg (get the dose in 2–4 gastramet tablets)*	Phosphatidylcholine 750–1,500 mg
	Chlorella 1/2–1 tsp
Liquorice root extract 1–2 capsules	Kava extract 1–2 capsules
Gamma-oryzanol 450–900 mg	Gotu kola extract 1–2 capsules
Pantethine 600–900 mg†	Reishi extract 1–2 capsules

Note: All of these agents should be taken just before or at the start of each meal.
* Vitamin U is the name given to cabbage juice extract, an Eastern European folk remedy that has proven extremely beneficial for relieving stomach distress. I have found very little in the way of supporting scientific studies.
† See the discussion of pantethine supplements on page 371.

Ulcers Thought for a century to be the result of stress, ulcers are more accurately attributed to the bacterium *Helicobacter pylori*. These lesions that form on the stomach walls do not occur among people on primitive diets, leading to the conclusion that they are caused at least in part by refined carbohydrates like sugar and flour. Of this I am certain: reducing one's intake of dietary carbohydrates is a major part of the treatment for ulcers. Adding fibre to the diet is important, along with beneficial bacteria supplements. Moreover, the following nutrients are marvellous for helping the two most common types of ulcer – duodenal and gastric – to heal:

Most Important	Moderately Important
Gamma-oryzanol 450–900 mg	Chlorella 1–2 tsp
Glutamine 1,500–3,000 mg	Vitamin C (nonacidic) 1–3 grams
Zinc 50–100 mg	Folic acid 5–10 mg*
Vitamin U 120–240 mg	Essential oils formula 3–6 grams
Pantethine 600–1,200 mg†	Aloe vera 1–2 capsules
Liquorice 1–2 capsules	Propolis 1/2–1 dropper tincture
Vitamin E 400–800 IU	Capsaicin extract 1–2 capsules
Cat's claw extract 1–2 capsules	Kava extract 1–2 capsules
Vitamin A 15,000–30,000 IU	Gotu kola extract 1–2 capsules

* Women who need to shrink uterine fibroids, prevent breast cancer recurrences or deal with endometriosis or fibrocystic breasts should keep supplemental folic acid below 600 mcg.
† See the discussion of pantethine supplements on page 371.

Inflammatory Bowel Diseases The inflammatory bowel diseases (IBD) – Crohn's and ulcerative colitis – bear such similarities that they are best considered together. Both have a poor prognosis when treated by mainstream medicine. However, at the Atkins Center we have obtained dramatic improvements within two weeks using vita-nutrient therapy. Often patients on our programme are able to overcome their illnesses entirely. How? By pinpointing and combating glucose intolerance, from which the majority of IBD patients suffer. IBD patients generally consume inordinate quantities of simple sugars. In addition, there is a high frequency of candida overgrowth in patients with any form of IBD. The following nutritional therapy is crucial for recovery:

Most Important	Moderately Important
Pantethine 900–1,800 mg*	Curcuminoids 50–300 mg
Folic acid 30–60 mg†	Grape seed/pycnogenol 150–300 mg
Essential oils formula 3,600–7,200 mg	Vitamin E 400–800 IU
Glutamine 5–12 grams	Vitamin C (nonacidic) 1–3 grams
Vitamin D₃ 600–1,200 IU	Quercetin 600–1,200 mg
Vitamin A 15,000–30,000 IU	Selenium 200–400 mcg
Beneficial bacteria 1–2 tsp	Chlorella 1/2–1 tsp
Natural-source beta-carotene 25,000–50,000 IU	Manganese 20–40 mg
Gamma-oryzanol 450–900 mg	PABA 750–1,500 mg
Zinc 50–100 mg	Propolis 1/2 dropper of tincture in water
Aloe vera powder 1–2 tsp	Phosphatidylcholine 750–1,500 mg
Cat's claw extract 2–4 capsules	

* See the discussion of pantethine supplements on page 371.
† Women who need to shrink uterine fibroids, prevent breast cancer recurrences or deal with endometriosis or fibrocystic breasts should keep supplemental folic acid below 600 mcg.

ENERGY ENHANCEMENT

Without a doubt, the most common complaint I hear from my patients is fatigue. There are many reasons for this condition, including a chronic debilitating illness, a viral overload, an accumulation of external and internal toxic by-products, an underactive thyroid and a stressed immune system. But the most common cause of tiredness is diet – and, more specifically, unstable blood sugar. In other words, a diet high in protein and fat and low in simple sugars is usually the best approach for overcoming fatigue. However, other dietary practices can also help: optimizing digestive health, avoiding metabolic poisons such as margarine and junk foods, eating three meals a day, and avoiding coffee and other stimulants as a temporary solution.

Here are the basic nutrients to provide an energy-optimizing effect:

Most Important	*Moderately Important*
B complex 50–150 mg*	Glutamine 1,500–3,000 mg
CoQ$_{10}$ 50–100 mg	Thiamine 100–150 mg
NADH 2.5–5 mg	ALT 1,000–2,000 mg
Phenylalanine 500–1,500 mg	Germanium 25–75 mg
Octacosanol 12–24 mg	Siberian ginseng 150–300 mg
DMG 125–250 mg	Royal jelly 1/4–1/2 tsp non-freeze-dried
L-carnitine 500–1,000 mg	Inosine 400–800 mg
Vitamin B$_{12}$ injections or	Lipoic acid 100–200 mg
2,000–4,000 mcg sublingual	Methionine 400–800 mg
PABA 1,500–3,000 mg	Acetyl carnitine 500–1,000 mg

* The coenzymes of the B complex should be tried if the fatigue does not respond to regular B complex. These coenzymes are active forms of the B vitamins, and they are available at health food stores in sublingual tablets.

CHRONIC FATIGUE SYNDROME

Although this term is often applied to people who are always tired, it actually describes a specific kind of fatigue. Chronic fatigue syndrome (CFS) is a condition where a person's immune system is compromised enough to render him defenceless against chronic relapsing viruses. This, in turn, impairs his ability to ward off other infectious agents like yeast, parasites, viruses and occasionally virulent bacteria, which are normally kept in check by a vigorous immune system. The usual scenario is a sudden onset of a flulike syndrome with a dramatic drop in energy from one week to the next, brain fog or some failure of mental performance and, often, muscle aches.

The nutritional treatment for chronic fatigue may involve the protocols listed for energy enhancement, for acute and chronic infections, for candida overgrowth, for depression or for all of the above. It really depends on which elements are most prominent. An experienced doctor will be able to help you determine the nature of your illness. At the Atkins Center we succeed with most cases by administering our vita-nutrient therapy intravenously in large quantities. The usual combination is 50 grams of vitamin C, along with oxygen-delivering compounds such as ozone. Such treatments help clear up other viral illnesses like chronic hepatitis and can also bring about dramatic improvements in AIDS patients.

FIBROMYALGIA

Similar to chronic fatigue syndrome, this is an illness that mostly attacks women. It is characterized by pain in the muscles throughout the body, but it is not due to inflammation of the tissues. Many people respond to treatments similar to those for chronic fatigue syndrome. Adequate rest and stress management are extremely important. The Atkins Center protocol centres around vitamin C and ozonelike compounds (we use chlorine dioxide) intravenously. In addition, the following nutrients can be helpful:

Most Important	May Prove Valuable
Magnesium 400–800 mg	Acetyl carnitine 1,000–3,000 mg
Essential oils formula 3,600–7,200 mg	NADH 2.5–5 mg
Beneficial bacteria 1–2 tsp	Chlorella 1/2 tsp
B complex 50–100 mg	Panax ginseng 2–4 capsules
Phosphatidyl serine 300–600 mg	Black cohosh extract 1–2
Reduced glutathione 0.5–1 gram	capsules
Natural-source beta-carotene 25,000–50,000 IU	Reishi extract 1–3 capsules per day

(CONTINUED)

Most Important	Moderately Important
Vitamin C 3–5 grams	Barley/wheat grass 1–2 capsules
Zinc 50–100 mg	Glutamine 1–3 grams
Cetyl myristoleate 300–600 mg	Liquorice root extract 1–3 capsules*

* Not indicated during pregnancy unless deglycyrrhyzinated licorice (DLG) is used.

INFECTIOUS DISEASES

Certain nutrients like zinc, vitamin A and vitamin C have a favourable effect on viral and bacterial infections with few exceptions, especially when administered during the illness's onset. Because of this, my medical staff and I have been able to devise a strategy to prevent such illnesses from even developing. Simultaneous administration of high doses of the following nutrients at the very onset of the infection has produced an impressively high percentage of dramatic benefits.

	Initial Dose	Maintenance Dose
Vitamin A	40,000–80,000 IU	10,000–20,000 IU
Beta-carotene	60,000–120,000 IU	15,000–30,000 IU
B complex	100 mg	25–50 mg
Vitamin C	10–20 grams	2–4 grams
Garlic	2,400–3,200 mg	2,400–3,200 mg
Zinc	200–400 mg	50–100 mg
Bioflavonoids	800–1,600 mg	200–400 mg

For those unfortunate individuals who can't nip their illness in the bud, the foregoing formula still decreases the severity of acute infections. Meanwhile there are other vita-nutrients and herbs worth considering when trying to overcome bacterial and viral illnesses. All of them work to support our immune defences and are therefore appropriate treatments for any infectious disease:

Most Important	Moderately Important
Olive leaf extract 500–2,000 mg*	St-John's-wort 300–600 mg
Oil of oregano 2–4 drops	Astragalus 1–2 droppers in water
Glycerol monolaurate 1,200–2,400 mg	Flaxseed oil 1–2 tbsp
Echinacea 1–2 capsules	Reishi extract 3–4 capsules
Goldenseal 1–2 capsules	Panax ginseng 2–4 capsules
Pantethine 600–1,200 mg†	Propolis 1/2 tsp tincture in water
Quercetin 900–1,800 mg	Liquorice 1–2 capsules
Selenium 200–400 mcg	Barley/wheat grass 1–3 servings/day
Vitamin E 400–1,200 IU	Cat's claw extract 1–2 capsules

* Start at 500 and build slowly to 2,000 mg. There can be a 'die-off', where the very success of the treatment leads to uncomfortable symptoms due to the killing of yeast.
† See the discussion of pantethine supplements on page 371.

Urinary Tract Infections

The major symptoms of urinary tract infections (UTI) are urinary frequency and burning plus fever, and white blood cells in urine specimens confirm the diagnosis of this painful condition. These infections can often be treated by adding cranberry extract (six capsules daily) to the infectious disease regimen. In addition, be sure that candida overgrowth is not present, because a) candida can mimic a bacterial infection and b) the antibiotics usually prescribed for recurrent UTIs will aggravate the yeast condition (see page 388). The treatment for each is quite distinct.

Allergy

In addition to the stuffy nose and watery, itchy eyes that most people identify with allergy (or hay fever), important illnesses like asthma, eczema and hives are largely caused by allergy. Complexes called 'immunoglobulins' mediate the allergic reaction, and certain nutrients help control its various manifestations.

Whether you are battling airborne or food allergies, an inflammatory component is always involved. If you have food allergies, you should use elimination diets or blood tests to determine the foods to which you may be sensitive. If your allergies are airborne based, you should use air filters or other systems to make the air you breathe as pure as possible. Making sure your home has wood floors without carpets is another helpful benefit. The following programme is helpful for both food and airborne allergies:

Most Important	Moderately Important
Pantethine 600–900 mg*	Essential oils formula 3,600–7,200 mg
Quercetin 600–1,200 mg	Bioflavonoids 1,000–3,000 mg
Vitamin C at least 3 grams	B₆ 100–200 mg.
Magnesium 400–600 mg	Natural-source beta-carotene
Grape seed extract 50–300 mg	25,000–50,000 IU
Liquorice extract 100–300 mg	Bromelain 400–800 mg
DHEA 30–100 mg	Vitamin A 15,000–30,000 IU
Pregnenolone 30–100 mg	Selenium 150–300 mcg
B₁₂ 1–3 mg	Vitamin E 400–800 IU
	Zinc 25–50 mg

* See the discussion of pantethine supplements on page 371.

PULMONARY HEALTH: ASTHMA, BRONCHITIS AND EMPHYSEMA

The lungs and bronchial airways of the body are amazing but delicate tissues. They are assaulted daily with both indoor and outdoor pollution, not to mention cigarette smoke and the toxic chemicals found throughout our environment. Compound these inflammatory insults with the lack of anti-inflammatory nutrients such as fish oils and antioxidants in our diets, and you'll understand why asthma and other pulmonary problems are continually on the rise. Food allergies can also be involved in triggering bronchial problems, particularly asthma. (Most asthma, in fact, is a result of some type of allergy.) However, the bottom line approach for inflammation of the bronchial passages is to relax them with magnesium, protect them with antioxidants and reduce their exposure to environmental insults as much as possible. Emphysema, pulmonary fibrosis and other chronic lung disorders can also be alleviated with a similar programme. For promoting optimal health of the lungs and bronchial area, I recommend the following:

Most Important	Moderately Important
Vitamin C 3–6 grams	Natural-source beta-carotene
Vitamin A 15,000–30,000 IU	25,000–50,000 IU
Essential oils formula 3,600–7,200 mg	Quercetin 600–1,200 mg
N-acetyl cysteine 500–1,000 mg	Selenium 200–400 mcg
Magnesium 400–800 mg	Taurine 500–1,000 mg
Pantethine 300–600 mg*	Vitamin E 400–800 IU
	CoQ_{10} 50–100 mg

* See the discussion of pantethine supplements on page 371.

For asthma and emphysema, add the following nutrients or increase the following dose ranges:

Most Important	Moderately Important
Vitamin A 25,000–50,000 IU	Molybdenum 500–1,000 mcg
Fish oils 3,600–7,200 mg	*Coleus forskohlii* extract 150–300 mcg
Pantethine 600–1,200 mg*	*Ginkgo biloba* extract 240–360 mg
Magnesium 500–1,000 mg	Taurine 750–1,500 mg
Quercetin 1,000–2,000 mg	B_6 75–150 mg
Grape seed/pycnogenol 150–300 mg	*Aloe vera* 1–2 tbsp
Liquorice root extract 300–600 mg	N-acetyl cysteine 1,000–2,000 mg
DHEA 75–150 mg	B_{12} 5,000–10,000 mcg
Pregnenolone 60–120 mg	

* See the discussion of pantethine supplements on page 371.

If you decide to use either DHEA or pregnenolone as an alternative to the drug prednisone, please do so under a doctor's supervision.

For bronchitis or pneumonia, use the following nutrient doses only for the duration of your illness:

Most Important	Moderately Important
Vitamin C 5–40 grams	Selenium 300–600 mcg
Vitamin A 50,000–150,000	Lipoic acid 100–200 mg
(not during pregnancy)	N-acetyl cysteine 1,000–2,000 mg
Zinc 60–120 mg	Astragalus 1–2 droppers
Oil of oregano 2–4 drops	Propolis 1–2 droppers
Quercetin or citrus bioflavonoids	Natural-source beta-carotene
1,000–2,000 mg	25,000–50,000 IU
Echinacea 3–6 capsules	Vitamin E 800–1,600 IU
Goldenseal 750–1,500 mg	Olive leaf extract 2–4 capsules*
(not during pregnancy)	
Pantethine 600–1,200 mg†	

* See page 395 for caveat.
† See the discussion of pantethine supplements on page 371.

CANCER PREVENTION

The epidemic of cancer that has gripped the civilized world still rages unchecked. We need to take a more aggressive approach towards preventing cancer, beyond the recommendation that we all stop smoking. Foods sprayed with pesticides or herbicides should be avoided, and we should make every effort to clean up our living and working environments from pollutants. Targeted Nutrition can also play an enormous role in preventing cancers of many kinds, and I recommend the following regimen to all those who want to lower their risk of cancer. This programme is also useful for cancer survivors who want to avoid a recurrence:

Most Important	Moderately Important
Selenium 200–400 mcg	Lycopene 6–12 mg (take with
Natural-source beta-carotene	dietary oil)
20,000–40,000 IU	Modified citrus pectin 8–16 grams
Vitamin E 400–1,200 IU	Beneficial bacteria 1/2–1 tsp
Lipoic acid 50–100 mg	Vitamin A 10,000–25,000 IU
Mixed tocotrienols 200–400 mg	Cat's claw 2–4 capsules
Essential oils formula 3,600–7,200 mg	Vitamin D₃ 400–800 IU

(CONTINUED)

Most Important	Moderately Important
Vitamin C 5–10 grams	Barley/wheat grass 2–4 capsules
Folic acid 5–10 mg*	Chlorella 1–2 tsp
Zinc 50–100 mg	B complex 50–100 mg
N-acetyl cysteine 500–1,000 mg	Milk thistle extract 150–300 mg
CoQ$_{10}$ 200–400 mg	Panax ginseng 2–4 capsules
Quercetin 300–600 mg (and other flavonoids)	Arginine 1,500–4,000 mg
	Magnesium 400 mg
Mushrooms (reishi, shiitake and maitake) 20–40 drops	Manganese 10 mg
	Squalene 1–3 grams

*Women who need to shrink uterine fibroids, prevent breast cancer recurrences, or deal with endometriosis or fibrocystic breasts should keep supplemental folic acid below 600 mcg.

Because excess iron can increase the risk of cancer, remember to avoid iron supplements and foods fortified with iron unless you are iron-deficient. Also be sure to avoid the use of the polyunsaturates such as safflower, sunflower and corn oil, since they contain fats that can also promote tumours.

CANCER THERAPY

Treatments using natural nontoxic therapies for overcoming existing cancer are light-years ahead of conventional drug- and surgery-based treatments. The nutritional approaches are valuable largely because they provide an alternative to toxic doses of chemotherapy. And unlike chemo, nutrition can often stabilize the cancer growth in its early stages as well as yield a complete remission. Although I would love to disclose this lifesaving treatment option, I am unable to outline the complete Atkins Center cancer therapy for several reasons. First, with the exception of the essential fats, antioxidant nutrients, medicinal mushrooms and some of the herbs, the treatment requires more than just the nutrients described in this book. Second, the therapy must be customized for each patient's biochemistry and particular form of cancer. Finally, I don't want to compromise the value of complementary cancer therapy by offering a do-it-yourself solution. If this is your problem, I beseech you to find a complementary doctor or nutritionally aware health professional who has the experience to use the treatments effectively. (The best resource to help you find such a doctor is to read *Alternative Medicine: The Definitive Guide to Cancer* by John Diamond, MD, Lee Cowden, MD and Burton Goldberg, published by Future Medicine Publishing in 1997 and available through amazon.com.

MEN'S HEALTH PROBLEMS

Benign Enlargement of the Prostate This condition, in which the prostate gland becomes swollen enough to obstruct urine flow, makes urination difficult and causes frequent trips to the bathroom during the night. It strikes most men as they age, usually by the time they reach sixty or sixty-five. Billions of dollars are spent annually managing benign enlargement of the prostate, mostly with medication and surgical procedures. However, prostate enlargement responds so well to nutritional and herbal medicine that mainstream solutions are in fact completely unnecessary. Many complementary doctors recommend a procedure called hyperthermia, which involves applying enormous amounts of heat (around 42°C/108°F) to the enlarged prostate. This practice, along with the following regimen, allows patients to avoid complication-laden surgery.

I have found the treatment programme below to be remarkably effective in treating men with benign enlargement of the prostate. It is also excellent for supporting male reproductive health in general. Plan on taking the supplements for at least three months.

Most Important	*Moderately Important*
Saw palmetto 250–500 mg of standardized extract	Zinc 50–100 mg
	B₆ 100–200 mg
Pygeum africanum 100–200 mg of standardized extract	Selenium 200–400 mcg
	Gamma-oryzanol 300–600 mg
Glutamic acid 500–1,000 mg	Bee pollen 1/4–1/2 tsp*
Glycine 250–500 mg	Vitamin E 400–800 IU
Alanine 250–500 mg	
Manganese 20–40 mg	
Essential oils formula 3,600–7,200 mg	

* Use carefully if sensitive to pollens.

Low Libido For those with an especially low libido or those who suffer from impotence, I recommend the following treatment programme for the specific purpose of increasing a man's sex drive:

Most Important	*Moderately Important*
DHEA*	Boron 6–12 mg
Androstenedione 150–300 mg†	Folic acid 15–30 mg
Arginine 2–5 grams	Saw palmetto 250–500 mg
Siberian ginseng 300–600 mg	Panax ginseng 250–1,000 mg
Ginkgo biloba 240–360 mg	B complex 50–100 mg
Zinc 50–100 mg	*Avena sativa* 750–1,500 mg‡
Yohimbe	

* Start with 20–40 mg and then adjust dosage until the blood level of DHEA is that of an average thirty-year-old male.
† A metabolite of DHEA, it should be used in a similar way. It allows testosterone levels to build up.
‡ An herb from green oats not mentioned in part two, but with considerable word-of-mouth affirmation of effectiveness.

WOMEN'S HEALTH PROBLEMS

Cervical Dysplasia Cervical dysplasia is a precancerous condition that can signal an increased risk of cervical cancer. It can be detected when the cells of the cervix begin to reproduce abnormally, because it causes an abnormal Pap smear reading. High doses of certain nutrients, especially prescription doses of folic acid, have reversed the majority of abnormal Pap smear readings caused by cervical dysplasia. However, you must use the following treatment programme in conjunction with the cancer prevention protocol for three to six months, even up to one year, to make certain that a delayed benefit has not been overlooked:

Most Important	Moderately Important
Folic acid 15–30 mg*	B$_{12}$ 1–5 mg
Natural-source beta-carotene 50,000–100,000 IU	Grape seed extract/pycnogenol 150–300 mg
Vitamin A 20,000–40,000 IU	Gotu kola extract 1–2 capsules
Vitamin C 1–3 grams	Green tea extract 1–3 capsules
Vitamin E 400–800 IU	
Selenium 200–400 mcg	

*Women who need to shrink uterine fibroids, prevent breast cancer recurrences or deal with endometriosis or fibrocystic breasts should keep supplemental folic acid below 600 mcg.

Endometriosis and Fibrocystic Breast Disease Endometriosis (uterine lining tissue growing elsewhere in the abdomen), fibrocystic breast disease (the benign lumpy breast condition often mistaken for early breast cancer) and uterine fibroids (the nonmalignant tumours that grow so large that hysterectomies are often recommended) are all conditions that often occur because of imbalanced female hormones; oestrogen predominates over progesterone. Supporting the liver with methionine, choline and inositol helps the body better balance the hormones by converting oestradiol to the weaker oestrogen, oestriol. With the following regime, I have seen these problems disappear over a period of six months to a year:

Most Important	Moderately Important
Methionine 500–1,000 mg	Zinc 25–50 mg
Choline 1,000–1,500 mg	Vitamin C 1–3 grams
Inositol 1,000–1,500 mg	Vitex 1–2 capsules
Essential oils formula 3,600–7,200 mg	Milk thistle extract 150–300 mg
B$_6$ 100–200 mg	Beneficial bacteria 1–2 tsp
Vitamin E 200–400 IU*	Flaxmeal fibre 1–3 tbsp
	Vitamin A 30,000–60,000 IU

* Natural-source beta-carotene 25,000 IU (for fibrocystic breast disease, higher doses may backfire).
Note: Folic acid, PABA and boron, three nutrients that help overcome menopausal symptoms by increasing oestrogen levels, must be eliminated from the list of supplements.

Premenstrual Syndrome Premenstrual syndrome (PMS) has symptoms such as anger, breast tenderness, food cravings and depression that come just before the bleeding phase of the female cycle. They can often be alleviated by optimizing nutrition. Elimination of sugar and caffeine is a must, and consuming adequate protein throughout the day – not just at one meal – is essential. The following nutrients and herbs will also greatly reduce symptoms of PMS:

Most Important	Moderately Important
Essential oils formula 3,200–7,600 mg	Milk thistle extract 150–300 mg
B$_6$ 100–200 mg	Vitamin C 1–5 gm
Choline 1,000–1,500 mg	Zinc 50–100 mg
Inositol 1,000–1,500 mg	Vitex extract 1–2 capsules
Methionine 500–1,000 mg	Phosphatidyl serine 300–600 mg
Magnesium 300–600 mg	Flaxmeal 1–3 tsp in morning
Chromium 200–600 mcg	Calcium 1,000–1,500 mg
Beneficial bacteria 1–2 tsp	Manganese 15–30 mg
GABA 500–3,000 mg	Vitamin A 20,000–40,000 IU
Black cohosh extract 12–24 mg	L-tryptophan 1,000–2,000 mg

Refer to the following for special PMS problems:

Heavy bleeding: add grape seed/pycnogenol
2,000–4,000 mg
Menstrual cramps: add magnesium up to 1,000 mg daily
for entire month
Depression: add St-John's-wort 1/2 dropperful of
tincture in water one to two times per day plus
GABA 1,000–2,000 mg
Anxiety: add kava extract 200–400 mg and GABA
1,000–2,000 mg
Sugar cravings: add L-glutamine 2–3 grams
Water retention: add L-taurine 1,000–2,000 mg

Menopausal Symptoms Women are often told that any discomforts of menopause, such as hot flushes or dry skin, can be fixed only by hormonal replacement therapy. Not so. These symptoms are in fact the first and foremost signs that the body needs optimal nutrition. While oestrogen replacement therapy carries with it significant increased risk for cancer, nutrient therapy has only positive benefits and should always be the first defence against menopause symptoms. The nutritional therapy should be centred around large doses of folic acid as well as the hormone precursors pregnenolone and DHEA. Here is an example of an effective nutritional programme:

Most Important	*Moderately Important*
Folic acid 20–60 mg*	Vitamin C 2,000–4,000 mg
Boron 6–18 mg	PABA 1,500–3,000 mg
Pregnenolone 30–60 mg†	Black cohosh extract 15–30 mg
DHEA 20–40 mg†	Magnesium 400–800 mg
Essential oils formula 3,600–7,200 mg	Vitex extract 1–2 capsules
Vitamin E 400–1,200 IU	Vitamin A 20,000–40,000 IU
B₆ 150–300 mg	Calcium 750–1,500 mg
Gamma-oryzanol 150–450 mg	Phosphatidyl serine 200–400 mg
B complex 50–100 mg	Kava extract 1–2 capsules
Chromium 200–600 mcg	Flaxmeal 1–3 tsp in the morning

*Women who need to shrink uterine fibroids, prevent breast cancer recurrences or deal with endometriosis or fibrocystic breasts should keep supplemental folic acid below 600 mcg.

† Pregnenolone and DHEA dosages should be prescribed according to their blood levels. The objective is to reach the norms for a healthy thirty-year-old woman.

Note: Topical progesterone creams made from wild yams that are also enhanced with natural progesterone make an extremely useful therapy. They should be administered in doses of 1/3–1/2 teaspoon for three weeks of each month.

OSTEOPOROSIS

Osteoporosis – the well-known bone-thinning disease that leads to easily broken bones, especially in women – is best prevented by regular weight-bearing exercise combined with upper-body exercise (particularly if begun in the teenage years). Women with a history of bulimia or anorexia are at particular risk. Avoiding caffeine, smoking, sugar and soft drinks is another crucial safeguard, along with keeping female hormone levels high. However, this is not always accomplished through oestrogen replacement therapy; nutrients can achieve the same goal with greater safety.

The following nutrients should also help to prevent and treat osteoporosis:

Most Important	*Moderately Important*
Folic acid 20–60 mg*	Chondroitin sulfate 50–150 mg
Boron 6–12 mg	Copper 2–4 mg
Calcium 800–1,600 mg	Manganese 10–20 mg
Vitamin D 400–800 IU	Zinc 20–50 mg
Magnesium 400–800 mg	Essential oils formula 3,600–7,200 mg
Vitamin K 150–300 mcg	Black cohosh extract 15–30 mg
Silicon 100–300 mg	Glucosamine 1,000–2,000 mg
Lysine 500–1,000 mg	Vitamin C 1–3 grams
B complex 50–100 mg	Natural-source beta-carotene 10,000–20,000 IU

*Women who need to shrink uterine fibroids, prevent breast cancer recurrences or deal with endometriosis or fibrocystic breasts should keep supplemental folic acid below 600 mcg.

GOUT

Gout is an age-old disease of dietary excess, so you can imagine how nutritional changes will make a big difference. The disease is an acute inflammation of the joints that typically leads to symptoms such as pain in the big toe. Although acute flare-ups may be successfully managed by conventional medications, nutrition serves as a good line of defence.

Gout is characterized by an excess of uric acid, which is one of the body's major antioxidants. This has led many complementary doctors to theorize that uric acid is produced as a response to excess free radical production and that other antioxidants would signal the body to stop producing surplus uric acid. That's why I use high doses of the antioxidant vitamin C (5 grams or higher) in my gout-afflicted patients. Here are the nutrients I find helpful:

Vitamin C 5–10 grams
Folic acid 10–30 mg (women who need to shrink uterine
    fibroids, prevent breast cancer recurrences or deal with
    endometriosis or fibrocystic breasts should keep supple-
    mental folic acid below 600 mcg)
L-cysteine 1,000–2,000 mg
Pantethine 600–1,200 mg (see the discussion of pantethine
    supplements on page 325)
Chondroitin sulfate 750–1,500 mg
Essential oils formula 3,600–7,200 mg
Germanium 150–300 mg

ARTHRITIS

Arthritis affects more than eight million Britons and is one of our most mismanaged health conditions. The disease consists of two different mechanisms for causing pain and deformity in your joints: inflammation (rheumatoid is the best example) and degeneration (exemplified by osteoarthritis, the most common form). Early use of Targeted Nutrition has fostered remarkable results, particularly for osteoarthritis. Obviously, if there is no cartilage left in your joints, there is little natural medicine can do.

As different as osteo- and rheumatoid arthritis are, a considerable number of people have both; therefore there is considerable overlap in the nutritional approach used for both kinds. For all arthritics, I strongly recommend the following regime. It has helped the majority of arthritis patients at the Atkins Center reduce or eliminate their need for side effect-laden arthritis medication:

Most Important	*Moderately Important*
Cetyl myristoleate 18 grams per course (400–600 mg divided over 30–45 days)	Calcium AEP 4–6 tablets*
	PABA 500–1,500 mg
Chrondroitin sulfate 750–1,500 mg†	Curcuminoids (from turmeric)
Glucosamine sulfate 1,250–2,500 mg†	1,200–2,400 mg
Copper sebacate 8–16 mg†	Ginger 800–1,600 mg
Sea cucumber 1,000–2,000 mg†	Beneficial bacteria 1/4–1/2 tsp
Essential oils formula 3,600–7,200 mg	Selenium 200–400 mcg
Pantethine 900 mg‡	Quercetin 600–1,200 mg
Niacinamide 1,500–2,000 mg	Liquorice root extract 2–4
B₆ 150–300 mg	capsules
Pregnenolone 30–100 mg**	Grape seed extract 50–150 mg
DHEA 30–100 mg**	Manganese 25–50 mg
Bovine/shark cartilage 6–12 grams	DMSO (rub on affected area)
Vitamin E 400 IU	B₁₂ 1,000–2,000 mcg
Bromelain 600 mg*	Bilberry 250–500 mg
Vitamin C 1–3 grams	Methionine 1–2 grams
Folic acid 5–15 grams††	Zinc 50–100 mg
	Cat's claw extract 1,000– 2,000 mg
	Molybdenum 500–1,000 mcg

* Indicates use for rheumatoid arthritis.

† Indicates primary use is for osteoarthritis.

‡ See the discussion of pantethine supplements on page 371.

** Dosage regulation requires doctor management.

†† Women who need to shrink uterine fibroids, prevent breast cancer recurrences or deal with endometriosis or fibrocystic breasts should keep supplemental folic acid below 600 mcg.

CARPAL TUNNEL SYNDROME

Carpal tunnel syndrome (CTS), an inflammation in the wrist leading to the palm, is a widespread condition common among office workers and computer users. It is best treated by taking in one hundred times the RDA for B_6. While over half of those with CTS respond well to B_6 therapy alone, in my treatment programme I usually include the following nutrients, which also help to alleviate symptoms. Use the therapy for two to three months before you assess whether or not it has worked for you. If not, use the osteoarthritis protocol, maintaining the high dose of pyridoxal-5-phosphate.

Pyridoxine (B_6) 200–400 mg; or
Pyridoxal-5-phosphate 50–100 mg
B_2 75–150 mg
B complex 100 mg

AUTOIMMUNE DISEASE

Complementary doctors often use nutritional medicine to correct the mechanism that cause illnesses. A good example is autoimmune disease, a condition in which the body begins to attack itself. Food allergies or sensitivities are usually involved and should be investigated by a nutritionally oriented doctor. While each autoimmune illness is unique – from autoimmune thyroiditis to lupus and rheumatoid arthritis – I find the following nutrients helpful in virtually all instances. Perhaps the success of this nutritional treatment programme for a variety of autoimmune problems means that a nutrient deficiency may trigger our immune system on a self-destructive path.

Most Important	*Moderately Important*
Calcium AEP 1,500–4,000 mg	Vitamin E 400–800 IU
Pantethine 600–1,200 mg*	Vitamin B_6 100–200 mg
Essential oils formula 3,600–7,200 mg	Selenium 200–400 mcg
Pregnenolone 30–100 mg†	Vitamin A 20,000–40,000 IU
DHEA 30–100 mg†	PABA 500–1,500 mg

(CONTINUED)

Most Important	Moderately Important
Vitamin C 3–6 grams	Liquorice root extract 1–2 capsules
Beneficial bacteria 1–2 tsp	Milk thistle 150–300 mg
Natural-source beta-carotene 25,000–50,000 IU	

* See the discussion of pantethine supplements on page 371.
† Dosage regulation requires doctor management.

Several of the autoimmune conditions have unique features that require other nutrients as well.

Scleroderma Scleroderma is a Greek-derived word for 'hardened skin', and this indeed is a feature of this autoimmune illness. In addition to the above programme, the following nutrients can soften the fibrous tissue that causes the hardening:

Frozen shark cartilage extract 1 vial daily (or bovine cartilage 6–12 capsules)
PABA 10–20 grams
Gotu kola 4–6 capsules
DMSO Consult health care practitioner

Multiple Sclerosis Multiple sclerosis is an autoimmune demyelinating disease. This means the body mistakenly identifies and destroys the protective sheath of nerves, made of myelin. The most common cause of demyelinization is the accumulation of toxic minerals like mercury, the toxic element that largely constitutes the 'silver' dental fillings. Because the immune system considers mercury-saturated brain tissue to be a foreign substance, it begins to destroy it. While conventional medicine considers multiple sclerosis a progressive advancing illness, our experience at the Atkins Center has been very different. Based on hundreds of successful clinical cases, we believe that the illness will reverse itself once the cause has been identified and removed. The treatment of choice is intravenous calcium AEP, one vial every two days. Though there are no scientific papers, five thousand case histories confirm the power of this treatment.

The following nutrients are valuable supplements to calcium AEP and to the autoimmune protocol:

Most Important	*Moderately Important*
AEP salts of magnesium, potassium, and calcium 3–6 capsules	Folic acid 5–15 mg*
Octacosanol 15–30 mg	DHEA and pregnenolone as directed
B₁₂ as methylcobalamin 30–60 mg	Phosphatidyl serine 200–400 mg
Vitamin D₃ 800–1,600 IU	Inositol 500–1,000 mg
Sphingomyelin 3–6 capsules†	Lecithin 1–3 tsp
EPA/DHA fish oil 1,800–3,600 mg	Methionine 1,500–3,000 mg
Pancreatic enzymes 3–6 grams‡	CoQ₁₀ 100–200 mg

* Women who need to shrink uterine fibroids, prevent breast cancer recurrences or deal with endometriosis or fibrocystic breasts should keep supplemental folic acid below 600 mcg.

† The lost myelin sheath is made of this substance, and it seems to be more valuable after the illness is stabilized.

‡ Valuable treatment during a flare-up.

Many doctors caution those with autoimmune disease to avoid immune-stimulating herbs for fear of empowering the immune system to act against the body; but others, I among them, feel that autoimmunity is really a response of a weakened immune system.

Skin Problems

The skin is the largest organ of the body and is incredibly responsive to nutrition. Usually the manifestations of internal imbalances, skin problems as diverse as acne, eczema and psoriasis respond well to a programme of diet and vita-nutrients. Removing margarine and other sources of trans-fats in the diet, such as partially hydrogenated oils, is crucial. Many dermatologists say that sweets don't cause acne. But avoiding sugar helps more skin conditions than any other therapy, based on the fact that sugar fuels the bad bacteria in the intestinal tract that can cause many skin problems.

Here is my basic protocol for optimizing skin health:

Most Important	Moderately Important
Vitamin A 20,000–40,000 IUs	B$_6$ 100–200 mg
Natural-source beta-carotene 25,000–	B complex 50–100 mg
50,000 IU	Selenium 200–400 mcg
Vitamin C 1–3 grams	Calcium 800–1,200 mg
Zinc 50–100 mg	Manganese 25–50 mg
Beneficial bacteria 1/4–1/2 tsp	Gotu kola 1–3 capsules of
Essential oils formula 3,600–7,200 mg	standardized extract
Magnesium 400 mg	Liquorice 1–3 capsules
Pantethine 300–600 mg*	

* See the discussion of pantethine supplements on page 371.

However, you should also be aware that each skin condition has a unique treatment programme consisting of certain key nutrients. For acne, I occasionally prescribe increased doses of vitamin A for a month or so – sometimes as high as 100,000 IU. (For me, vitamin A is the skin vitamin, zinc is the skin mineral, and together they are the two most important nutrients for the treatment of acne.) Women who have the slightest chance of being pregnant should avoid vitamin A supplements, as high doses of A can cause foetal malformations. Eczema also responds well to the targeted programme above and occasionally requires higher doses of GLA and EPA. For psoriasis, topical vitamin D$_3$ cream in addition to the foregoing regime speeds up healing, along with daily 220 and 660 mg doses of a compound called fumaric acid esters. I also recommend the topical fumaric acid cream. This compound, used both internally and externally, is a major part of our successful psoriasis programme.

PERIODONTAL DISEASE

Gum health is very responsive to vita-nutrient therapy, which could explain why many of the great pioneers of the twentieth century have been dentists. Periodontal disease, or the deterioration of the gums, is a condition that requires more than just good dental hygiene; you have to give the body the right nutrients to heal gum tissue. Because the bacteria that cause periodontal disease are fuelled by carbohydrates, I recommend reducing carbohydrate intake and eliminating sweets (even natural ones like fruit). I also like to use herbs like hawthorn and gotu kola, because of their ability to strengthen and heal tissues like those found in the gums. My recommendations:

Most Important	Moderately Important
CoQ_{10} 100–200 mg	Gotu kola extract 2–4 capsules
Beneficial bacteria 1–2 tsp	Hawthorn extract 2–4 capsules
Vitamin A 10,000–20,000 IU	Propolis for gums*
Folic acid 5–10 mg (used topically)†	Chlorella 1/2–1 tsp
Zinc 50–100 mg	Calcium 750–1,500 mg
Vitamin C 2–5 grams	

* Test sensitivity on skin first.
† Women who need to shrink uterine fibroids, prevent breast cancer recurrences or deal with endometriosis or fibrocystic breasts should keep supplemental folic acid below 600 mcg.

Vision Health

Eye problems such as cataracts, glaucoma and macular degeneration respond in varying degrees to nutritional therapy. One thing is clear: prevention, as always, is your strongest card. Antioxidant nutrients are particularly important for cataract prevention.

My general programme for maximizing eye health is as follows:

Most Important	Moderately Important
Natural-source beta-carotene 25,000–50,000 IU	Bilberry extract 250–500 mg
Lutein 6–12 mg	Vitamin A 10,000–30,000 IU
Vitamin C 1–3 grams	B complex 50–75 mg
Zinc 50–100 mg	Vitamin E 400–800 IU
Selenium 200–400 mcg	Lysine 500–1,000 mg
Taurine 1–2 grams	N-acetyl cysteine 500–1,000 mg

Cataracts If your vision is blurring, you may be developing a cataract, or a clouding of the lens of the eye. For treatment, I recommend a stronger dosage of certain nutrients, as follows:

Most Important	*Moderately Important*
Vitamin C 3–10 grams	DMG 250–500 mg
Zinc 50–100 mg	*Ginkgo biloba* 240–360 mg
Lipoic acid 100–200 mg	Vitamin E 600–1,200 IU
Bilberry 250–500 mg	Manganese 25–50 mg
N-acetyl cysteine 1,000 mg	

Glaucoma Glaucoma is an eye disease involving increased pressure of the fluid within the eyeball. The effect can be to damage the optic disk and cause a gradual loss of vision – and ultimately blindness. Early treatment is important, and I recommend using the various eyedrops prescribed by your ophthalmologist and increasing the general treatment programme as follows:

Vitamin A 25,000–50,000 IU
Vitamin C 6–12 grams
Bee pollen 1/4–1/2 tsp
Rutin 50–100 mg

Macular Degeneration I receive more inquiries about macular degeneration, a breakdown of the highly vascular centre of vision in our retinas, than any other eye condition. This is because the problem is considered untreatable by conventional medicine. In fact, it is quite responsive to nutritional therapy. I start off with an intravenous dose of taurine, which I feel is the best available treatment for the condition. My oral support programme includes these nutrients:

Most Important	Moderately Important
Zinc 60–120 mg (adjust dose according to zinc taste test)	Grape seed/pycnogenol 80–160 mg
	Lipoic acid 100–200 mg
Natural-source beta-carotene 40,000–80,000 IU	N-acetyl cysteine 500–1,000 mg
	Vitamin A 20,000–40,000 IU
Lutein 10–20 mg	Vitamin E 600–1,200 IU
Ginkgo biloba extract 240–360 mg	Selenium 100–200 mcg
Bilberry 250–500 mg	
Taurine 1,500–3,000 mg	

As you may have noted, all the conditions that respond to vita-nutrient therapy may not be covered in this survey. Don't despair until you have used the index; you may find that your problem is discussed in part two of the book.

A FINAL REMINDER

One point bears repeating: my vita-nutrient solutions are usually powerful enough to replace conventional medications. However, when combined with these medications, they can turn a safe medication into an overdose. Because vita-nutrients are many times safer than drugs, the drugs are the logical target for dosage reduction. This should certainly be done under a doctor's supervision, but it is mandatory that the decision-making doctor be as knowledgeable about vita-nutrients as about pharmaceuticals. Should your doctor not have the requisite vita-nutrient knowledge, your health may be jeopardized by this shortcoming. I strongly advise that you make sure your doctor is well versed in nutrition; otherwise you should find another doctor. Should you not wish to change doctors, you should then try to convince your doctor to familiarize himself with this information.

GAUNTLET THROWING MAKES FOR A WIN-WIN SITUATION

I hope you will understand the method in my militancy. More and more doctors are beginning to show a genuine interest in using nutritional therapies. If enough people can supply a little tender loving marketplace motivation, even more of our caregivers will begin practising this safe, natural and more comprehensive kind of medicine.

So with your urging, you become a winner – your health decisions are made by someone who understands the full range of options you really have. And your doctor wins, too. He or she gets to experience the heady satisfaction of knowing that he or she is *really* helping patients get well. Maybe this trend will put us back on the path that Hippocrates planned for us when he wrote, 'First, do no harm'.

Supplement Guidelines

Here are some of the most commonly asked questions – and answers – about supplementation.

Where should I buy my supplements? From my nutritionist, health food store or from a mail order catalogue?

The real answer is, 'Wherever you will get the best quality'. I have seen high- and low-quality supplements from all three sources, so you should buy where you feel the most comfortable. You may seek a direct recommendation from your nutritionist or a knowledgeable health food store assistant, but if you know exactly what you want, you may prefer mail order. Do whatever is most convenient, as long as you are getting high-quality supplements from a reputable manufacturer.

How do I know which supplements are the best quality and which manufacturers are reputable?

One thing is certain: quality is not indicated on the label. The decision requires an industry insider such as a nutritionally oriented doctor or nutritionist. Such professionals learn about quality by seeing the results of various products they have recommended in treating their patients. If you ever consult with one, be sure to ask this very question.

Should supplements be taken with or away from meals?

Most supplements should be taken with meals for the simple

reason that you tolerate them better when food is in your stomach. Herbs should ideally be taken about twenty minutes before eating, but they can also be taken with food if that is more convenient. Buffered vitamin C powders and amino acids involved in mood enhancement should be taken before meals. Minerals such as calcium and magnesium should be taken with only water on an empty stomach before bed, preferably in a capsule form that will dissolve easily. This will help you take advantage of their natural relaxant properties. The following supplements are best taken with a meal that contains some fat or oil: vitamins A, E, D, tocotrienols, carotenoids, lycopene, lutein and CoQ_{10}. Why? All are fat-soluble, and eating them with fat helps you absorb them better.

I started taking a high-potency multivitamin, and my urine is a bright yellow. Is this Okay?

Yes, it's perfectly normal. The phenomenon comes from a metabolite of a B-complex vitamin, riboflavin, and is a sign that your body is metabolizing vitamins well and that you are taking enough B complex.

If I take only one supplement per day, what should it be?

It is difficult for me to give this answer, because I believe that for optimal health we should take a minimum of four to five supplements per day. (Combining the essential nutrients in one pill would make that pill the size of an ice hockey puck.) However, if I were forced to pick just one, it would be a high-quality multivitamin rich in vitamins B, C and E, with adequate amounts of trace minerals like zinc, selenium and chromium.

Can I take my supplements all at once, or should I try to spread them out throughout the day?

If you follow my programme to its logical conclusion, you will be taking too many supplements to ingest comfortably at one sitting. Therefore it should not be surprising that my advice is to spread out your supplement intake over the course of the day. The GI tract can absorb only so much at once, and certain nutrients compete for absorption, so the more you spread out your supplement intake, the better.

My doctor told me that I can get all the nutrients I need from my diet. What should I tell him?

Tell him, respectfully, that you have great difficulty accepting his premise, and offer three responses. First, how does he know you are getting all the nutrients you need? Has he ever performed nutrient blood tests or mineral challenge tests? Second, how does he know how much enough is? Heart disease- and cancer-preventing amounts of vitamin E, for example, are not available from any food. If you do not take a supplement of E, you cannot get optimal amounts of this potent heart and immune system protector no matter what you eat. Third, show him this book as proof of the thousands of scientific studies that affirm the value of these nutrients. Fortunately the discussion among doctors today is becoming more and more pro-nutrient. It is not whether to take supplements, but how much to take.

I am on many medications, and my doctor told me not to take supplements. What should I do?

As one of my mentors, Dr Carlton Fredericks, so often said, 'Why do doctors advise people against supplements when they still let them eat food?' Supplements are concentrated, therapeutic amounts of nutrients – that's all – and if you can eat food, you can take supplements. If anything, taking medications increases the need for nutrients, particularly vitamin C, the B complex and liver-supporting herbs like milk thistle.

There are occasions, however, when supplements interfere with the active mechanism of some medications. For example, you do not want to take calcium, magnesium or other minerals at the same time as the antibiotic tetracycline, because minerals will bind to the drug and render it inactive. You should avoid vitamin K if you are depending on warfarin's anticoagulant effect. And limit folic acid if you depend on methotrexate to help you. (However, taking a limited amount of folic acid when using this drug is not only harmless, but also helps counter some of its side effects.)

By and large, however, adverse drug-nutrient interactions are actually quite rare. The overwhelming majority of interactions are positive. Vitamin C has been found to enhance the benefits of many drugs, including chemotherapy. Niacin enhances the benefits of cholesterol-lowering medications. And in some cases, using drugs increases the need for nutrients. It is well known that oral contraceptives increase the need for B vitamins. Drugs like sulfasalazine, used to treat colitis, deplete folic acid. Even using aspirin regularly depletes nutrients like vitamin C and folic acid. Diuretics deplete minerals. The list goes on, so your best bet is to find a doctor well versed in complementary practices who can give you the best of both conventional and nutritional medicine.

Should I keep my supplements in the refrigerator?

Only a few supplements need to be refrigerated, such as fish oil liquids and capsules, flaxseed oil and other essential fatty acid supplements like borage and evening primrose oil. CoQ_{10} should also be kept refrigerated to preserve potency. Keep all other supplements in a cool dark place (refrigeration may have negative effects because the moisture in the refrigerator may cause a decline in the supplement's potency).

EPILOGUE

◈

THE GRASS-ROOTS SOLUTION

Now that you have read this book, I hope you will agree with me that vita-nutrients can and should replace pharmaceuticals. If you or family members have actually *used* the treatment formulations given here, you'll know firsthand how powerful vita-nutrient therapy really is. Understandably you may wonder why the rest of the world has not yet caught up to your way of thinking. Here's the answer: if vita-nutrients can replace drugs, then the pharmaceutical companies, appropriately interested in their own economic fortunes, must play the role of adversary – a part they are reluctant to assume. Therefore they must find spokespeople to discredit the vita-nutrient movement.

With plenty of doctors and nutritionists willing to go with the economic power core, their strategy is rather straightforward, and it has been overwhelmingly successful. When asked about the medical feasibility of a certain nutrient, the authority figures in question simply say that the benefit is 'unproven'. Meanwhile charitable foundations that welcome pharmaceutical industry donations publish a list of unproven therapies (which, ironically, is startlingly similar to my list of 'most valuable nutritional therapies'). Then the media, whom the pharmaceutical companies support with lots of advertising money, proclaim that 'unproven' is not really different from 'disproven'. Therefore, they conclude, doctors who use unproven therapies are committing health fraud, and their licences to practice medicine should be revoked.

Heartening News

Happily, more and more doctors are adopting some of the nutritional techniques you have read about here. Millions more Britons and Americans are taking vitamins, and many have learned that they are able to replace their medications. Several medical centres have even set up departments of alternative medicine. But before you begin to celebrate, remember that the notion that vita-nutrient therapy can replace medication is generally frowned upon in hospitals. Strange, isn't it? The most science-based alternative modality is the only one considered unworthy. And despite the encouraging fact that some insurance carriers cover alternative medicine, their networks often do not have complementary doctors who treat with nutrients.

The Road to Change

If we want to challenge the drug industry's stranglehold and reap the medical benefits (for example, insurance coverage for the vita-nutrient treatments), we are going to have to fight for it. And that fight may very well take the shape of a grass-roots movement. However, a crusade like this takes many devoted participants to achieve its goals.

If you think the movement is worth your efforts, here are some suggestions. Talk up the issue with friends and family, or call in on talk radio. (Talk show hosts seem to like this mixture of self-help and controversy.) Give health suggestions to fellow employees. You may want to sound off on the Internet. But you can strike a real blow for the cause when you convince your doctor to use nutrition in his practice. Whenever you benefit from taking vita-nutrients, let your doctor know about it. A good way, of course, would be to get him interested in this book.

To be an effective grass-roots crusader, you may have to do some convincing and perhaps win some debates. The opposition is formidable and includes many in the medical establishment, both in the United States and in the United Kingdom. I have studied the position papers of many of the organizations that are opposed to the use of vita-nutrients; though the excerpts that follow happen to come from the American Dietetic Association, all groups use the same arguments. It is interesting to analyze the overall platform.

To begin with, the establishment organizations feel that 'the best nutritional strategy for optimal health is to obtain adequate nutrients from a wide variety of foods. Supplementation is not appropriate unless scientific evidence of safety and effectiveness is well-accepted.' In other words, they continue to reject all the scientific evidence I've shown you in which vita-nutrients have proven effective in dosages beyond those in a normal diet.

Knowing that the insider groups have all endorsed the same positions allows them to fall back on the term 'scientific agreement', which they recognize as the basis for the RDAs and which they insist should serve as the *maximum* dosage, should a person wish to take supplements. They also want 'scientific agreement' to determine what can be stated on your vitamin bottle label. My answer would be: 'Just how would one go about agreeing scientifically?' I presume it means having the agreement of scientists who cooperate with them. In any event, it most certainly does *not* mean 'scientifically performed research', because that is what they seem to be fighting against.

Then there is the universal endorsement of the food pyramid, which, as I've mentioned several times, makes white flour, a form of junk food and an antinutrient, a basic staple.

The position statements indicate a greater concern for the *risk* of taking vita-nutrients than with their value. Dietary counselling should be 'to prevent excessive intakes' and, of course, that supplements must not have 'adverse interactions with medical treatment'. I don't think we will hear mainstream medicine say in our lifetimes that medical treatment might have adverse effects on our nutrition.

I, my family, and tens of thousands of my patients have been taking vitamins, with great benefit, for decades – yet the organizations insist that even when dietary levels are low and no adverse effects have been discovered, 'long term nutrient consumption at levels found in usual diets cannot be assumed to be safe'. Their bias is reflected in their concern with 'nutrition misinformation', which they define as 'misinterpretation of nutrition science'. Of course, we are not told who the arbiters of these interpretations would be, but we do know that membership in this insider group has never been open to vita-nutrient enthusiasts. But the future may bring change; I expect a new group of leaders to emerge from the ranks of these organizations. It is my fervent hope that these words will help them see the fallacies in the positions their predecessors held and that the conflict will simply vanish.

No matter how the struggle will be resolved, I feel certain that we are going to convince a lot of people about the importance of nutritional medicine. The one pillar of certainty is that the vita-nutrient solution works.

The Never-Ending Solution

We are at the crest of an information explosion about vita-nutrients as treatments for illness. If this positive trend continues, the orthomolecular school of thought will be swept to the forefront of health care practice and policy. Hopefully this book will be part of that trend, by teaching doctors of the future to prescribe vita-nutrients before prescription drugs when treating their patients. I plan for this book to be a living, growing instrument, one that will serve not only to bring vita-nutrient therapy to the heart of modern medical practice, but to continue to show how you can best do it. I trust you see that these pages are chock full of cutting-edge information. I want that kind of information always to be readily available.

There are many ways to carry out my pledge to keep you current in this dynamic, exciting field. At present I publish a monthly newsletter, *Dr Atkins' Health Revelations;* I have a website (http://www.atkinscenter.com); and, if you are in America, I have a toll-free number for 'Dr Atkins'-branded vita-nutrient product information, 1-800-6-ATKINS. I have a nationally syndicated weekday radio programme as well. The most effective way to keep in touch will be the website; there you will learn of symposia, radio and TV appearances I'll be making, and ways to access new vita-nutrient information. I hope that each and every one of you will use one of these modalities to keep in contact with my staff. If you create the demand, I will appoint a task force to keep this book's bibliography updated.

In fact, this reference source, which currently is updated monthly and is considerably larger than the abridged version printed here, contains the titles of each paper so that the reader will know the scope of each study. I believe health care professionals and nutrition students will find it extremely useful. Ideally you will use these outlets to stay informed.

I also hope each of you show your doctors, by your very success, just how worthwhile vita-nutrient therapy is. Simply let them know what you've been doing, and don't feel intimidated if they don't seem receptive. Rejecting these cutting-edge ideas can only serve to weaken the doctor's ability to maintain patient loyalty. No health professional can afford to be so out of touch with the new reality. Finally, remember that one of complementary medicine's most exciting assets is how quickly it is progressing. I urge you not to miss out on the excitement.

My passion for the ideas I have set forth here does not allow me to say, 'I have made my statement; the book speaks for itself.' It allows me only to say, 'Let this book be the beginning of a dialogue.' Let this book be an event in which you and I are players, and let that event be the enactment of Hippocrates' prophetic dictum: 'Let food be your medicine.'

REFERENCES

◄O►

CHAPTER 3: VITAMINS

VITAMIN A

1. O'Keefe, J., et al., *Mayo Clinic Proceedings*, 1995; 70: 69–79.
2. Glaszia, P., et al., *British Medical Journal*, 1993; 306: 366–70.
3. Ozsoylu, S., *Journal of Pediatrics*, 1994; 125(6): 1017–18.
4. Velasquez-Melendez, G., et al., *European Journal of Clinical Nutrition*, 1995; 49(5): 379–84.
5. Jolly, P. E., et al., *AIDS*, 1996; 10(1): 114.
6. Semba, R. D., et al., *Journal of Infectious Diseases*, 1995; 171(5): 1196–202.
7. Dochao, A., et al., *Actas Dermo-sifiliograficas*, 1975; 66(3–4): 121–30.
8. Paiva, S. A. R., *American Journal of Clinical Nutrition*, 1996; 64: 928–34.
9. Aldoorli, W. L., et al., *American Journal of Epidemiology*, 1997; 145: 42–50.
10. Scheef, W., *Combined Tumor Therapy: Basic Possibilities and Related Adjuvant Therapeutic Methods*, 1995, Heinrich Wrba, ed.; Stuttgart: Hippocrates.
11. Pastorino, A., et al., *Journal of Clinical Oncology*, 1993; 11: 1216–22.
12. Hsing, Ann W., et al., *Journal of the National Cancer Institute*, 1990; 82(11): 941–46.
13. Kune, G. A., et al., *Nutrition and Cancer*, 1992; 18: 237–44.
14. Lithgow, D., and W. Politzer, *South African Medical Journal*, 1977; 51: 191–93.
15. Band, P., et al., *Preventive Medicine*, 1984; 13: 549–54.
16. Ghebremeskel, K., et al., *Early Human Development*, 1994; 39: 177–88.
17. Panth, M., et al., *International Journal of Vitamin and Nutrition Research*, 1991; 61: 17–19.
18. Mazzotta, M., *Journal of the American Podiatric Medical Association*, 1994; 84(9): 456–62.
19. Facchini, F., et al., *American Journal of Clinical Nutrition*, 1996; 63(6): 946–49.

CAROTENOIDS

1. Yeum, K., et al., *Journal of the American College of Nutrition*, 1995; 14: 536, Abstract 48.
2. Stahelin, H. B., *British Journal of Clinical Practice*, Dec. 1990; 44(11): 543–45.
3. Palan, P. R., et al., *American Journal of Obstetrics and Gynecology*, Dec. 1989; 161(6): 1649–52.
4. Dorgan, J. F., et al., *Hematology/Oncology Clinics of North America*, Feb. 1991; 5(1): 43–68.
5. Kritchevsky, D., *Cancer*, Sept. 15, 1990; 66(6): 1321–24.
6. Bankhead, C. D., *Medical World News*, Aug. 1991; 37.
7. Singh, V. N., and S. K. Gaby, *American Journal of Clinical Nutrition*, 1991; 53: 386S–390S.
8. Garewal, H., *American Journal of Clinical Nutrition*, 1995; 62S: 1510–16.
9. *Medical Tribune*, Nov. 29, 1990; 2.
10. Gester, H., *International Journal of Vitamin and Nutrition Research*, 1991; 61: 277–91.
11. Jialal, Z., *Circulation*, Oct. 1991; 84(4): 449.
12. Canfield, L. M., et al., *Proceedings in the Society of Experimental Biology and Medicine*, 1992; 200: 260–65.
13. Branowitz, S. A., et al., *AIDS*, 1996; 10: 115.
14. Omene, J. A., *Journal of National Medical Association*, 1996; 88: 789–93.
15. Jacques, P., et al., *American Journal of Clinical Nutrition*, 1991; 53: 352S–355S.
16. Watson, R. R., et al., *American Journal of Clinical Nutrition*, 1991; 53: 90–94. See also: Landrum, J., et al., *Advances in Pharmacology*, 1997; 38: 537–53.
17. Snodderly, D., *American Journal of Clinical Nutrition*, 1995; 62S: 1448–61.
18. Levy, J., et al., *Nutrition and Cancer*, 1995; 24: 257–66.
19. *Medical Tribune*, May 22, 1997; 32.
20. Giovanucci, E., et al., *Journal of the National Cancer Institute*, 1995; 87: 1767–76.

VITAMIN B$_1$

1. Nichols, H., et al., *Journal of the American College of Nutrition*, 1994; 10(1): 57–61.
2. Pfitzemeyer, P., *International Journal of Vitamin and Nutrition Research*, 1994; 64: 113–18.
3. Shimon, I., et al., *American Journal of Medicine*, 1995; 98: 485–90.
4. Harrell, R., *Effect of Added Thiamin on Learning*, 1973; New York: AMS Press.
5. Brotzman, G. L., *Journal of the American Board of Family Practice*, May–June 1992; 5(3): 323–25.
6. Benton, D., et al., *Psychopharmacology*, 1997; 129: 66–71.
7. Carney, M. W. P., *British Journal of Psychiatry*, 1990; 156: 878–82.

8. Nolan, K. A., et al., *Archives of Neurology,* Jan. 1991; 48: 81–83.
9. Frydl, V., et al., *Medwelt,* 1989; 40: 1484–86.
10. Quinn H., *Bibliotheca Nutritio et Dieta,* 1986: 38: 110–11.
11. Blakely, B. R., et al., *Journal of Applied Toxicology,* 1990; 10(2): 93–97.
12. Lonsdale, D., *A Nutritionist's Guide to the Clinical Use of Vitamin B_1,* 1987; Tacoma, Wash.: Life Sciences Press.

VITAMIN B_2

1. Weisburger, J. H., *American Journal of Clinical Nutrition,* 1991; 53: 226S–237S.
2. Eckhert, C., et al., *Experientia,* 1993; 49(12): 1084–87.
3. *Nutrition Reviews,* 51(5): 149–50.
4. Bell, I. R., et al., *Acta Psychiatrica Scandinavica,* 1992; 85: 360–63.
5. Shenkin, S. D., et al., *Clinical Nutrition,* 1989; 8: 269–71.
6. Shenkin, S. D., et al., *Clinical Nutrition,* 1989; 8: 269–71.

VITAMIN B_3

1. Luria, M. H., *Medical Hypothesis,* 1990; 32: 21–28.
2. Berge, K., and P. Canner, *European Journal of Clinical Pharmacology,* 1991; 40: S49–S51.
3. O'Keefe, J. H., *Mayo Clinic Proceedings,* 1995; 70: 69–79.
4. Martin-Jadraque, R., et al., *Archives of Internal Medicine,* 1996; 156: 1081–88.
5. Gibbons, L. W., et al., *American Journal of Medicine,* Oct. 1995; 99: 378–85.
6. Hoffer, A., and M. Walker, *Putting It All Together,* 1996; New Canaan, Conn.: Keats Publishing.
7. Aronov, A., et al., *Archives of Family Medicine,* 1996; 5: 567–75.
8. Chait, A., et al., *American Journal of Medicine,* 1993; 94: 350–56.
9. Holvoet, P., et al., *Circulation,* 1995; 92: 698–99.
10. Hoffer. A., and M. Walker, *Putting It All Together,* 1996; New Canaan, Conn.: Keats Publishing.
11. Jacobson, E., *Journal of the American College of Nutrition,* 1993; 12(4): 412–16.
12. Garg, A., et al., *Journal of the American Medical Association,* Aug. 8, 1990; 264(6): 723–26.
13. Rubin, R. A., *Cortlandt Forum,* March 1992; 124: 49–117.
14. Elliot, R., et al., *Annals of the New York Academy of Sciences,* 1993; 696: 333–41.
15. Pozzilli, P., et al., *Diabetologia,* 1995; 38: 848–52.
16. Murray, M., et al., *Biochemical and Biophysical Research Communications,* 1995; 210(3): 954–59.

VITAMIN B$_6$

1. Rogers, K., and C. Mohan, *Biochemical Medicine and Metabolic Biology,* 1994; 32: 10–17.
2. Selhub, J., *New England Journal of Medicine,* Feb. 2, 1995; 332: 286–91.
3. Robinson, K., et al., *Circulation,* 1995; 92(28): 25–30.
4. Chasen-Taber, L., et al., *Journal of the American College of Nutrition,* 1996; 15(2): 136–43.
5. Meydani, S. N., et al., *American Journal of Clinical Nutrition,* 1990; 53: 1275–80.
6. Vutyavanich, T., et al., *American Journal of Obstetrics and Gynecology,* 1995; 173: 881–84.
7. Galland, L. D., *1986: A Year in Nutritional Medicine,* 1986; New Canaan, Conn.: Keats Publishing, 10–12.
8. Smith, L. H., *American Journal of Kidney Diseases,* April 1991; 17(4): 370–75. See also: Ruml, L., *Urologic Clinics of North America,* Feb. 1997; 24: 117–33.
9. Baumeister, F., et al., *Pediatrics,* 1994; 94(3): 318–21. See also: Nakagawa, E., *Neurology,* 1997; 48: 1468–69.
10. Rimland, B., *Autism Research Review International,* 1996; 10(3): 3.
11. Riggs, K. M., et al., *American Journal of Clinical Nutrition,* 1996; 53: 306–14.
12. *Nutrition Report,* Oct. 1994; 12: 10, 75.
13. Ellis, J. M., *Vitamin B$_6$: The Doctors Report,* 1973; New York: Harper & Row.
14. Kremer, J., et al., *Journal of Rheumatology,* 1996; 23: 990–94.

FOLIC ACID

1. Super, M., *Lancet,* Sept. 21, 1991; 755–56.
2. The MRC Vitamin Study Research Group, *Lancet,* July 20, 1991; 338: 131–37.
3. Stampfer, M. J., et al., *New England Journal of Medicine,* 1995; 332: 328–29.
4. Verhoef, P., *American Journal of Epidemiology,* May 1996; 143(9): 845–59.
5. Boers, G. H. J., *Netherlands Journal of Medicine,* 1994; 45: 34–41.
6. Rodier, M., et al., *Diabetes and Metabolism,* 1993; 19: 560–65.
7. Cuskelly, G. J., et al., *Lancet,* March 9, 1996; 347: 657–59.
8. Maurer, K., *Family Practice News,* June 1, 1996; 20.
9. Joosten, E., *Journal of Gerontology: Medical Sciences,* 1997; 52(2): M76–M79.
10. Jancin, B., *Family Practice News,* March 1, 1996; 4.
11. Wouters, M. G. A. J., et al., *European Journal of Clinical Nutrition,* 1995; 25: 801–05.
12. Morgan, S. L., et al., *Arthritis and Rheumatism,* Jan. 1990; 33(1): 9–18.
13. Nehler, M. R., *Cardiovascular Pathology,* 1997; 6: 1–9.

14. Lennard, J. E., *Annals of the Royal Journal of England*, 1990; 72: 152–54.
15. Caruthers, L. G., *Lancet*, 1946; 1: 849.
16. Carney, M. W. P., et al., *Journal of Affective Disorders*, 1990; 9: 207–13.
17. Fava, M., *American Journal of Psychiatry*, 1997; 154: 426–28.
18. Crellin, R., et al., paper presented at the Annual Meeting of the Royal College of Psychiatrists, Dublin, July 24–27, 1992.
19. Butterworth, C. E., Jr., *Journal of the American College of Nutrition*, 1993; 12(4): 438–41.
20. Haile, R. W., et al., *Cancer Epidemiology, Biomarkers and Prevention*, 1995; 4: 709–14.
21. Flynn, M., et al., *Journal of the American College of Nutrition*, 1994; 13(4): 351–56.
22. Cuskelly, G., et al., *Lancet*, 1996; 347: 657–59.
23. Tucker, K., et al., *Journal of the American Medical Association*, 1996; 276: 1879–85.

VITAMIN B$_{12}$

1. Carmel, R., *Annals of Internal Medicine*, 1996; 124: 338–39.
2. Al-Momen, A. K., *Journal of Internal Medicine*, 1995; 231: 551–55.
3. Scarlett, J. D., et al., *American Journal of Hematology*, 1992; 39: 79–83.
4. Sumner, A., et al., *Annals of Internal Medicine*, 1996; 124: 469–75.
5. Salzman, J., et al., *Journal of the American College of Nutrition*, 1994; 13: 584–91.
6. Bell, I., *Nutrition Report*, 1991; 9: 1–8.
7. Narang, R., et al., *Trace Elements in Medicine*, 1992; 9: 43–44.
8. Herzlich, B. C., et al., *American Journal of Gastroenterology*, 1992; 87(12): 1781–88.
9. Kira, J., et al., *Internal Medicine*, 1994; 33: 82–86.
10. Ohta, T., et al., *Japanese Journal of Psychiatry and Neurology*, 1991; 45: 167–68.
11. Honma, K., et al., *Experientia*, 1992; 48: 716–20.
12. Caruselli, M., *Riforma Medica*, 1952; 66: 841–64.
13. Yaqub, B., et al., *Clinical Neurology and Neurosurgery*, 1992; 94: 105–11.
14. Fahey, J., et al., *New England Journal of Medicine*, 1990; 322: 166–72. See also: Tang, A., et al., *Journal of Nutrition*, 1997; 127: 345–51.
15. Shemesh, J. et al., *American Journal of Otolaryngology*, 1994; 14: 94–96.
16. Brodsky, J. B., *New England Journal of Medicine*, Jan. 28, 1993; 284–85.
17. Saito, M., et al., *Chest*, 1994; 106: 496–99.

CHOLINE AND LECITHIN

1. Growden, J., et al., *New England Journal of Medicine*, 1977; 297: 524–27.
2. Canty, D., *Nutrition Reviews*, 1994; 52(10): 327–39.
3. Sitaram, N., et al., *Science*, July 21, 1978; 201: 274–76.
4. Arsenio, L., *La Clinica Therapeutica*, 1985; 114: 117–27.
5. Sitaram, N., et al., *Science*, July 21, 1978; 201: 274–76.

6. Dodson, W., and D. Sachen, *American Journal of Clinical Nutrition*, 1996; 63: 904–10.
7. Cowen, R., *Science News*, 1990; 138: 340.
8. Canty, D., *Nutrition Reviews*, 1994; 52(10): 327–39.
9. Buchman, A. L., et al., *Hepatology*, 1995; 22(5): 1399–1403.

INOSITOL

1. Levine, J., et al., *American Journal of Psychiatry*, 1995; 152(5): 792–94.
2. Benjamin, J., et al., *Psychopharmacology Bulletin*, 1995; 31: 167–75.
3. Fux, M., et al., *American Journal of Psychiatry*, 1996; 153: 1219–21. For an excellent review, see also: Vadnal, R., et al., *CNS Drugs*, 1997; 7: 6–16.
4. Barak, Y., et al., *Progress in Neuropsychopharmacology and Biological Psychiatry*, 1996; 20: 729–35.
5. Salway, J., et al., *Lancet*, 1978; 2: 1282–84.
6. Hallman, M., et al., *New England Journal of Medicine*, May 7, 1992; 326(19): 1233–39.

PANTETHINE/PANTOTHENIC ACID

1. Gensini, G., et al., *International Journal of Clinical Pharmacology Research*, 1985; 5(5): 309–18.
2. Arsenio, L., et al., *Clinical Therapeutics*, 1986; 8(5): 537–45.
3. Coronel, F., *Nefrologia*, 1995; 15: 68–73.
4. Prisco, D., et al., *Angiology*, 1987; 38(3): 241–47.
5. Truss, C., *Journal of Orthomolecular Psychiatry*, 1984; 13: 66–93.
6. Ellestad-Sayed, J., et al., *American Journal of Clinical Nutrition*, 1976; 29: 333–38.
7. Davis, V., and M. Walsh, *Science*, 1970; 167: 1005–07.
8. Shimuzu, S., et al., *Chemistry and Pharmacology Bulletin*, 1965; 13: 2–4.
9. Leung, L., *Medical Hypotheses*, 1995; 44: 490–92.
10. Vaxman, F., et al., *European Surgical Research*, 1996; 28: 306–14.
11. Friedman, B., *Cortlandt Forum*, May 1990; 19–26.
12. Leung, L., *Medical Hypotheses*, 1995; 44: 403–05.

PABA

1. Zarafonetis, C., et al., *Journal of Clinical Epidemiology*, 1988; 193–204.
2. Zarafonetis, C., et al., *American Journal of Medical Sciences*, 1964; 550–61.
3. Sieve, B., *Virginia Medical Monthly*, 1945; 72: 6–17.
4. Hughes, C., *Journal of the American Academy of Dermatology*, 1983; 9: 770.
5. Sagone, A., et al., *Free Radicals in Biology and Medicine*, 1993; 14(1): 27–45.
6. Levine, M., et al., *Archives of Environmental Health*, 1972; 24: 243–47.

BIOTIN

1. Noda, H., et al., *Journal of Nutritional Sciences and Vitaminology,* 1994; 40: 181–88.
2. Maebashi, M., et al., *Journal of Clinical Biochemical Nutrition,* 1993; 14: 211–18.
3. Koutsikos, D., et al., *Biomedical Pharmacotherapy,* 1990; 44: 511–14.
4. Hochman, L., *Cutis,* 1993; 51: 303–37.

VITAMIN C

1. Levine, M., et al., *Annals of the New York Academy of Sciences,* 1987; 498: 424–44.
2. Levine, M., et al., *Annals of the New York Academy of Sciences,* 1987; 498: 424–44.
3. Levine, M., et al., *American Journal of Clinical Nutrition,* 1995; 62: 1347S–1356S.
4. Bendich, A., et al., *Journal of the American College of Nutrition,* 1995; 14(2): 124–36.
5. Bendich, A., *Food Technology,* 1987; 41: 112–14.
6. Levy, R., et al., *Journal of Infectious Disease,* 1996; 173: 1502–05.
7. Cathcart, R., *Medical Hypotheses,* 1984; 14: 423–33.
8. Klenner, F., *Journal of Applied Nutrition,* 1971; 23: 61–88.
9. Harakeh, S., et al., *Journal of Nutritional Medicine,* 1994; 4: 393–401.
10. Hunt, C., et al., *International Journal of Vitamin and Nutrition Research,* 1994; 64: 212–19.
11. Peters, E., *International Journal of Sports Medicine,* 1997; 18: 569–77.
12. Hemila, H., et al., *Journal of the American College of Nutrition,* 1995; 14: 116–23.
13. Johnston, C. S., et al., *Journal of the American Dietetic Association,* Aug. 1992; 92(8): 988–89.
14. Hatch, G., et al., *American Journal of Clinical Nutrition,* 1995; 61: 625S–630S.
15. Bucca, C., et al., *New York Academy of Sciences,* Feb. 9–12, 1992; 16.
16. McKinney, M., *Medical Tribune,* June 5, 1997; 6.
17. Henson, D. E., et al., *Journal of the National Cancer Institute,* April 17, 1991; 83(8): 547–50.
18. Cohen, M., et al., *Journal of the American College of Nutrition,* 1995; 14(6): 576–78.
19. Howe, G. R., et al., *Journal of the National Cancer Institute,* 1990; 82: 561–69.
20. Block, G., *Epidemiology,* 1992; 3(3): 189–91.
21. Cameron, E., et al., *Cancer Research,* 1979; 39: 663–81.
22. Cameron, E., and A. Campbell, *Chemical-Biological Interactions,* 1974; 9: 285–315.
23. Block, G., *American Journal of Clinical Nutrition,* 1991; 53(1): 270S–282S.
24. Manson, J., et al., *Circulation,* 1992; 85: 865.

25. Simon J. A., *Journal of the American College of Nutrition*, 1992; 11(2): 107–25.
26. Iswarlel, J., et al., *Atherosclerosis*, 1996; 119:139–50.
27. Kritchevsky, S. B., et al., *Circulation*, 1995; 92(8): 2142–50.
28. Hallfish, J., *American Journal of Clinical Nutrition*, 1994; 60: 100–05.
29. Levine, G. N., et al., *Circulation*, March 15, 1996; 93(6): 1107–13.
30. Rath, M., *Journal of Applied Nutrition*, 1996; 48: 22–33.
31. Tomoda, H., et al., *American Journal of Cardiology*, 1996; 1284–86.
32. Eriksson, J., *Annals of Nutrition and Metabolism*, 1995; 39: 217–23.
33. Feldman, E. B., *New York Academy of Sciences*, Feb. 9–12, 1992; 9.
34. Cohen, L., et al., *American Journal of Clinical Nutrition*, 1990; 18: 512.
35. Naylor, G., et al., *Nutrition and Health*, 1985; 4: 25–28.
36. Stein, H., et al., *Archives of Internal Medicine*, 1976; 84(4): 385–88.
37. Gustafsson, U., et al., *European Journal of Clinical Investigation*, 1997; 27: 387–91.
38. Lane, B., *Journal of the American College of Nutrition*, 1991; 10(5): 536.
39. Free, N., et al., *Journal of Orthomolecular Psychiatry*, 1978; 7: 264–70.

BIOFLAVONOIDS

1. *Lancet*, 1993; 341: 454–57.
2. Reidenberg, M. M., *Clinical Pharmacology and Therapeutics*, 1996; 59: 62–71.
3. Hertog, M., et al., *Lancet*, 1993; 342: 1007–11.
4. Hertog, M., et al., *Archives of Internal Medicine*, 1995; 155: 381–86.
5. Fischer, M., et al., *Carcinogenesis*, 1982; 3: 1243–45.
6. Singhal, R., et al., *Biochemical and Biophysical Research Communications*, 1995; 208(1): 425–31.
7. Agullo, G., et al., *Cancer Letters*, 1994; 87(1): 55–63.
8. *Brain Research*, 1994; 635: 1127–31.
9. Knekt, P., et al., *British Medical Journal*, 1996; 312: 478–81.

VITAMIN D

1. Haug, S., et al., *Journal of Infectious Disease*, 1994; 169: 889–92.
2. Bell, N. H., *Journal of Clinical Endocrinology and Metabolism*, 1995; 80(4): 1051.
3. Dawson-Hughes, B., et al., *Annals of Internal Medicine*, Oct. 1, 1991; 115(7): 505–12.
4. Fogh, K., et al., *Experimental Dermatology*, 1996; 5(1): 24–27.
5. Elwood, M., *New Zealand Medical Journal*, Dec. 8, 1993; 517–18.
6. Baynes, K., *Diabetologia*, 1997; 40: 344–47.
7. Ito, M., et al., *International Journal of Gynecology and Obstetrics*, 1994; 47(2): 115–20.
8. Gloth, F. M., et al., *Archives of Internal Medicine*, 1991; 151: 1662–64.
9. Lefkowitz, E., et al., *International Journal of Epidemiology*, 1994; 23(6): 1133–36.

10. Feldman, D., et al., *Advances in Experimental Medicine and Biology*, 1995; 375: 53–63.
11. Shabahang, M., et al., *Annals of Surgical Oncology*, 1996; 3(2): 144–49.

VITAMIN E

1. Losonczy, K., et al., *American Journal of Clinical Nutrition*, 1996; 64: 190–96.
2. Stephens, N., et al., *Lancet*, 1996; 347: 781–86.
3. Ghatak, A., et al., *International Journal of Cardiology*, 1996; 57: 119–27.
4. Steiner, M., et al., *American Journal of Clinical Nutrition*, 1995; 62: 1381S–1384S.
5. Salonen, J., et al., *British Medical Journal*, 1995; 311: 1124–27.
6. Jain, S. K., et al., *Journal of the American College of Nutrition*, 1996; 15: 458–61.
7. Wald, N., et al., *British Journal of Cancer*, 1984; 49: 321–24.
8. Knekt, P., et al., *American Journal of Clinical Nutrition*, 1991; 53: 283S–286S.
9. Gridley, G., et al., *American Journal of Epidemiology*, 1992; 135: 1083–92.
10. Hoshino, E., et al., *Journal of Parenteral and Enteral Nutrition*, May–June 1990; 14(3): 300–05.
11. Fahn, S., *Annals of Neurology*, 1992; 32: S128–S132.
12. Sano, M., *New England Journal of Medicine*, 1997; 336(17): 11–12.
13. Dow, L., et al., *American Journal of Respiratory Critical Care Medicine*, 1996; 154: 1401–04.
14. Kolarz, G., et al., *Akta Rheumatologica*, 1990; 15: 233–37.
15. Meydani, S., et al., *American Journal of Clinical Nutrition*, 1990; 52: 557–63.

TOCOTRIENOLS

1. Serbinova, E., et al., *Oxidative Damage and Repair*, 1991; 77–80.
2. Tomeo, A. C., et al., *Lipids*, 1995; 30(12): 1179–83.
3. Qureshi, A., et al., *American Journal of Clinical Nutrition*, 1991; 53(suppl. 4): 1021S–1026S.

VITAMIN K

1. Vermeer, C., et al., *Annual Review of Nutrition*, 1995; 15: 1–22.
2. Vermeer, C., et al., *Journal of Nutrition*, 1996; 126(suppl. 4): 1187S–1191S.
3. Kim, J. H., *Vitamins in Cancer Therapy*, 1995; 363–72.
4. Noto, V., et al., *Cancer*, 1989; 63: 901–06.
5. Merkel, R. L., *American Journal of Obstetrics and Gynecology*, 1952; 62(2): 416–18.
6. Hansen, M. U., et al., *Acta Neurologica Scandinavica*, 1992; 85: 39–43.
7. Krasinski, S. D., et al., *American Journal of Clinical Nutrition*, 1985; 41(3): 639–43.

Chapter 4: Minerals

CALCIUM

1. Reid, I. R., et al., *American Journal of Medical Sciences*, 1996; 312: 278–86.
2. Toss, G., *Journal of Internal Medicine*, 1992; 231: 181–86.
3. Strause, L., et al., *Journal of Nutrition*, July 1994; 124: 1060–64.
4. Osborne, C., et al., *Nutritional Review*, 1996; 54: 365–81. See also: Bucher, H. *Journal of the American Medical Association*, 1996; 275: 1016–22.
5. Schardt, D., *Nutrition Action Health Letters*, 1993; 20(5): 5–7.
6. Sanchez-Ramos, L., et al., *Obstetrics and Gynecology*, June 1995; 85(6): 915–18.
7. Bacquer, D., et al., *Atherosclerosis*, 1994; 108: 193–200.
8. Arbman, G., et al., *Cancer*, April 15, 1992; 69(8): 2042–48.
9. Garland, C. F., et al., *American Journal of Clinical Nutrition*, 1991; 54: 193S–201S.

MAGNESIUM

1. Smetena, R., et al., *Magnesium Bulletin*, 1991; 13(4): 125–27.
2. Keller, P. K., and R. S. Aronson, *Progress in Cardiovascular Diseases*, May–June 1990; 32(6): 433–48.
3. Sanjuliani, A., *International Journal of Cardiology*, 1996; 56: 177–83.
4. Seelig, M. S., *American Journal of Cardiology*, 1991; 1221–22.
5. Ravn, H., *Thrombosis and Hemostasis*, 1996; 76: 88–93.
6. Rabbani, L., et al., *Clinical Cardiology*, 1996; 79: 841–44.
7. Seelig, M., *American Heart Journal*, 1996; 132, Part 2: 471–77. See also: Shechter, M., *Coronary Artery Disease*, 1996; 7: 352–58.
8. Seelig, M., *American Heart Journal*, 1996; 76: 88–93.
9. Tosiello, L., *Archives of Internal Medicine*, June 10, 1996; 156: 1143–48.
10. Kisters, K., et al., *Trace Elements and Electrolytes*, 1995; 12(4): 169–72.
11. Wirell, M., et al., *Journal of Internal Medicine*, Aug. 1994; 236: 189–95.
12. Zarcone, R., et al., *Panminerva Medica*, Dec. 1994; 36(4): 168–70.
13. Abu-Osba, Y. K., et al., *Archives of Disease in Children*, 1992; 67: 31–35.
14. Skobeloff, E., *Journal of the American Medical Association*, 1989; 262: 1210–13.
15. Mauskop, A., et al., *Clinical Science*, 1995; 89: 633–36.
16. Abraham, G., et al., *Journal of Nutritional Medicine*, 1991; 3: 49–58.
17. Yasui, M., et al., eds., *Mineral and Metal Neurotoxicology*, 1997; Boca Raton, Fla.: CRC Press, 22: 217–26.
18. Abraham, G., et al., *Journal of Nutritional Medicine*, 1991; 2: 165–78.
19. Tanimura, A., et al., *Experimental Pathology*, 1986; 2(4): 261–73.
20. Boschert, S., *Family Practice News*, March 1, 1996; 33.

POTASSIUM

1. Hoes, A., et al., *Drugs*, 1994; 47(5): 711–33.

2. Bourke, E., et al., *Heart Disease and Stroke,* March–April 1994; 2: 63–67.
3. Nordrehaug, J., et al., *Circulation,* 1985; 71(4): 645–49.
4. Horowitz, N., *Medical Tribune,* Aug. 17, 1989; 6.
5. Brancati, F., et al., *Archives of Internal Medicine,* 1996; 156(1): 61–67.
6. Krishna, G. G., et al., *Annals of Internal Medicine,* 1991; 115(2): 77–83.
7. Geleijnse, J. M., et al., *British Medical Journal,* 1994; 309: 436–40.
8. Whelton, P. K., et al., *Annals of Epidemiology,* 1995; 5: 85–95.
9. Whelton, P., et al., *Journal of the American Medical Association,* 1997; 277: 1624–32.
10. Shaw, D., et al., *American Journal of Medical Sciences,* 1962; 243: 758–69.
11. Smith, B. L., *Journal of Applied Nutrition,* 1993; 45(1): 35–39.

IRON

1. Beard, J. L., et al., *American Journal of Clinical Nutrition,* 1990; 52: 813–19.
2. Bruner, A., et al., *Lancet,* 1996; 348: 992–96.
3. Vreugdenhil, G., *Annals of Rheumatic Diseases,* 1990; 49: 93–98.
4. Salonen, J., et al., *Circulation,* 1992; 86: 803–11.
5. Reizenstein, P., *Medical Oncology and Tumor Pharmacology,* 190; 7(1): 1–2.
6. Youdim, M. B. H., *Acta Neurologica Scandinavica,* 1989; 126: 47–54.
7. Cutler, P., *American Journal of Geriatrics,* Jan. 1991; 148: 147–48.
8. Corti, M. C., et al., *American Journal of Cardiology,* 1997; 79: 120–27.
9. Sweeten, M. K., et al., *Journal of Food Quality,* 9: 263–75.
10. *Geriatric Consultant,* March–April 1990; 6.
11. Lauffer, R., *American Heart Journal,* June 1990; 199(6): 1448.

ZINC

1. McClain, C. J., *Journal of the American College of Nutrition,* 1990; 9(5): 545.
2. Wood, R., et al., *American Journal of Clinical Nutrition,* 1997; 65: 1803–09.
3. Heimburger, D. C., et al., *American Journal of Medicine,* Jan. 1990; 88: 71–73.
4. Godfrey, J. C., et al., *Journal of International Medical Research,* June 1992; 20(3): 234–46.
5. Mossad, S. B., et al., *Annals of Internal Medicine,* 1996; 125(2): 81–88.
6. Mochegiani, E., *International Journal of Immunopharmacology,* 1995; 7: 719–27.
7. Melichar, B., et al., *Clinical Investigations,* 1994; 72: 101–04.
8. Harden, J. W., *International Journal of Immunopharmacology,* 1995; 17: 697–701.
9. Chandra, R. K., et al., *Nutrition,* 1994; 10.
10. Honnorat, J., et al., *Biological Trace Element Research,* 1992; 32: 311–16.
11. Faure, P., et al., *Biological Trace Element Research,* 1992; 32: 305–10.
12. Winterberg, B., et al., *Trace Elements in Medicine,* 1989; 6(4): 173–77.

13. Dreno, B., et al., *Acta Dermato-venereologica*, 1992; 72: 250–52.
14. Prasad, A. S., et al., *Nutrition*, 1996; 12: 344–48.
15. Goldenberg, R., et al., *Journal of the American Medical Association*, 1995; 274: 463–68.
16. Favier, A., *Biological Trace Element Research*, 1992; 32: 363–82.
17. Lansdown, A., et al., *Lancet*, 1996; 347: 706–07.
18. Rogers, S. A., et al., *International Clinical and Nutrition Review*, 1990; 10: 253–58.
19. Sturniolo, G. C., et al., *Journal of the American College of Nutrition*, 1991; 4: 372–75.
20. Birmingham, C., et al., *International Journal of Eating Disorders*, 1994; 15.
21. *Nutrition Reviews*, July 1990; 40(7): 286–87.
22. Christen, W. G., et al., *Annals of Epidemiology*, 1996; 6: 60–66.
23. Sazawal, S., et al., *New England Journal of Medicine*, 1995; 333: 839–44. See also: Ruel, M., et al., *Pediatrics*, 1997; 99: 808–13.
24. Rogers, S., *International Clinical and Nutrition Review*, 1990; 10: 253–58.
25. Taneja, S. K., et al., *Experientia*, 1996; 52: 31–33.

COPPER

1. Olivares, M., et al., *American Journal of Clinical Nutrition*, 1996; 63: 791S–796S.
2. Payar, L., *Medical Tribune*, Oct. 18, 1990; 14.
3. Medieros, D. M., *Nutrition Report*, 1993; 89: 96.
4. Klevay, L. J., *Trace Elements and Electrolytes in Health and Disease*, 1993, 7(2): 63–69.
5. Salonen, J., et al., *American Journal of Epidemiology*, 1991; 134: 268–76.
6. Reunanen, A., et al., *European Journal of Clinical Nutrition*, 1996; 50: 431–37.
7. Conlan, D., et al., *Age and Aging*, 1990; 19: 212–14.
8. Sorenson, J., in *Progress in Medicinal Chemistry*, 1989, Ellis and West, eds.; New York: Elsevier, 26.
9. Vaughn, V. J., et al., *Mycopathologica*, 1978; 64(1): 39–42.
10. Kelley, D. S., *American Journal of Clinical Nutrition*, 1995; 62: 412–16.
11. Gahlot, D. K., and K. S. Ratnakar, *Indian Journal of Ophthalmology*, 1981; 29(4): 351–53.
12. Brophy, M., et al., *Clinical Chimica Acta*, 1985; 145: 107–12.
13. Yenisey, C., *Biochemical Society Transactions*, 1996; 24: 321S.
14. Rosas, R., *Revista Investigacion Clinica*, 1995; 47: 447–52.

MANGANESE

1. Rubenstein, A. H., et al., *Nature*, 1962; 194: 188–89.
2. Zidenberg-Cherr, S. K., et al., *Trace Elements, Micronutrients and Free Radicals*, 1992, I. E. Dreosti, ed.; Totowa, N.J.: Humana Press, 107–27.

3. Masonari, T. Y. Y., *Free Radical Biology and Medicine*, 1992; 13: 115–20.
4. Mangus, O., et al., *Archives of Andrology*, 1990; 24: 159–66.
5. Carl, G. F., et al., *Neurology*, 1988; 36: 1584.
6. Campbell, M. J., et al., *Journal of Allergy and Clinical Immunology*, 1991; 89.

IODINE

1. Xue-Yi, C., et al., *New England Journal of Medicine*, 1994; 331(26): 1739–44.
2. Tiwari, B., et al., *American Journal of Clinical Nutrition*, 1996; 63(5): 782–86.
3. Tomlinson, R., *British Medical Journal*, 1995; 310(6973): 148.
4. Edward, J., *Manitoba Medical Review*, 1954; 34(6): 337–39.
5. Ghent, W., et al., *Canadian Journal of Surgery*, 1993; 36: 453–60.
6. Ghent, W., and B. Eskin, *Proceedings of the Annual Meeting of the American Association of Cancer Research*, 1986; 27: 189.
7. Wright, J., *International Clinical Nutrition Reviews*, 1991; 11(3): 144–45.

CHROMIUM

1. Anderson, R., *Biological Trace Element Research*, 1992; 32: 19–24.
2. Anderson, R., *American Diabetes Association 56th Scientific Session*, June 9, 1996; San Francisco.
3. Anderson, R., et al., *Diabetes*, 1996; 45(supp. 2): 124A/454.
4. Evans, G. W., *Nutrition Report*, Oct.–Nov. 1989; 7(10–11): 73, 81.
5. Bahadori, B., et al., *International Journal of Obesity*, 1995; 19: 38.
6. Hallmark, M., et al., *Medicine and Science in Sports and Exercise*, 1993; 25: S101.
7. Lefavi, R., et al., *Nutrition Report*, July 1991; 53.
8. Evans, G., et al., *FASEB Journal*, 1995; 9: 525.

VANADIUM

1. Brichard, S., et al., *Trends in Pharmacological Sciences*, 1995; 16(8): 265–70.
2. Harland, B., et al., *Journal of the American Dietetic Association*, 1994; 94(8): 891–94.
3. Meyerovitch, J., et al., *Biological Chemistry*, 1987; 262: 6658–62.
4. Heyliger, C., et al., *Science*, 1985; 227: 757–59.
5. Orvig, C., et al., *Metabolic Ions in Biological Systems*, 1995; 31: 575–94.
6. Boden, G., et al., *Metabolism*, 1996; 45(9): 1130–35.
7. Yuen, V., et al., *Canadian Journal of Physiology and Pharmacology*, 1995; 73: 55–64.
8. Cohen, N., et al., *Journal of Clinical Investigation*, 1995; 95(6): 2501–09.
9. Halberstam, M., et al., *Diabetes*, 1996; 45(5): 659–66.

10. McNeill, J., et al., *Journal of Medicinal Chemistry*, 1992; 35(8): 1489–91.
11. Cohen, N., et al., *Journal of Clinical Investigation*, 1995; 95(6): 2501–09.

SELENIUM

1. Look, M., *Biological Trace Element Research*, 1997; 56: 31–41.
2. Schrauzer, G., et al., *Chemical and Biological Interactions*, 1994; 19: 199–205.
3. *Nature Medicine*, 1995; 1: 433–36.
4. For a recent review, see: Rayman, M., *British Medical Journal*, 1997; 314: 387–88.
5. Oster, O., and W. Prellwitz, *Biological Trace Elements*, 1990; 24: 91–103.
6. Zbigneiw, B., et al., *International Journal of Immunopathology and Pharmacology*, 1992; 5(1): 13–21.
7. Clark, L. C., et al., *Journal of the American Medical Association*, Dec. 25, 1996; 276(24): 1957–63.
8. Suadicani, P., et al., *Atherosclerosis*, 1992; 96: 33–44.
9. Neve, J., *Experientia*, 1991; 47: 187–93.
10. Lehr, D., *Journal of the American College of Nutrition*, 1994; 13(5): 496–98.
11. Hampel, G., et al., *Biochemica et Biophysica Acta*, 1989; 1006: 151–58.
12. Oster, O., et al., *Biological Trace Elements*, 1990; 24: 91–103.
13. Peretz, A. M., et al., *Seminars in Arthritis and Rheumatism*, April 1991; 20(5): 305–16.
14. Jameson, S., et al., *Nutrition Research*, 1985; 1: 391–97.
15. O'Dell, J. R., et al., *Annals of Rheumatic Diseases*, 1991; 50: 376–78.
16. Flatt, A., et al., *Thorax*, 1990; 45: 95–99.
17. Broglund, E., et al., *British Journal of Dermatology*, 1987; 117(5): 665–66.
18. Berry, M. J., et al., *Endocrine Reviews*, 1992; 13(2): 207–20.
19. Olivieri, O., et al., *Clinical Sciences*, 1995; 89(6): 637–42.
20. Hu, Y., *Biological Trace Element Research*, 1997; 56: 331–42.
21. Mai, J., et al., *Biological Trace Element Research*, 1990; 24: 109–17.
22. Guvenc, H., et al., *Pediatrics*, 1995; 95(6): 879–82.
23. Fitzherbert, J. C., *New Zealand Medical Journal*, July 24, 1991; 321.
24. Kuklinski, B., et al., *Zeitschrift für die Gesamte innere Medizen*, 1991; 46: S1–S52.

MOLYBDENUM

1. Wright, L., et al., *International Clinical Nutrition Review*, 1989; 9: 118–19.
2. Moss, M., *Journal of Nutritional and Environmental Medicine*, 1995; 5(1): 55–61.
3. Wright, L., et al., *International Clinical Nutrition Review*, 1989; 9: 118–19.
4. Slot, H., et al., *Neuropediatrics*, 1993; 24(3): 139–42.
5. Nakadaira, H., et al., *Archives of Environmental Health*, 1995; 50(5): 374–80.
6. Turnland, J., et al., *American Journal of Clinical Nutrition*, 1995; 62: 790–96.

BORON

1. Travers, R. L., et al., *Journal of Nutritional Medicine,* 1990; 1: 127–32.
2. Kidd, P. M., *Townsend Letter for Doctors,* May 1992; 400–05.
3. Hunt, C., et al., *American Journal of Clinical Nutrition,* 1997; 65: 803–13.
4. Ferrando, A., and N. Green, *FASEB Journal,* 1992; 6(4): A1945.
5. Naghii, M., and S. Samman, *Biological Trace Element Research,* 1997; 56: 273–86.
6. Travers, R. L., et al., *Journal of Nutritional Medicine,* 1990; 1: 237–32.
7. Penland, J., *Environmental Health Perspectives,* 1994; 7: 102.

SILICON

1. Seaborn, C. D., et al., *Nutrition Today,* July–Aug. 1993; 13–18.
2. Calomme, M., et al., *Biological Trace Element Research,* 1997; 56. 153–65.
3. Moukaizel, A., et al., *Journal of the American College of Nutrition,* 1992; 11(5): 601.
4. Nielsen, F., *FASEB Journal,* 1991; 5: 2661.
5. Schwartz, K., et al., *Lancet,* 1977; 1: 538.
6. Jacquin-Gadda, H., *Epidemiology,* 1996; 7: 281–85.

GERMANIUM

1. Asai, K., *Miracle Cure: Organic Germanium,* 1980; Tokyo: Japan Publications, Inc.
2. Kidd, P., *International Clinical Nutrition Review,* 1987; 7(1): 11–19.
3. Goodman, S., *Medical Hypotheses,* 1988; 26(3): 207–15.
4. Schauss, A., *Renal Failure,* 1991; 13(1): 1–4.
5. Hess, B., et al., *American Journal of Kidney Diseases,* 1993; 21(5): 548–52.

CHAPTER 5: AMINO ACIDS

ARGININE

1. Snyder, S., et al., *Scientific American,* 1992; 266(5): 68–77.
2. Drexler, H., et al., *Lancet,* 1991; 1546–50.
3. Wolf, A., et al., *Journal of the American College of Cardiology,* 1997; 29: 479–85.
4. Loscalzo, J., *New England Journal of Medicine,* 1995; 333(4): 251–53.
5. Clarkson, P., et al., *Journal of Clinical Investigation,* April 1996; 97(8): 1989–94.
6. Koifman, B., et al., *Journal of the American College of Cardiology,* Nov. 1, 1995; 26(5): 1251–56.
7. Egashira, K., et al., *Circulation,* July 15, 1996; 94(2): 130–34. See also: Tousoulis, D., *Lancet,* 1997; 349: 1812–13.

8. Korbonits, M., et al., *European Journal of Endocrinology*, 1996; 135: 543–47.
9. Hurson, M., et al., *Journal of Parenteral and Enteral Nutrition*, 1995; 19(3): 227–30.
10. Park, K., *Lancet*, 1991; 337: 645–46.
11. Azzara, A., et al., *Drugs in Experimental and Clinical Research*, 1995; 21(2): 71–78.
12. Green, S., *Nature Medicine*, 1995; 1(6): 515–17.
13. Brittenden, J., et al., *Surgery*, 1994; 115: 205–12.
14. *International Journal of Impotence Research*, 1994; 6: 33–36.
15. Aydin, S., et al., *International Urology and Nephrology*, 1995; 27(2): 199–202.
16. Steed, D., et al., *Diabetes Care*, 1995; 18(1): 39–46.
17. Cestaro, B., *Acta Neurologica Scandinavica*, 1994; 154: 32–41.
18. Visser, J., et al., *Medical Hypotheses*, 1994; 43(5): 339–42.
19. Visek, W., *Journal of Nutrition*, 1985; 115: 532–41.

GLUTAMINE

1. Shabert, J., *The Ultimate Nutrient: Glutamine*, 1994; Garden City Park, N.Y.: Avery.
2. Shive, W., et al., *Texas State Journal of Medicine*, 1957; 53: 840–43.
3. Skubitz, K., et al., *Journal of Laboratory and Clinical Medicine*, 1996; 127(2): 223–38.
4. Jensen, G. L., et al., *American Journal of Clinical Nutrition*, 1996; 64: 615–21.
5. MacBurney, M., et al., *Journal of the American Dietetic Association*, 1994; 94: 1263–66.
6. Goldin, E., et al., *Scandinavian Journal of Gastroenterology*, 1996; 31: 345–48.
7. Klimberg, V., et al., *Journal of Parenteral and Enteral Nutrition*, 1992; 16(6): 83S–87S.
8. Parry-Billings, M., et al., *Lancet*, 1990; 336: 523–25.
9. Greig, J., et al., *Medical Journal of Australia*, 1995; 163(7): 385, 388.
10. Ziegler, T., et al., *Annals of Internal Medicine*, 1992; 116: 821–28.
11. Teran, J. C., et al., *American Journal of Clinical Nutrition*, 1995; 62: 897–900.
12. Rogers, L., and R. Pelton, *Quarterly Journal of Studies of Alcohol*, 1957; 18(4): 581–87.
13. Goodwin, F., *APA Psychiatric News*, Dec. 5, 1986.
14. Nurjhan, N., et al., *Journal of Clinical Investigation*, 1995; 95(1): 272–77.
15. Curthoys, N., et al., *Annual Review of Nutrition*, 1995; 15: 133–59.
16. Keast, D., et al., *Medical Journal of Australia*, 1995; 162(1): 15–18.
17. Varnier, M., et al., *American Journal of Physiology*, 1995; 269: E309–E315.

LYSINE

1. Hurrell, R., et al., *British Journal of Nutrition,* 1977; 38: 285–97.
2. Furst, P., *Nutrition,* 1993; 9(1): 71–72.
3. Griffith, R., et al., *Chemotherapy,* 1981; 27: 209–13.
4. Azzara, A., et al., *Drugs in Experimental and Clinical Research,* 1995; 21(2): 71–78.
5. Rath, M., *Journal of Applied Nutrition,* 1996; 48: 22–33.
6. Schmeisser, D., et al., *Journal of Nutrition,* 1983; 113(9): 1777–83.
7. Flodin, N., *Journal of the American College of Nutrition,* 1997; 16: 7–21.

PHENYLALANINE

1. Spetz, H., et al., *Biological Psychiatry,* 1975; 10: 235.
2. Braverman, E. R., with C. C. Pfeiffer, *The Healing Nutrients Within,* 1987; New Canaan, Conn.: Keats Publishing, 37–39.
3. Kravitz, H., et al., *Journal of the American Osteopathic Association,* 1984; 84: 119.
4. Budd, K., *Advances in Pain Research and Therapy,* 1983; 5: 305.
5. Walsh, N., et al., *Archives of Physical Medicine and Rehabilitation,* 1986; 67: 436.
6. Siddiqui, A., et al., *Dermatology,* 1994; 188(3): 215–18.
7. Antoniou, C., et al., *International Journal of Dermatology,* 1989; 28(8): 545–47.
8. Winter, A., *Journal of Neurological and Orthopedic Medicine and Surgery,* 1984; 5: 1.
9. Heller, B., et al., *Arzneim-Forschstellung,* 1976; 26: 577.

TYROSINE

1. Braverman, E. R., with C. C. Pfeiffer, *The Healing Nutrients Within,* 1987; New Canaan, Conn.: Keats Publishing, 44–45.
2. Reimherr, D., et al., *American Journal of Psychiatry,* 1987; 144: 1071–73.
3. Nutt, J., et al., in *Therapy of Parkinson's Disease,* 1990, W. C. Koller and G. W. Paulson, eds.; New York: Marcel Dekker, chap. 28.
4. Tennant, F., *Postgraduate Medicine,* 1988; 84: 225–35.
5. Nutt, J., et al., in *Therapy of Parkinson's Disease,* 1990, W. C. Koller and G. W. Paulson, eds.; New York: Marcel Dekker, chap. 28.

GABA

1. Petty, F., et al., *Biological Psychiatry,* 1995; 38(9): 578–91.
2. Petty, F., et al., *Biological Psychiatry,* 1995; 38(9): 578–91.
3. Halbreich, U., et al., *American Journal of Psychiatry,* May 1996; 153(5): 718–20.

4. Braverman, E. R., with C. C. Pfeiffer, *The Healing Nutrients Within,* 1987; New Canaan, Conn.: Keats Publishing, 417.
5. Braverman, E. R., with C. C. Pfeiffer, *The Healing Nutrients Within,* 1987; New Canaan, Conn.: Keats Publishing, 198–200.
6. Gillis, R., et al., *Federal Proceedings,* 1984; 43(1): 32–38.
7. DeFeudis, F., *Experientia,* 1983; 39: 845–49.

METHIONINE

1. Mato, J., et al., *The Liver: Biology and Pathobiology,* 1994; 27: 461–69.
2. Kagan, B., et al., *American Journal of Psychiatry,* 1990; 147(5): 591–95.
3. Criconia, A., et al., *Current Therapeutic Research,* 1994; 55(6): 666–74.
4. Di Padova, C., et al., *American Journal of Gastroenterology,* 1984; 79: 941–44.
5. Schenker, S., et al., *Seminars in Liver Disease,* 1993; 13(2): 196–207.
6. Plasencia, A. M. Caballero, et al., *Drug Investigation,* 1991; 3(5): 333–35.
7. Di Padova, C., *American Journal of Medicine,* 1987; 83(5A): 60–65.
8. Meininger, V., et al., *Revue Neurologique,* 1982; 138(4): 297–303.
9. Carrieri, P., et al., *Current Therapeutic Research,* 1990; 48(1): 154–59.
10. Surtees, R., et al., *Lancet,* Dec. 21–28, 1991; 338: 1550–54.
11. Grassetto, M., and A. Varotto, *Current Therapeutic Research,* 1994; 55(7): 797–806.
12. Eaton, K. K., and A. Hunnisett, *Journal of Nutritional Medicine,* 1991; 2: 369–75.

GLUTATHIONE, N-ACETYL CYSTEINE

1. Wrigley, E., *British Journal of Cancer,* 1996; 73(6): 763–69.
2. Julius, M., *Journal of Clinical Epidemiology,* 1994; 47(9): 1021–26.
3. Vallis, K., *Lancet,* 1991; 337: 918–19.
4. *Lancet,* March 15, 1997; 349: 781.
5. Martin, D., et al., *Journal of the American Board of Family Practice,* 1990; 3: 293–96.
6. Harrison, P., *Lancet,* 1990; 335: 1572–73.
7. Stalenhoef, A., et al., *Lancet,* 1991; 337: 491.
8. Ardissino, D., et al., *Journal of the American College of Cardiology,* 1997; 29: 941–47.
9. Chirkov, Y. Y., et al., *Journal of Cardiovascular Pharmacology,* 1996; 28: 375–80.
10. Millman, M., et al., *Annals of Allergy,* 1985; 54(4): 294–96.
11. Meyer, A., *European Respiratory Journal,* 1994; 7: 431–36.
12. Bernard, G., *Chest,* 1997; 112: 164–72.
13. Ruan, E., et al., *Nutrition Research,* 1997; 17: 463–73.

TAURINE

1. Trachtman, H., et al., *Amino Acids*, 1996; 11: 1–13.
2. Azuma, J., et al., *Japanese Circulation Journal*, 1992; 56(1): 95–99.
3. Chapman, R. A., et al., *Cardiovascular Research*, 1993; 27: 358–63.
4. Franconi, F., et al., *American Journal of Clinical Nutrition*, 1995; 61: 1115–19.
5. Lombardini, J. B., *Brain Research Reviews*, 1991; 16: 151–69.
6. Gerster, H., *Age and Aging*, 1991; 20: 60.
7. Franconi, F., et al., *American Journal of Clinical Nutrition*, 1995; 61: 1115–19.
8. Smith, L. J., et al., *American Journal of Diseases in Children*, 1991; 145: 1401–04.
9. Huxtable, R., and D. V. Michalk, *Taurine in Health and Disease*, 1994; New York: Plenum Press, 31–39.
10. Huxtable, R., and D. V. Michalk, *Taurine in Health and Disease*, 1994; New York: Plenum Press, 413–17.

VALINE, LEUCINE, ISOLEUCINE

1. Grant, J., *Annals of Surgery*, 1994; 220: 610–16.
2. Louard, R. J., et al., *Metabolism*, April 1995; 44(4): 424–29.

HISTIDINE

1. Gerber, D., *Arthritis and Rheumatism*, 1969; 12: 295.
2. Cai, Q., et al., *Journal of Cardiovascular Pharmacology*, 1995; 25: 147–55.
3. Braverman, E. R., with C. C. Pfeiffer, *The Healing Nutrients Within*, 1987; New Canaan, Conn.: Keats Publishing, 314–22.

TRYPTOPHAN

1. Jaffe, R., *Journal of Nutritional Medicine*, 1994; 4: 133–39.
2. Sullivan, E., et al., *Archives of Internal Medicine*, 1996; 156(9): 973–99.
3. Menkes, D. B., et al., *Journal of Affective Disorders*, 1994; 32: 37–44.
4. Cleare, A. J., *Archives of General Psychiatry*, 1994; 51: 1004–05.
5. Pilar, S., *Journal of Psychiatry and Neuroscience*, 1994; 19(2): 114–19.
6. Lam, R., et al., *Canadian Journal of Psychiatry*, 1997; 42: 303–06.
7. Weltzin, T., et al., *American Journal of Psychiatry*, 1995; 152(11): 1668–71.
8. Farren, C., and T. Dinan, *Acta Psychiatrica Scandinavica*, 1996; 50: 457–61.
9. Sandyk, R., *International Journal of Science*, 1992; 67: 127–44.
10. Sharma, R., *Neuropsychobiology*, 1997; 35: 5–10.
11. Werbach, M., *Journal of the American College of Nutrition*, 1989; 15: 539 /A95.
12. Hartmann, E., et al., *Journal of Nervous and Mental Disease*, 1979; 167(8).
13. Newsholme, E. A., et al., *Experientia*, 1996; 52: 413–15.

CARNITINE

1. Singh, R. B., et al., *Postgraduate Medical Journal,* 1995; 71.
2. Reitz, V., et al., *American Journal of Cardiology,* March 1990; 755–60.
3. Reitz, V., et al., *American Journal of Cardiology,* March 1990; 755–60.
4. Kobayashi, A., et al., *Japanese Circulation Journal,* Jan. 1992; 56: 86–94.
5. Cerretelli, P., et al., *International Journal of Sports Medicine,* 1990; 11: 1–4.
6. Giamberardino, M. A., *International Journal of Sports Medicine,* 1996; 17: 320–24.
7. Swart, I., *Nutrition Research,* 1997; 17: 405–14.
8. Cederblad, G., et al., *Scandinavian Journal of Clinical Laboratory Investigation,* 1976; 36: 547–52.
9. Rebouche, C. J., et al., *Biochimica et Biophysica Acta,* 1980; 106: 295–300.
10. Chapoy, P. R., et al., *New England Journal of Medicine,* 1980; 303: 1389–94.
11. Rebouche, C. J., et al., *Annual Review of Nutrition,* 1986; 6: 41–66.
12. Arduini, A., *American Heart Journal,* June 1992; 123(6): 1726–27.

ACETYL L-CARNITINE

1. Patti, F., et al., *Clinical Trials Journal,* 1988; 25(supp. 1): 87–101.
2. Pettegrew, J. W., et al., *Neurobiology of Aging,* 1995; 16(1): 1–4.
3. Spagnoli, A., et al., *Neurology,* Nov. 1991; 41: 1726–32.
4. Salvioli, G., *Drugs in Experimental Clinical Research,* 1994; 20: 169–76.
5. Bodis-Wollner, I., et al., *Journal of Neural Transmission,* 1991; 3: 63–72.
6. Kuratsune, H., et al., *Clinical Infectious Diseases,* 1994; 18(suppl. 1): S62–S67.
7. Jirillo, E., et al., *Immunopharmacology and Immunotoxicology,* 1991; 13(1–2): 135–46.

CHAPTER 6: FATTY ACIDS

ESSENTIAL FATS

1. Willett, W., et al., *Lancet,* 1993; 341(8845): 581–85.
2. Katan, M., et al., *Annual Review of Nutrition,* 1995; 15: 473–93.
3. Hodgoson, J., et al., *Atherosclerosis,* 1996; 120(1–2): 147–54.
4. Jenkins, D., *Canadian Journal of Cardiology,* 1995; 11: 118G–122G.
5. Kummorow, F., *Journal of the American College of Nutrition,* 1993; 12: 12–13.

THE OMEGA-3S

1. Dyerberg, J., et al., *American Journal of Clinical Nutrition,* 1975; 28: 958–66.

2. Dyerberg, J., *World Review of Nutrition and Dietetics,* 1994; 76: 133–36.
3. Kromhout, D., et al., *New England Journal of Medicine,* 1985; 312: 1205–09.
4. Siscovick, D., et al., *Journal of the American Medical Association,* 1995; 274: 1363–67.
5. Burr, M., et al., *Lancet,* 1989; 2: 756–61.
6. Berg, E., and J. Dyerberg, *Drugs,* 1994; 47: 405–24. See also: Simopoulos, A., *Canadian Journal of Physiology and Pharmacology,* 1997; 75: 234–39; Dyerberg, J., *Omega-3, Lipoproteins and Atherosclerosis,* 1996; 27: 251–58.
7. Seidelin, K. N., et al., *American Journal of Clinical Nutrition,* 1992; 55: 1117–19.
8. Gerster, H., *Journal of Nutrition and Environmental Medicine,* 1995; 5: 281–96.
9. Booyens, J., and C. V. Van Der Merwe, *South African Medical Journal,* 1991; 79(4): 568.
10. Kinsella, J., et al., *American Journal of Clinical Nutrition,* 1990; 52: 1–28.
11. Harris, W. S., et al., *American Journal of Clinical Nutrition,* 1990; 51: 399–406.
12. Harris, W. S., et al., *American Journal of Clinical Nutrition,* 1997; 65: 1645S–1654S.
13. Sellmayer, A., et al., *American Journal of Cardiology,* 1995; 76: 974–77.
14. Simopoulos, A., *Canadian Journal of Physiology and Pharmacology,* 1997; 75: 234–39.
15. Salachas, A., et al., *Angiology,* 1994; 45(12): 1023–31.
16. Radack, K., et al., *Archives of Internal Medicine,* June 1991; 151: 1173–80.
17. Toft, I., et al., *Annals of Internal Medicine,* Dec. 1995; 123(12): 911–18.
18. Vessby, B., and M. Boberg, *Journal of Internal Medicine,* 1990; 228: 165–71.
19. Landgraf-Leurs, M. M. C., et al., *Diabetes,* March 1990; 39: 369–75.
20. Zambon, S., et al., *American Journal of Clinical Nutrition,* 1992; 56: 447–54.
21. Connor, W. E., *Annals of Internal Medicine,* Dec. 1995; 123(12): 950–51.
22. Hamazaki, T., et al., *Lipids,* 1990; 25(9): 541–45.
23. Brown, J. E., and K. W. J. Wahle, *Clinica Chimica Acta,* 1990; 193: 147–56.
24. Bang., O., et al., *Acta Medica Scandinavica,* 1976; 200: 69.
25. Cave, W. T., *Nutrition,* 1996; 12: 530–41.
26. Kromhout, D., *Medical Oncology and Tumor Pharmacotherapy,* 1990; 7(2–3): 173–76.
27. Zhu, Z. R., et al., *Nutrition and Cancer,* 1995; 24: 151–60.
28. *Nutrition Reviews,* 1994; 8(51): 241–43.
29. Caygill, C., and M. Hill, *European Cancer Prevention Organization,* 1995; 6–7.
30. Gogos, C. A., *Cancer Detection and Prevention,* 1995; 19: 415–17.
31. Wigmore, S., et al., *Nutrition,* 1996; 12: S27–S30.
32. Kremer, J., et al., *Arthritis and Rheumatism,* 1995; 38: 1107–14.
33. Kim, D. N., et al., *Atherosclerosis,* 1990; 81: 209–16.
34. Van Der Tempel, H., et al., *Annals of Rheumatic Diseases,* 1990; 49: 76–80.

35. Lau, B. S., et al., *British Journal of Rheumatology,* 1993; 32: 982–89.
36. Geusens, P., et al., *Arthritis and Rheumatism,* 1994; 37: 824–29.
37. Mohan, I., and V. N. Das, *Prostaglandins, Leukotrines and Essential Fatty Acids,* 1997; 56: 193–98.
38. Aslan, A., and G. Triadafilopoulos, *American Journal of Gastroenterology,* April 1992; 87(4): 342–433.
39. Stenson, W. F., et al., *Annals of Internal Medicine,* 1992; 116(8): 609–14.
40. Belluzi, A., et al., *New England Journal of Medicine,* 1996; 334: 1557–60.
41. Grimminger, F., et al., *Clinical Investigator,* 1993; 71: 634–43.
42. Knapp, H. R., et al., *Journal of the American College of Nutrition,* 1995; 14: 18–23.
43. Hodge, S., et al., *Australia and New Zealand Journal of Medicine,* 1984; 24: 727.
44. Shahar, E., et al., *New England Journal of Medicine,* 1994; 331: 228–33.
45. Van Der Heide, J. J., et al., *Transplantation,* 1992; 54(2): 257–63.
46. Scharschmidt, L., et al., *Journal of Laboratory and Clinical Medicine,* 1990; 115: 405–14.
47. Donadio, J. V. Jr., *Mayo Clinic Proceedings,* 1991; 66: 1018–28.
48. Holman, R. T., et al., *American Journal of Kidney Disease,* 1994; 23: 648–54.
49. Behan, P. O., et al., *Acta Neurologica Scandinavica,* 1990; 82: 209–16.

DHA

1. Makrides, M., et al., *Lancet,* 1995; 345: 1463–48.
2. Carlson, S. E., et al., *Pediatric Research,* 1996; 39: 88–888.
3. Taylor, B., and J. Wadsworth, *Developmental Medicine and Child Neurology,* 1984; 26: 73–80.
4. Laugharne, J. D. E., et al., *Lipids,* 1996; 31: 163–65.
5. Davidson, M., et al., *Journal of the American College of Nutrition,* 1997; 16: 236–43.
6. Connor, W. E., et al., *Lipids,* 1996; 31: 5183–87.

GAMMA-LINOLEIC ACID

1. Bjerve, M., et al., *Nutrition,* 1992; 8: 130–32.
2. Horrobin, D. F., *Journal of Nutritional Medicine,* 1990; 1: 145–51.
3. Horrobin, D., and M. Manku, *Lipids,* 1983; 18: 558–62.
4. Pullman-Mooar, S., et al., *Arthritis and Rheumatism,* Oct. 1990; 33(10): 1526–32.
5. Zurier, R. B., *Arthritis and Rheumatology,* Nov. 1996; 39: 1808–17.
6. Horrobin, D., *Journal of Reproductive Medicine,* 1983; 28(7): 465–68.
7. Pashby, N., et al., *British Journal of Surgery,* 1981; 68: 801–24.
8. Keen, H., et al., *Diabetes Care,* 1993; 16: 8–15.
9. Jamal, G., *Diabetic Medicine,* 1994; 11(2): 145–49.
10. Stewart, J. C., et al., *Journal of Nutritional Medicine,* 1991; 2: 9–15.
11. Horrobin, D. F., and A. Campbell, *Medical Hypotheses,* 1980; 6: 225–32.

12. Vaddadi, K., and D. Horrobin, *Journal of Medical Science,* 1979; 7: 52.
13. Tulloch, I., et al., *Urology Research,* 1994; 22: 227–30.
14. Wagner, W., *Cephalalgia,* 1997; 17: 127–30.

CHAPTER 7: FAT-BASED NUTRITION

MEDIUM-CHAIN TRIGLYCERIDES

1. Scalfi, L., et al., *American Journal of Clinical Nutrition,* 1991; 53(5): 1130–33.
2. Bach, A., and V. Babayan, *American Journal of Clinical Nutrition,* 1982; 36(5): 950–62.

SQUALENE

1. *Lancet,* 1990; 336: 1313.
2. Chan, P., et al., *Journal of Clinical Pharmacology,* 1996; 36(5): 422–27.
3. *Cancer Letters,* 1996; 101(1): 936.
4. *Archives of Pharmaceutical Research,* 1992; 15: 20–29.
5. Storm, H., et al., *Lipids,* 1993; 28(6): 555–59.

GLYCEROL MONOLAURATE

1. Sands, J., et al., *Antimicrobial Agents and Chemotherapy,* 1979; 15: 67–73.
2. Temme, E., et al., *American Journal of Clinical Nutrition,* 1996; 63(6): 897–903.

ALKYLGLYCEROLS

1. Palmblad, J., et al., *Scandinavian Journal of Clinical Laboratory Investigation,* 1990; 50: 363–70.
2. Brohult, A., et al., *Acta Obstetrica Gynecologica Scandinavica,* 1978; 57(1): 79–83.
3. Weber, N., *Progress in Biochemistry and Pharmacology,* 1988; 22: 48–57.

CETYL MYRISTOLEATE

1. Diehl, H. W., and E. L. May, *Journal of Pharmaceutical Sciences,* 1994; 83(3): 296–99.

CHAPTER 8: DIGESTIVE AIDS

FIBRE

1. Burkitt, D., *PCRM Update*, May–June, 1990; 1–9.
2. Bennett, W., et al., *Postgraduate Medicine*, 1996; 99(2): 153–6.
3. Pietinen, P., et al., *Circulation*, 1996; 94: 2720–27.
4. Chan, E., et al., *Annals of Pharmacotherapy*, 1995; 29(6): 625–27. See also: Jenkins, D., *American Journal of Clinical Nutrition*, 1997; 65: 1524–33.
5. *Nutrition Week*, Sept. 20, 1996; 26(36): 7.
6. Truswell, A., *Nutrition Reviews*, 1977; 35: 51.
7. Brown, R. C., Kelleher, J., et al., *British Journal of Nutrition*, 1979; 42: 357–65.
8. Bereza, V., et al., *Vrach Delo*, 1993; 8: 21.
9. Cummings, J. H., et al., *British Journal of Nutrition*, 1979; 41: 477–85.
10. Adlercreutz, H., and W. Mazur, *Annals of Medicine*, 1997; 29: 95–120.
11. Cunnane, S. C., and L. U. Thompson, *Flaxseed in Human Nutrition*, 1995; Champaign, Ill.: AOCS Press, 219–36.
12. Todd, P. A., et al., *Drugs*, 1990; 36(6): 917–28.
13. Vnorinen-Markkola, H., et al., *American Journal of Clinical Nutrition*, 1992; 56: 1056–60.
14. Groop, P., et al., *American Journal of Clinical Nutrition*, 1993; 58: 513–18.
15. Landin, K., et al., *American Journal of Clinical Nutrition*, 1992; 56: 1061.
16. Kirby, R. W., et al., *American Journal of Clinical Nutrition*, 1981; 34: 824–29.
17. Lia, A., et al., *American Journal of Clinical Nutrition*, 1995; 62(6): 1245–51.
18. Behall, K. M., *Journal of the American College of Nutrition*, 1997; 16: 46–51.
19. Rose, D. E., et al., *American Journal of Clinical Nutrition*, 1991; 54: 520–25.
20. Pienta, K., et al., *Journal of the National Cancer Institute*, 1995; 87(5): 348–53.
21. Platt, D., et al., *Journal of the National Cancer Institute*, 1992; 84(6): 438–42.

BENEFICIAL BACTERIA

1. Hughes, V., et al., *Obstetrics and Gynecology*, 1990; 75(2): 244.
2. Hilton, E., et al., *Annals of Internal Medicine*, 1992; 116(5): 353–57.
3. Rasic, J., Kurman, J., et al., *Bifidobacteria and Their Role*, 1983; Boston: Birkhauser.
4. Passerat, B., et al., *Nutrition Research*, 1995; 15: 1287–95.
5. Bogdanov, I., *Digest*, Sofia, Bulgaria, 1982; 3–19.
6. Bocci, V., *Perspectives in Biology and Medicine*, 1992; 2: 251–60.
7. Isolauri, E., *Journal of Allergy and Clinical Immunology*, 1997; 99: 179–85.

8. Hazenburg, M., *Scandinavian Journal of Rheumatology,* 1995; 24(101): 207–11.
9. *Lancet,* 1992; 239: 1263–64.
10. Babbs, C. F., *Free Radicals in Biology and Medicine,* 1990; 8(2): 191–200.

DIGESTIVE AIDS

1. Bray, G., *Quarterly Journal of Medicine,* 1931; 24: 181–97.
2. Recker, R., *New England Journal of Medicine,* 1985; 313(2): 70–73.
3. Bolivar, R., et al., *Candidiasis,* New York: Raven Press, 1985.
4. Giannella, R. A., et al., *Annals of Internal Medicine,* 1973; 78: 271–76.
5. Howitz, J., et al., *Lancet,* 1971; 1: 1331–35.
6. Ayers, S., *Archives of Dermatology and Syphiology,* 1929; 20: 854–57.
7. Lechago, J., et al., *Gastroenterology,* 1993; 105: 1591–92.
8. Humbert, P., et al., *Gut,* 1994; 35(9): 1205–08.
9. Pizzorno, J., and M. Murray, *Textbook of Natural Medicine,* 1993; Bothell, Wash.: Bastyr University Press.
10. *Oral Enzymes: Basic Information and Clinical Studies,* 1992; Geretsried, Germany: Mucos Pharma and Co.
11. Maver, R. W., *On the Risk,* 1991; 7(2).

FOS

1. Gibson, G., and M. Roberfroid, *Journal of Nutrition,* 1995; 125: 1401–12.
2. Yamashita, K., et al., *Nutrition Research,* 1984; 4: 961–66.
3. Hidaka, H., et al., *Bifidobacteria Microflora,* 1991; 10(1): 65–79.

CHARCOAL

1. Lamminpaa, A., et al., *Human Experimental Toxicology,* 1993; 12(1): 29–32.

CHAPTER 9: NUTRIENT-DENSE SUPERFOODS

BARLEY AND WHEAT GRASS JUICE

1. Lai, C., et al., *Nutrition and Cancer,* 1978; 1: 27–30.
2. Lau, B., et al., *International Clinical Nutrition Review,* 1992; 12: 147–55.

CHLORELLA

1. Horkoshi, et al., *Radioisotopes,* 1979; 28(8): 485–86.
2. Okuda, M., et al., *Japanese Journal of Nutrition,* 1975; 33(1): 3–8.

SPIRULINA

1. Matthew, B., et al., *Nutrition and Cancer*, 1995; 24(2): 197–202.
2. Hayashi, O., et al., *Journal Nutritional Science and Vitaminology*, 1994; 40(5): 431–41.
3. Schwartz, J., and Shklar, G., *American Academy of Oral Pathology Abstracts*, 1986; 40: 23.

BEE PRODUCTS

1. Chauvin, R., *General Clinical Pathology Review*, April 1957; 687.
2. Bauer, L., et al., *Journal of Allergy and Clinical Immunology*, 1996; 97(1): 65–73.
3. Rugendorff, E., et al., *British Journal of Urology*, 1993; 71(4): 433–38.
4. Amoros, M., et al., *Journal of Natural Products*, 1994; 57(5): 644–47.
5. Serkedjieva, J., et al., *Journal of Natural Products*, 1992; 55: 294–97.
6. Focht, J., et al., *Arzneimittelforschung*, 1993; 43(8): 921–93.
7. Huang, M., et al., *Carcinogenesis*, 1996; 17(4): 761–65.
8. O'Connor, K. J., et al., *Comparative Biochemistry and Physiology*, 1985; 81: 755–60.
9. Vittek, J., *Experientia*, 1995; 51: 927–35.
10. Townsend, G. F., et al., *Nature*, May 2, 1959, 183: 1270–71.

CHAPTER 10: VITA-NUTRIENTS WITH UNIQUE ROLES

COENZYME Q_{10}

1. Greenburg, S. and W. H. Frishman, *Journal of Clinical Pharmacology*, 1990; 30: 596–608.
2. Mortensen, S. A., et al., *Clinical Investigator*, 1993; 71: S116–S123.
3. Morisco C., et al.; Baggio, E, et al.; Lampertico, M., et al., *Clinical Investigator*, 1993; 71: S129–S149.
4. Langsjoen, P. H., et al., *International Journal of Tissue Research*, 1990; 12(3): 163–68.
5. Langsjoen, P. H., et al., *International Journal of Tissue Research*, 1990; 12(3): 169–71.
6. Langsjoen, P. H., et al., *American Journal of Cardiology*, 1990; (65): 521–23.
7. Folkers, K., et al., *Journal of Optimal Nutrition*, 1993; 2(4): 264–74.
8. Mohr, D., et al., *Biochimica et Biophysica Acta*, 1992; 1126: 247–54.
9. Esterbauer, H., et al., *Free Radical Research Communications*, 1989; 6: 67–75.
10. Digiesi, V., et al., *Current Therapeutic Research*, 1992; 51(5): 668–72.
11. Shimora, Y., et al., *Japanese Journal of Clinical and Experimental Medicine*, 1981; 58: 1349–53.
12. Folkers, K., and Y. Yamamura, eds., *Biomedical and Clinical Aspects of CoEnzyme Q_{10}*, 1984; 4: 369–73.

13. Lockwood, K., et al., *Biochemical and Biophysical Research Communications,* 1995; 212: 172–77.
14. *Biochemical and Biophysical Research Communications,* 1994; 199: 1504–08.
15. Imagawa, M., et al., *Lancet,* Sept. 12, 1992; 340: 671.
16. Folkers, K., et al., *Biochemical and Biophysical Research Communications,* 1995; 1271(1): 281–86.
17. Beal, M., *Current Opinion in Neurology,* 1994; 7(6): 542–47.
18. Mancini, A., et al., *Journal of Andrology,* 1994; 15(6): 591–94.
19. Folkers, K., *Biomedical and Clinical Aspects of CoQ_{10},* 1981; 1: 294–311.
20. Vanfracchi, J. H. P., *Biomedical and Clinical Aspects of CoQ_{10},* 1981; 3: 235–41.
21. Sobriera, C., et al., *Neurology,* 1997; 48: 1238–43. See also: Chen, R., et al., *European Neurology,* 1997; 212–18.

LIPOIC ACID

1. Packer, L., et al., *Free Radical Biology and Medicine,* 1995; 19(2): 227–50.
2. Ziegler, D., et al., *Diabetische Stoffwechsel,* 1993; 2: 443–48.
3. Hamdorf, G., *Experimental Clinical Endocrinology and Diabetes,* 1995; 104: 126–27.
4. Ziegler, D., et al., *Diabetologica,* 1995; 38: 1425–33.
5. Frolich, L., et al., *Drug Research,* 1995; 45(1): 443–46.
6. Wickramasinghe, S. N., and R. Hasan, *Biochemical Pharmacology,* 1992; 43(3): 407–11.

PHOSPHATIDYL SERINE

1. Crook, T., et al., *Neurology,* 1991; 41: 644–49.
2. Funfgeld, E., et al., *Progress in Clinical Biological Research,* 1989; 317: 1235–46.
3. Monteleone, P., et al., *European Journal of Clinical Pharmacology,* 1992; 41: 385–88.

DMSO

1. Muir, M., *Alternative and Complementary Therapies,* 1996; 2(4): 230–35.
2. Evans, M. S., et al., *Neuroscience Letters,* 1993; 150: 145–48.
3. Lockie, L., and B. Norcross, *Annals of the New York Academy of Sciences,* 1967; 141: 599–602.
4. Salim, S., *American Journal of Medical Sciences,* 1990; 300(1): 1–6.
5. Scherbel, A., et al., *Annals of the New York Academy of Sciences,* 1967; 141: 613–29.
6. Ravid, M., et al., *Annals of the Rheumatic Diseases,* 1982; 41: 587–92.
7. Wein, A. J., et al., *Urology Clinics of North America,* Feb. 1994; 21(1): 153–61.

CREATINE

1. Dawson, B., et al., *Australian Journal, Science Medicine for Sport*, 1995; 27(3): 56–61.
2. Greenhaff, P., *British Journal of Sports Medicine*, 1996; 30: 276–81.
3. Ekblom, B., *American Journal of Sports Medicine*, 1996; 24: S38–S39.
4. Chambers, D., et al., *Annals of Thoracic Surgery*, 1996; 61(1): 67–75.
5. Field, M., *Cardiovascular Research*, 1996; 31: 174–75.
6. Miller, E., et al., *Proceedings of the National Academy of Sciences*, 1993; 90(8): 3304–08.

OCTACOSANOL

1. Cureton, T., et al., *The Physiological Effects of Wheat Germ Oil on Humans in Exercise*, 1972; Springfield, Ill.: Charles C Thomas.
2. Rabinovitch, R., et al., *Journal of Neurology, Neurosurgery and Psychiatry*, 1951; 14: 95–100.
3. Snider, S., *Annals of Neurology*, 1984; 16(6): 723.
4. Norris, F., et al., *Neurology*, 1986; 36(9): 1263–64.
5. Stone, S., *Journal of the American Medical Association*, 1941; 18: 310–12.

GAMMA-ORYZANOL

1. Takemoto, T., et al., *Shiyaku To Rinsho*, 1977; 26: 25–27.
2. Yoshino, G., *Current Therapeutic Research*, 1989; 45: 543–52.
3. Ishihara, M., *Asia Oceania Journal of Obstetrics and Gynecology*, 1984; 10: 317.
4. Bucci, L., et al., *Journal of Applied Sports Science Research*, 1990; 4: 104–09.

DMG

1. Graber, C. D., et al., *Journal of Infectious Diseases*, 1981; 143(1): 101–05.
2. Harpaz, M., et al., *Medicine and Science in Sports and Exercise*, 1985; 17(2): 287.
3. Roach, E., and L. Carlin, *New England Journal of Medicine*, 1982; 307: 1081–82.
4. Freed, W. J., *Archives of Neurology*, 1984; 41(11): 1129–30.
5. Rimland, B., *Autism Research Review International*, 1991; 5(2): 7. 1994; 8(2): 6. 1996; 10(3): 7.
6. Todd, G., *Nutrition, Health, and Disease*, 1985; Norfolk, Conn.: Donning.

TRIMETHYLGLYCINE

1. *Medical Letter*, Jan. 31, 1997; 39: 12.

NADH

1. Birkmayer, J., et al., *Acta Neurologica Scandinavica*, 1993; 87(146): 32–35.
2. Vrecko, K., et al., *Journal of Neural Transmission*, 1993; 5: 147–56.
3. Birkmayer, J., *Annals of Clinical and Lab Science*, 1996; 26: 1–9.
4. Birkmayer, J., *New Trends in Clinical Neuropharmacology*, 1992; 1–7.

CHAPTER 11: CARTILAGE-BUILDING NUTRIENTS

SHARK AND BOVINE CARTILAGE

1. Prudden, J., and J. Allen, *Journal of the American Medical Association*, 1965; 192: 352–56.
2. Prudden, J., *American Journal of Surgery*, 1970; 199: 560.
3. Prudden, J., et al., *Seminars in Arthritis and Rheumatism*, 1974; 3: 287–321.
4. Prudden, J., *Journal of Biological Response Modifiers*, 1984; 4: 551–84.

GLUCOSAMINE

1. Brooks, P., et al., *Journal of Rheumatology*, 1982; 9: 3–5.
2. Bucci, L., *Nutrition Report*, 1996; 14(1): 8.
3. Newman, M. L., *Lancet*, 1985; 2: 11–13.
4. Tapadinhas, M., et al., *Pharmatherapeutica*, 1982; 3(3): 157.
5. Drovanti, A., et al., *Clinical Therapeutics*, 1980; 3: 260–72.

CHONDROITIN SULFATE

1. Oliverieri, U., et al., *Drugs in Experimental and Clinical Research*, 1991; 17(1): 45.
2. Pipitone, V., *Drugs in Experimental and Clinical Research*, 1991; 17(1): 3.
3. Bradford, R., et al., Bradford Research Institute, Chula Vista, Calif., 1992.
4. Tsubura, E., et al., *Chemical Abstracts*, 1977; 86: 65688a.
5. Jurkiewicz, E., et al., *AIDS*, 1989; 3(7): 423–27.

CHAPTER 12: HORMONES AND GLANDULARS

DHEA

1. Morales, A., et al., *Journal of Clinical Endocrinology and Metabolism*, 1994; 78: 1360–67.
2. Ebeling, P., et al., *Lancet*, 1994; 343: 1470–81.
3. Herbert, J., et al., *Lancet*, May 13, 1995; 345: 1193–94.
4. Van Vollenhoven, R., et al., *Arthritis and Rheumatism*, 1994; 37: 1305–10.
5. Wilder, R. L., *Journal of Rheumatology*, 1996; 23(suppl. 44): 10–12.
6. Gordon, G., et al., *Cancer Research*, March 1, 1991; 51: 1366–69.

7. Newcomer, L., et al., *American Journal of Epidemiology*, 1994; 140: 870–75.
8. Hata, T., et al., *American Journal of Perinatology*, March 1995; 12(2): 135–37.
9. Wolkowitz, O., et al., *Annals of the New York Academy of Sciences*, 1995; 774: 337–39.

PREGNENOLONE

1. *Proceedings of the National Academy of Sciences*, 1995; 92: 10806–10.

MELATONIN

1. Reiter, R., *Brazilian Journal of Medical and Biological Research*, 1993; 26: 1141–55.
2. Reiter, R., et al., *Trends in Endocrinology and Metabolism*, 1996; 7(1): 22–27.
3. Wurtman, R. J., et al., *Lancet*, Dec. 2, 1995; 346: 1491.
4. Croughs, R., et al., *Netherlands Journal of Medicine*, 1996; 49: 164–66.
5. Petrie, K., et al., *Biological Psychiatry*, 1993; 33(7): 526–30.
6. Garfinkel, D., *Lancet*, 1995; 346(8974): 541–44.
7. Webb, S. M., et al., *Clinical Endocrinology*, 1995; 42: 221–34.
8. Morrey, K., et al., *Immunology*, 1994; 153: 2671–80.
9. Wichman, M., et al., *Journal of Surgical Research*, 1996; 63(1): 256–62.
10. Maestroni, G., *Journal of Pineal Research*, 1993; 14: 1–10.
11. Reiter, R., et al., *Trends in Endocrinology and Metabolism*, 1996; 7(1): 22–27.
12. Reiter, R., *Frontiers of Hormone Research*, 1996; 21: 160–66.
13. Leone, M., et al., *Cephalalgia*, 1996; 16: 494–96.
14. Cagnoni, M. L., et al., *Lancet*, Nov. 4, 1995; 346: 1229–30.

GLANDULAR EXTRACTS (PROTOMORPHOGENS)

1. Gardener, M., *Annual Review of Nutrition*, 1988; 8: 329–50.
2. Bortolotti, F., et al., *Current Therapeutic Research*, 1988; 43: 67–72.
3. Britton, S., et al., *Science*, 1931; 74: 440.

CHAPTER 13: HERBS

MULTIPURPOSE HERBS

1. Hopfenmuller, W., *Arzneimittelforschung*, 1994; 44: 1005–13.
2. Kanowski, S., et al., *Pharmacopsychiatry*, 1996; 29: 49–56.
3. Sotaniemi, E., et al., *Diabetes Care*, 1995; 18: 1373–75.
4. Farnsworth, N. R., et al., *Economic and Medicinal Plant Research*, 1985; 1: 156–215.

5. Yun, T., et al., *Cancer Epidemiology,* 1995; 4: 401–08.
6. D'Angelo, L., et al., *Journal of Ethnopharmacology,* 1986; 16: 15–22.
7. Scaglione, F., et al., *Drugs in Experimental and Clinical Research,* 1996; 22: 65–72.
8. Endo, K., et al., *Planta Medica,* 1983; 49: 188.
9. Blitz, J., et al., *Journal of the American Osteopathic Society,* 1963; 62: 731–35.
10. Shida, T., et al., *Planta Medica,* 1985; 51: 273–5.
11. Beppu, H., et al., *Phytotherapeutic Research,* 1993; 7: 537–42.
12. McDaniel, H., et al., *Antiviral Research,* 1990; 13(suppl. 1): 117.
13. Ikegami, N., et al., *International Conference on AIDS,* 1993; 9(1): 234.
14. Chen, M. F., *Endocrinology Japan,* 1990; 37: 331–41.
15. Morgan, A. G., et al., *Gut,* 1985; 26: 599–602.
16. Fogarty, M., *British Journal of Clinical Practice,* March–April 1993; 47(2): 64–65.
17. Dorant, E., et al., *British Journal of Cancer,* 1993; 67: 424–29.
18. Steiner, M., et al., *American Journal of Clinical Nutrition,* 1996; 64: 866–70.
19. Bordia, T., et al., *Prostaglandins, Leukotrienes, and Essential Fatty Acids,* 1996; 183–86.
20. Srivastafa, K., et al., *Medical Hypothesis,* 1992; 39: 342–48.
21. Mowrey, D., et al., *Lancet,* 1982; 1: 655–57.
22. Fischer-Rasmussen, W., et al., *European Journal of Obstetrics, Gynecology and Reproductive Biology,* 1991; 38(1): 19.
23. Bone, M. E., et al., *Anesthesia,* 1990; 45: 669–71.
24. Grontved, A., et al., *Acta Oto-Laryngolica,* 1988; 105: 45–49.
25. Satoskar, R. R., et al., *International Journal of Clinical Pharmacological Therapy and Toxicology,* 1986; 24: 651–54.
26. Mazumder, A., et al., *Biochemical Pharmacology,* 1995; 49: 1165–70.
27. Hastak, K., *Cancer Letters,* 1997; 116: 265–69.

IMMUNE-ENHANCING HERBS

1. Taguchi, T., *Cancer Detection and Prevention,* 1987; 1(suppl.): 333–49.
2. Hayakawa, K., et al., *Anticancer Research,* 1993; 13(5C): 1815–20.
3. Torisu, M., et al., *Cancer Immunology and Immunotherapy,* 1990; 31(5): 261–68.
4. Nakazato, H., et al., *Lancet,* 1994; 343(8906): 1122–26.
5. Kobayashi, H., et al., *Cancer Epidemiology Biomarkers and Prevention,* 1993; 2(3): 271–76.
6. Heiny, B., *Krebsmedizin,* 1991; 12: 3–14.
7. Yang, Y. Z., et al., *Chinese Medical Journal,* 1990; 103: 304–07.
8. Hong, C., et al., *American Journal of Chinese Medicine,* 1992; 20: 289–94.
9. Awang, D., et al., *Journal of Herbs, Spices, and Medicinal Plants,* 1994; 2(4): 27–43.

INFECTION FIGHTERS

1. Bauer, R., et al., *Economics of Medicine and Plant Research*, 1991; 5: 253–321.
2. Dorn, M., et al., *Complementary Therapies in Medicine*, 1997; 5: 40–42.
3. Coeugniet, E., et al., *Therapiewoche*, 1986; 3352–58.
4. Werbach, M., and M. Murray, *Botanical Influences on Illness*, 1994; Tarzana, Calif.: Third Line Press, 23–24.
5. Rabbani, G. H., et al., *Journal of Infectious Diseases*, 1987; 155: 979–84.
6. Henize, J. E., et al., *Antimicrobial Agents and Chemical Therapy*, 1975; 8: 421–25.
7. Buck, D., et al., *Journal of Family Practice*, 1994; 38: 601–05.

CARDIOVASCULAR HERBS

1. Leuchtgens, I., *Fortschritte der Medezin*, 1993; 111: 352–54.
2. Schmidt, U., et al., *Phytomedicine*, 1994; 1: 17–24.
3. Kramer, W., et al., *Arzneimittelforschung*, 1987; 37: 364–67.
4. Bauer, K., et al., *Clinical Pharmacology and Therapeutics*, 1993; 53: 76–83.
5. Ammon, H., and A. Muller, *Planta Medica*, 1985; 51: 473–77.
6. Taussig, S., et al., *Journal of Ethnopharmacology*, 1988; 22: 191–203.
7. Bernstein, J., et al., *Journal of the American Academy of Dermatology*, 1987; 17: 93.
8. McCarty, D. J., *Seminars in Arthritis and Rheumatism*, 1984; 23: 41–47.
9. Baker, B., *Family Practice News*, May 15, 1997; 62.
10. Satyaviati, G., *Economic and Medicinal Plant Research*, 1991; 5: 47–81.
11. Felter, H., et al., *King's American Dispensatory*, 1983; 1: 374–76.

METABOLIC HERBS

1. Velussi, M., et al., *Current Therapeutic Research*, May 1993; 53(5): 533–45.
2. Frenci, P., et al., *Journal of Hepatology*, 1989; 9: 105–13.
3. Sharma, R., et al., *Phytotherapeutic Research*, 1991; 5: 145–47.
4. Shanmugasundaran, E. R. B., *Journal of Ethnopharmacology*, 1990; 30: 281–94.
5. Baskaran, K., *Journal of Ethnopharmacology*, 1990; 30: 295–305.

HERBS FOR MEN

1. Strauch, G., et al., *European Urology*, 1994; 26: 247–52.
2. Vahlensieck, V., et al., *Fortschritte der Medezin*, 1993; 18: 323–26.
3. Werbach, M., and M. Murray, *Botanical Influences on Illness*, 1994; Tarzana, Calif.: Third Line Press, 23–24.
4. Rowland, D., *Archives of Sexual Behavior*, 1997; 26: 49–62.

HERBS FOR WOMEN

1. Duker, E., *Planta Medica,* 1991; 57: 420.
2. Milewicz, A., et al., *Arzneimittelforschung,* 1993; 43: 752.

BRAIN STIMULANTS

1. Someya, H., *Journal of Tokyo Medical College,* 1985; 43: 815–26.
2. Lavie, G., et al., *Transfusion,* 1995; 35: 392–400.
3. Maquart, F., *Connective Tissue Research,* 1990; 24: 107–20.
4. Kartnig, T., *Journal of Herbs, Spices, and Medicinal Plants,* 1988; 3: 146–73.
5. Appa, M., et al., *Indian Journal of Psychiatry,* 1977; 19: 54–58.

MENTAL RELAXANTS

1. Volz, H., *Pharmacopsychiatry,* 1997; 30: 1–5.
2. Singh, Y., *Journal of Ethnopharmacology,* 1992; 37: 13–45.
3. Shide, C., et al., *Journal of Traditional Chinese Medicine,* 1984; 4(4): 297–300.
4. Bounthanh, C., et al., *Planta Medica,* 1981; 41: 21–28.

SINGLE-PURPOSE HERBS

1. Kuzminski, L., *Nutrition Reviews,* Nov. 1996; 587–90.
2. Light, I., et al., *Urology,* 1973; 1(1): 67–70.
3. *Annali di Ottalmologia e Clinica Oculistica,* 1989; 155.
4. *Annali di Ottalmologia e Clinica Oculistica,* 1988; 144.

ACKNOWLEDGMENTS

This book was a team effort, and I have never worked with a team so dedicated and so willing to give that extra effort. Because of my work schedule, much of the work was done on the weekends, and many of the following team members gave up lots of weekends.

My most heartfelt thanks goes to Robert Crayhon, who is a human nutrition source book. He uncovered and checked out thousands of references, then submitted a version of every vitanutrient chapter. He didn't hesitate to tell me when he thought I was wrong, and I listened. Without Robert, I would not have taken on this book assignment.

Thanks to Joe Wargo, who doubles as the managing editor of my newsletter, *Dr Atkins' Health Revelations*. He never lets me lose my writing style.

A key player is Jacqueline Eberstein, RN, for over two decades the chief of nursing at the Atkins Center, who painstakingly put the centre's protocols on paper and culled the case histories from our thousands of patients.

Thanks to Judith Newitz, who coordinated all of the chapters-in-progress, typed my longhand into the computer and provided valuable editorial advice.

From the very beginning, Nancy Hancock coordinated all of the book-related activities and helped make it a reality.

A big role was played by Wendy Olfenius, who took full responsibility for the bibliography.

Thanks to Lee Clifford, who kept the Atkins Center Library functioning at all times.

And to Mike Cohn, my literary agent, who found Fred Hills,

my Simon & Schuster editor, who conceived of the idea and convinced me that the world needed a Vita-Nutrient Solution.

Thanks also to the many employees of the Atkins Center, who supported me in my project and did whatever I asked of them.

And to my lovely wife, Veronica, who listened patiently to my reading of every chapter and told me in no uncertain terms what to keep and what to rewrite.

INDEX

ABOUT THE AUTHOR

◇

Robert C. Atkins, MD, is the founder and medical director of the Atkins Center, a world-renowned integrative medicine practice located in Manhattan. A graduate of the University of Michigan and Cornell University Medical School, Dr Atkins has been a practising physician, specializing in cardiology and internal medicine, for over thirty years. During his career, he has built an international reputation as a leader in the field of integrative medicine. He was the US National Health Federation's 'Man of the Year' and the recipient of the World Organization of Alternative Medicine's Recognition of Achievement Award. He is also cofounder and past president of the Foundation for the Advancement of Innovative Medicine. Dr Atkins is a professor of medicine at Capital University of Integrative Medicine. He also recently accepted an advisory position at the Columbia Miami Heart Institute's Center for Alternative Medicine and Longevity.

Dr Atkins first gained wide acclaim in 1972 with the publication of his initial book, *Dr Atkins' Diet Revolution*. This book, which first detailed how a low-carbohydrate diet combined with vitamin supplements and therapies could address most major health ailments, has become one of the top fifty best-selling books of all time, with worldwide sales of more than ten million copies. Dr Atkins has gone on to write several other best-selling books, including *Dr Atkins' Nutrition Breakthrough* and *Dr Atkins' Health Revolution*. His most recent book, *Dr Atkins' New Diet Revolution* has sold nearly two million copies and spent over one year on the *New York Times* Bestseller List.

In addition to his books, Dr Atkins reaches over one million people monthly via his nationally syndicated radio show, *Your Health Choices,* and newsletter, *Dr Atkins' Health Revelations.* He and other practitioners at the Atkins Center also appear at numerous health conferences, conventions and symposia annually.

Dr Atkins lives in New York City with his wife, Veronica.

ABOUT THE ATKINS CENTER

―◇―

Established in 1970, the Atkins Center for Complementary Medicine is an eighty-staff, six-storey medical facility in the heart of New York City. The Atkins Center's mission is to first address major health disorders through vita-nutrient therapies, diet modifications and lifestyle changes that can enhance the body's own restorative powers before patients resort to prescription drugs and/or surgical procedures. More than sixty thousand patients have been treated at the Atkins Center for a wide variety of disorders, including cancer, arthritis, asthma, diabetes, heart/cardiovascular disease, chronic fatigue, multiple sclerosis, as well as weight problems.

For information on becoming a patient at the Atkins Center, please visit us on the web at www.atkinscenter.com or contact us at the following address or telephone number:

Atkins Nutritionals, Inc.
2002 Orville Dr. North, Suite A
Ronkonkoma
NY 11779-7661
USA
001 631 738 7370

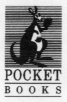

POCKET BOOKS

DR ATKINS
QUICK AND EASY
NEW DIET COOKBOOK

Dr Robert C. Atkins & Veronica Atkins

Companion to the bestselling
Dr Atkins New Diet Revolution

Forget about salad without dressing, dried-out skinless chicken breasts and tasteless steamed vegetables. Forget about tiny portions, no fat/no flavour food and no second helpings. Forget about spending hours in the kitchen. With the delicious new recipes in *Dr Atkins Quick and Easy New Diet Cookbook*, you'll feast on juicy steaks, succulent chops, savoury egg and cheese dishes and indulge in creamy sauces and desserts.

Based on the bestselling *Dr Atkins New Diet Revolution*, the recipes here will let you eat the Atkins way, whether you're beginning your diet, shedding pounds or maintaining your ideal weight.

PRICE £6.99
ISBN 0 7434 4064 1